Brooks

Health Care Policy

IN A CHANGING ENVIRONMENT

Edited by
Roger M. Battistella
and
Thomas G. Rundall
Cornell University

With an introduction by
Spencer C. Johnson

McCutchan Publishing Corporation
2526 Grove Street
Berkeley, California 94704

Library of Congress catalog card no. 78-57148
ISBN 0-8211-0131-5

Printed in the United States of America

To the memory of Harry J. Becker, a pragmatic idealist in his approach to health policy, who believed that career success conveyed a special obligation to assist and encourage junior colleagues, and who was, moreover, a counselor and friend to the Sloan Program of Hospital and Health Services Administration at Cornell.

Contents

Statement of Purpose

The aim of this collection of articles is to help consumers and nonhealth professionals, as well as students preparing for careers in personal health services administration and planning, to acquire an understanding of the factors underlying the mounting signs of crisis in the U.S. health care scene and of the range of choices available for making health services more responsive to both current and future needs. The instability now being experienced in the health sector is viewed as the consequence of changes in biomedical science, trends in demography, mortality, morbidity, and the availability of material resources, which have exceeded the adaptative capabilities of systems of health services finance and organization established over a quarter of a century ago, when medical technologies were simpler and demands on health services were fewer.

There is at present a state of confusion, bordering on chaos, characterizing health policy, which is the result of a process of ad hoc reexamination of concepts and assumptions intrinsic to the conventional wisdom which guided the enormous expansion of the health services in the postwar period. Orthodox ideas are being discarded and new notions pursued without benefit of sharply focused public discussion and systematic analysis and planning. Overall, the environment invites suboptimization in decisions for coping with problems, which results in inconsistent and contradictory programs and regulations. Thus, for example, the government is simultaneously pursuing strategies for economy and efficiency based on the application of conflicting principles of market competition and planning (i.e., HMOs, HSAs, and PSROs).

The absence of a sufficient consensus among vested interest groups, politicians, and the voting public as to the causes and solutions of the numerous problems in the health sector foster dependency upon quick solutions in which it is easy to lose sight of the forest for the trees. Moreover, the crisis atmosphere accompanying decision making is an invitation to pragmatic short-run solutions which have proven not only counterproductive, in that they create more problems than they solve, but also a source of continuing public confusion and futility.

The identification of the sources of confusion can provide an important means for alleviating confusion, together with a frame of reference more favorable to a consideration of alternative strategies for the restructuring of health services compatible with the political, social, and economic realities conditioning the future of health care in the United States and other highly developed industrial nations. Some of the more important obstacles to informed public opinion are due to the unspoken assumptions accompanying changes in health policy. A major aim of this collection is to make explicit these hidden assumptions, so that complex issues may be analyzed and choices for shaping the future may be clarified.

Foreword

We sail within a vast sphere,
ever drifting in uncertainty,
driven from end to end. —Pascal

One of the important features of the current American health care scene is the extent to which it is undergoing change. In a little over a decade we have observed significant, and at times dramatic, changes in both the environment affecting health care and the structure of the delivery system itself. One would hope that the changes occurring in these two areas are related—that as the environment is altered the health care system is adjusted appropriately to compensate for the change. Unfortunately there is a wealth of evidence to suggest that is not the case.

We are not foolish enough to attempt to identify all the environmental forces affecting the health care system. But certain characteristics of our society are currently undergoing significant change and seem to stand out. The prevalence and incidence of several leading causes of mortality and morbidity have changed significantly from their levels of only a decade ago. The social and demographic characteristics of our population are evolving. The migration of population in combination with changes in family structure has enormous implications for the utilization of health services including the potential for shifting illness care from institutions to the community. Also, we are becoming older as a nation and this, too, has important consequences for the need for and distribution of health resources, including a shift from acute-curative to chronic-carative services. Analyses of social and economic correlates of health services utilization suggest that while use of health services by the poor is increasing overall, residents of rural and inner city areas are experiencing an acute shortage of physicians. Finally, and perhaps most critically, we are experiencing an unprecedented rise in the cost of health services.

In the midst of these environmental changes heated debate has raged over the appropriate structure for the health care system. The debate has focused on three issues crucial to the development of health services in the United States: the mechanism for financing health care, the regulation of health care institutions, and control over physicians and other health services professionals. Indeed, we have witnessed considerable change in each of these areas in the past decade. But many critics of the health care system remain skeptical that the changes in financing, regulation, and control have been sufficient to adjust the system to changes in its environment: to put it simply, the fundamental problem is that large numbers of Americans are not receiving high quality medical care appropriate to the problems they have, when and where they need it, at a price they can afford.

In a pluralistic society such as ours, where public policy is largely the product of complex political processes, it would be well for us not to expect the health system and its environment to be tightly coupled. It would be unrealistic to require structure to perfectly match environment at any point in time. Competing social priorities, finite resources, and the organizational inertia inherent in social institutions will inevitably produce a lag between social and institutional change. But there is more to the problem than this. Current health care policy appears to be without a sense of direction (with the possible exception of controlling costs). We are drifting, in Pascal's terms, in a vast sphere of uncertainty, being driven from end to end. Suggested policy options range from introducing free market forces in the health sector to greater governmental regulation; from comprehensive national health insurance to proselytizing for greater personal responsibility for health; from strengthening the professional dominance enjoyed by physicians to implementing consumer control over medical practice. Confusion abounds from the pursuit of contradictory and inconsistent ideas derived from a reworking of old panaceas. The thrust of current policy is strikingly negative—marked more by a sense of failure of the conventional wisdom which directed the enormous growth of health services in the postwar years than by optimism in a body of innovative principles pointing the way to future aspirations and accomplishments.

Although interpreting the tentative efforts of policy makers to deal with this uncertainty is a hazardous business, it appears that certain patterns are emerging. First, old assumptions regarding the delivery of health care services are increasingly being questioned. Second, it is being recognized that to assert the poverty of old ideas is not enough to effect meaningful, constructive change. We need not only constructive ideas but a more comprehensive approach to decision making, guided both by a coherent national policy and a keener regard for the dysfunctionalities of piecemeal solutions.

It has been said that the decade of the 1960s constitutes a watershed era in the development of national health policy. Even if that is true, the considerably altered environment confronting today's health care system suggests that we embark on a new era of policy analysis and development. The purpose of this volume is to aid both students and professionals to identify the major issues which must be confronted in this process. We offer a collection of readings drawn from the work of a diverse set of scholars. The collection is divided into three interdependent sections: the current inconsistencies and contradictions of health policy in the United States; analyses of the underlying forces for change in the environment for health care services; and discussions of selected unresolved issues in the delivery of health care. In each case, we have attempted to select articles which describe and analyze the current status of the health care system, its environment, and the policy options available to us. We believe there are some useful ideas here. We intend the book to be both challenging and invigorating. We hope our readers will find it so.

Introduction: Perspectives on the Health Policy Process

Spencer C. Johnson

The forging of health care policy in the United States has become a full-time business, fraught with conflict and competition, in an arena that was once left to experts because of complexity and mystery. The Congress and public interest groups have put aside those laissez-faire attitudes of the golden age of medicine and are demanding an accounting of the stewardship of the scientific and medical communities, as well as a stronger role in the casting of health policy and the development and management of the nation's health care resources. The appetite of the new public health policy makers is unlimited, spanning the gap between such mega-issues as a national health policy and national health insurance, to such microconcerns as the safety standards of biomedical research facilities and fiduciary interests of individual hospital trustees.

This phenomenon began slightly over a decade ago when the federal government became heavily involved in the financing and delivery of personal medical care services by congressional enactment of Titles XVIII and XIX of the Social Security Act, Medicare and Medicaid, which provided health financing for the aged and medically indigent. Prior to that time federal involvement had been primarily in the support of biomedical research, health professions education, and health care delivery experimentation with a special emphasis on the funding of state public health programs. For example, between 1966 and 1978, the Department of Health, Education, and Welfare budget increased from $3.0 billion to $44.5 billion; of this increase, $37.3 billion has gone to pay for benefits under Medicare and Medicaid, with only $4.2 billion left over for the expansion of

This introduction includes contributions by Barbara A. Green.

other governmental health activities beyond their 1966 level (U.S. Senate, 1977, p. 6).

At the same time, public interest group and consumer activity and interest became more prevalent as federal legislation mandated lay involvement on advisory committees and policy-making boards. This, coupled with increased health concerns of labor unions, associations representing consumer oriented groups such as retired persons and minorities, and activist organizations such as Ralph Nader's Health Research Group and the Consumer Federation of America, has added dimension to the formulation of national health policies. With these thoughts in mind, it is important to develop the historical perspective in which today's health policy-making arena was molded.

GROWTH AND PATTERNS OF AMERICAN MEDICAL CARE*

The evolution of the American medical and health care system reflects a history that sprang primarily from concerns relating to public health and disease prevention programs. Such concerns dominated most thinking until the early 1900s for several pragmatic reasons: the state of medicine in the United States was generally primitive as a result of the absence of a sound, scientific base; although some individuals travelled to European medical schools to receive their training and therefore benefited from the experimental research taking place in those countries, most physicians trained through apprenticeships or received training in low or poor quality institutions within the U.S.; finally, the most pressing health problems facing the infant country were "public health" in nature, that is, diseases bred by poor sanitation, adverse living conditions, contaminated water supplies and imported products, and the like.

In response to widespread epidemics of smallpox, yellow fever, cholera, typhoid, typhus, tuberculosis, and malaria, many cities began establishing local boards of health to combat these problems. The first state boards of health were established in the mid-1800s and a National Board of Health was formed in 1879, although political pressures limited its effectiveness and finally forced it out of existence.

By the turn of the twentieth century, however, medicine began emerging as a scientific discipline as well as a developing political force. The American Medical Association, founded in 1847, asserted itself as the spokesman for physicians. Moreover, a newfound emphasis on experimental research reinforced the scientific foundation for the practice of medicine and promoted increasing specialization among physicians. Specialty societies began forming in the mid-1800s and the American Medical Association established scientific sections for educational purposes. While most physicians were primarily general practitioners,

*The factual information contained in this section was taken from Stevens (1973); Hanlon (1974); U.S. Department of Health, Education, and Welfare (1976a).

many adopted a specialty on which they focused part-time. This trend toward specialization intensified well into the 1900s and, although there is now growing political pressure for a reemphasis on general practice and primary care, this tendency still exists today.

In addition, the quality of medical school education was greatly upgraded as a result of the findings of a study on medical colleges conducted in 1910 by the American Medical Association and the Carnegie Foundation for the Advancement of Teaching. The Flexner report—named after the principal investigator, Abraham Flexner—was instrumental in revamping medical education in the United States. It revealed wide disparities in the quality of education and standards of performance among teaching institutions.

FEDERAL INVOLVEMENT IN HEALTH CARE

Notwithstanding the public health function developed by federal, state, and local governments during the early years of this country's history, public sector involvement in the health care system was virtually nonexistent until the 1900s. However, the twentieth century brought a dramatic transformation regarding the role of government in health care.

From the early 1900s to the 1960s, federal efforts were directed at providing financial assistance for research and development, direct patient services for limited groups of federal beneficiaries, construction of facilities, and manpower training support. In 1901, Congress established the Hygienic Laboratory which eventually evolved into the National Institutes of Health (NIH). As the NIH grew to include eleven separate Institutes—each of which is devoted to a specific disease or organ system—it quickly became the biomedical research center of the country and a favorite project among politicians. With increasingly generous appropriations from Congress, NIH has become the prime source of research grants to the majority of teaching institutions. This process has had a profound effect upon the medical care system: first, it has created an ever-growing dependence by medical schools on federal subsidies, since faculties and facilities have expanded to accommodate the research projects; second, it has greatly encouraged specialization, since the typical role model for students is a professor/researcher focusing upon a specific disease or part of the body; and, finally, it has developed a mindset among policy makers and the public that clinical medicine and technology is the answer to all health problems—in other words, good medicine is the key to good health.

Although the Public Health Service was formally established in 1912, its "public health" functions have become of less priority because it is now responsible for administering a wider range of health programs, many of which do not fall under the rubric of "health promotion and disease prevention."

Passage of the Social Security Act in 1935 significantly broadened federal participation in the health sector. Not only were funds provided for grants-in-aid programs to states and territories to carry out public health functions, but money was also earmarked for use in the development of maternal and child health programs and aid to crippled children. These "categorical programs" were the first of many created over the next thirty years to provide medical services to a wide range of distinctive population groups. Today, there are estimated to be about 1,000 such specifically targeted programs throughout the federal government with almost 300 in the Department of Health, Education, and Welfare.

In 1943, Congress passed its first law authorizing federal funds to be used in health manpower training. The scope of this legislation was narrow in that it provided monies for the training of nurses for the armed forces, government agencies, and private sector. In 1944, however, a provision was included in the Servicemen's Readjustment Act of 1944 (GI Bill) which made available public subsidies for the purposes of financing both undergraduate and graduate medical education to veterans. Manpower training again became the focus of political attention in the early 1960s. As the financial stability of medical schools became threatened due to the impact of advancing technology on the schools' resources, Congress stepped in to provide support in exchange for increasing medical school enrollments. This approach was designed to increase the supply of physicians in order to ward off what appeared to be an impending shortage. The first of these bills, passed in 1963, was called the Health Professions Educational Assistance Act. This law has been revised and extended in scope and authority several times since 1963, with the most recent amendments occurring in 1976.

Federal support for the construction of health facilities was initiated in 1946 with the passage of the Hospital Survey and Construction Act or Hill-Burton, as it was commonly called. The purpose of this program was to survey the need for and to construct hospitals in areas with a shortage of adequate facilities. Between 1947 and 1971, the Hill-Burton program provided $3.7 billion for the construction of facilities. In addition, the Defense Department, the Veterans' Administration, the Department of Housing and Urban Development, as well as numerous other federal agencies and programs, have each contributed millions of dollars to health facilities construction through grants, loans, loan guarantees, mortgage insurance, and tax subsidies.

As the federal government was expanding into the health care delivery system through greater and greater financial support, the nature of reimbursement for personal medical care services underwent a radical change in the 1940s with the introduction of private health insurance. Private health insurance or third-party coverage was spurred into existence for two reasons. First, hospitals, which, after barely weathering the Depression years, were growing wary of slowly rising health care costs, needed some degree of assurance that their patients' medical bills would be covered; thus, Blue Cross was born. Second, business and industry viewed health insurance as an attractive fringe benefit which they could offer their employees in lieu of wage increases; consequently, business quickly became a major purchaser of health insurance.

The federal government contributed to the rise of health insurance or third-party coverage by establishing the Federal Employees Health Benefits Program in 1959, which provides health insurance protection to employees of the federal government, and by enacting Medicare and Medicaid—programs designed to assure access to medical services for the aged and poor. Since the passage of these latter two programs in 1965, federal expenditures for health have jumped from 2 percent of total federal outlays in fiscal year 1966 to 9.5 percent in fiscal year 1977. The consequence of this rapid growth in expenditures has been a major change in the nature of federal involvement in the health sector—increasingly, the federal government has become more and more involved in health industry policy, management, and regulation.

THE GROWTH OF FEDERAL REGULATION

It is impossible to pinpoint an exact moment when the character of federal involvement in health care shifted from purely contributory to regulatory; in fact, from the earliest efforts to control public health hazards, regulation in some form has been a cornerstone of governmental activity. The important distinction to be made, however, is that as federal dollars have become a proportionately larger share of overall expenditures for health care, and as federal officials have become more concerned with the level of these expenditures, the focus of regulation has turned to the health care industry itself.

The three most notable examples of such regulation can be found in the Social Security Amendments of 1972 and the National Health Planning and Resources Development Act of 1974. The 1972 Social Security Amendments contained two provisions of significant consequence: the first established a nationwide system of Professional Standards Review Organizations, which are physician-controlled boards charged with developing norms of diagnosis and treatment of diseases for patients whose medical bills are reimbursed under Medicare and Medicaid. Among other responsibilities, these boards are authorized to review hospital lengths of stay and treatment procedures. The second provision established the "1122 Review Program," which is a voluntary program providing financial assistance to states which choose to designate a state agency for the review of capital expenditures. Under this program, payments authorized by Medicare and Medicaid for interest and depreciation are not allowed unless the project receives prior approval from the state-designated agency. Capital expenditures affected by this provision include any that exceed $100,000, that change the bed complement of a facility, or that add a service.

The National Health Planning and Resources Development Act of 1974 made sweeping changes in earlier efforts to allocate resources for health services. Basically, it combined and replaced three preexisting programs (the Comprehensive Health Planning and Public Health Service Amendments of 1966, which created a formal system for areawide planning and allocation of health resources;

the Regional Medical Program of 1965, which was designed to formulate regional networks for the cooperative treatment of heart disease, cancer, stroke, and, later, kidney diseases; and the Hill-Burton Program), and tightened requirements for the control of health care capital expenditures.

The new law authorized the designation of a nationwide network of Health Systems Agencies, each of which carries out planning and regulatory functions for its region. More importantly, however, the 1974 Act required each state to develop a certificate-of-need program—a program which makes prior approval for certain capital expenditures mandatory—by 1980.

Other regulatory measures enacted in recent years fall under the category of "public interest and protection." The scope of these laws is great, but the fundamental purpose of each is essentially the same—that is, to provide a safer working and living environment for Americans. Examples of these laws include the Occupational Safety and Health Act of 1970, the Radiation Control for Health and Safety Act of 1969, the Safe Water Drinking Act of 1974, the Medical Device Amendments of 1976, the Consumer Product Safety Act of 1972, and a variety of other laws which address such concerns as tobacco hazards, air quality conditions, pesticides, solid waste disposal, lead-based paint, and noise control.

The transition from a public health and prevention approach to an emphasis on curative medicine in a high-technology mode was influenced greatly by the intervention of the federal government. Enactment of legislation to finance the development of high technology biomedical research, train a myriad of health professionals and paraprofessionals, and construct facilities, has contributed significantly to today's national preoccupation with the quality, cost, and accessibility of personal medical care services.

Once committed to a firm policy of health resources development and planning, entry into the financing of services during the Great Society period of the mid-sixties was a logical step for federal policy makers. Thus, the regulatory function, or interest, of the government is a natural extension of these activities, especially when public funds are used to finance nearly 40 percent of the annual cost of health care. In the same manner the primary concerns of federal policy makers have become the agenda for future directions in the organization and development of the nation's health care delivery system.

THE HEALTH AGENDA

Health care has long enjoyed a special status in society. Perhaps this is so because of the very personal nature of health which allows no person, regardless of social class, income, heritage, or political influence, to escape the ultimate destiny of all living things—declining physical capability and eventual death. Perhaps it is a function of the fact that death, as mankind's greatest mystery, represents the unknown—a phenomenon which traditionally generates fear, hostility, and superstition. Perhaps it is simply due to the fact that illness and death are so often associated with discomfort, pain, violence, grief, and loss. Whatever the reason, people have, for centuries, searched for measures which will postpone death.

The quest to conquer illness and, by implication, death, has led to much irrational behavior in the health policy arena. Health, because of its unique importance to all persons, has traditionally been treated differently than other sectors of the economy. First, health care services have become a "right," an entitlement. As such, health policy makers have been governed by a "more is better" attitude—more resources, more facilities, more manpower, more of whatever it will take to provide better medical care. Secondly, until recently, little regard has been given to the cost of providing these services. In a society where human life is considered priceless, no amount of money has been considered too great to devote to health care.

Since the early 1970s, however, these fundamental governing principles have come under severe scrutiny for two basic reasons. First, expenditures for health care have increased dramatically; second, the return on investment appears, at best, to be marginal.

RISING HEALTH CARE COSTS

Expenditures for health care have risen dramatically over the last twenty-five years. In 1950, total expenditures for health equaled slightly more than $12 billion and represented 4.5 percent of the Gross National Product. By 1976, these expenditures had climbed to almost $140 billion or roughly 8.6 percent of the GNP. Over the last three years, outlays for health care have increased at an average rate of $20 billion per year.

Inflation in the health care sector is a result of the following factors:

—The increased demand for services, largely a result of the government programs, Medicare and Medicaid, as well as increased private health insurance coverage.

—A method of payment for medical services utilizing a third-party insurance mechanism which shields both the consumer and provider from the impact of the full cost of treatment at the time of utilization.

—The nature of the reimbursement system, which is primarily based on retrospective costs incurred, offers little incentive to restrain costs at the time services are provided.

—The uneven distribution and mix of health resources (facilities, services, and manpower).

—The introduction of high-level medical technology which is heavily capital and labor intensive.

—The excess capacity in the medical care system, especially hospital beds, which means that the consumer must bear the burden of paying for the fixed costs of underutilized facilities and equipment.

—The nature of the product, which makes any kind of consumer cost consciousness and comparative shopping difficult. Since consumers do not have the knowledge to diagnose or prescribe for themselves, they must rely upon the medical profession. Also, consumers have high expectations for medicine and urge physicians to provide the maximum possible amount of services.

—The impact of medical malpractice, which results in the increased practice of defensive medicine and increased malpractice insurance premiums reflected in higher professional charges.

The inflationary impact of these factors on the health care sector has produced widespread concern and debate over the expenditures. Some argue persuasively that there is nothing inherently wrong with the levels of these expenditures. For example, Professor Uwe Reinhardt of Princeton University, a prominent health economist, noted that expenditures for health care do not begin to rival what consumers spend on tobacco, alcohol, and clothing and further remarked:

Let me propose that, from a macro-economic viewpoint, the cause for limiting health care expenditures to 7 or 8 percent is certainly *not* compelling. Indeed, let me propose that the nation's economic survival is not really an issue in our current debate over the health care crisis. We should stop pretending that it is. We are rich enough as a nation to afford what we now spend, and to spend more." (National Leadership Conference, 1976, p. 70)

Unquestionably, this is true. However, the dilemma faced by policy makers arises from the fact that the nature of the health care system—as manifested in its reimbursement policies, the respective roles of its physicians and consumers, and the effects of an almost unregulated process of technology diffusion— impedes the ability of policy makers to rationally determine how much will be spent on health care. If how much this country spends on health care is simply a question of priorities, as some will argue, then the society must gain control over the process which determines that priority. Thus far, efforts in that direction have been limited; furthermore, those efforts which have been undertaken have achieved little success.

A CASE OF DIMINISHING RETURNS

A second, far more fundamental problem, centers around the question of resource allocation and return on investment. A review of the leading indicators of health status—morbidity, mortality, and disability—during the period 1950 through 1975 (when expenditures for health care grew tenfold) indicates that only modest improvements were experienced. This consequence is especially magnified when compared to the improvements made in the first half of this century.

Between 1900 and 1950, life expectancy for white males increased from forty-eight years to more than sixty-eight years; for white females, life expectancy grew from fifty-one years to more than seventy-six years. Major killers and disablers such as influenza, polio, tuberculosis, and gastric disorders were controlled or virtually eliminated during this period. At the same time, many health hazards associated with poor living and working conditions, food and water contamination, sanitation, and other public health problems were overcome.

In the last twenty-five years, these trends have tapered off. During this period, life expectancy for white males rose two years; for white females, it rose four years. Much of this improvement has been attributed to a dramatic decline in infant mortality rates rather than to better medical care for adults. Supportive evidence is obtained from studies which indicate that the death rate has scarcely changed during the past twenty-five years, ranging between 9.3 per 1,000 persons in 1950 to 9.7 in 1973.

Like mortality, morbidity exhibits little improvement. In examining acute illnesses for the years 1962 through 1969, the National Center for Health Statistics found that the number of conditions per capita remained virtually constant, not only overall but within the separate categories of respiratory, infective, parasitic and digestive conditions, and injuries.

Disability data on the limitation of activity due to chronic conditions actually show that more people suffered chronically induced disability in 1970 than in 1957. In 1957-58, 89.9 percent of the persons recorded showed no limitation of activity from chronic conditions; in 1969-70, the figure was 88.3 percent, an increase of 1.6 percent. (These statistics were developed from U.S. Department of Health, Education, and Welfare, 1976a, 1976b; U.S. House of Representatives, 1974.)

These changes appear to correspond to the rise of new types of killing and disabling diseases, including cancer, heart disease, and stroke. These particular diseases are representative of a new pattern, specifically:

—They are noninfectious and appear to be caused by environmental hazards, like pollution, or by life styles which lack exercise but include excessive smoking, drinking, and eating;

—They generally do not respond well to traditional forms of medical treatment (i.e., inoculation, surgery, and drug therapy); and,

—Their incidence has increased coincidentally with Americans' ability and tendency to effect a mass impact on the environment.

The medical care system operates essentially in two modes, curative and preventive. The curative model includes virtually all elements popularly associated with medical care delivery (biomedical research, surgery, drug therapy, etc.). It also includes an array of preventive programs that have become the province of those who deliver curative medical care. The preventive model, when broadly defined, includes medical and nonmedical interventions designed to prevent the onset of illness. This model encompasses such health factors as life style, environment, and living and working conditions.

With the caveat that some aspects of preventive medical care, such as annual checkups, well-baby care, inoculations, and pap smears, have been subsumed within the curative model, the preventive model is essentially represented by traditional public health activities. The emphasis in recent years, however, in terms of resource allocation, has been aimed almost exclusively at components of the curative model.

For example, in 1977, the federal government spent $2.4 billion for biomedical research. In comparison, the major "public health" arm of the federal government—the Center for Disease Control (CDC)—received $63.5 million to combat such major public health problems as venereal disease, lack of immunizations, rat control, and lead-based paint poisoning. Health education, viewed by many as the key to altering unhealthy life styles, received only $4.5 million. Clearly, the priorities established in these budget outlays suggest an extreme emphasis on the components of the curative model. In light of the marginal improvements in health status discussed previously, the fundamental question for health policy makers is, are the resources expended on health initiatives spent on efforts which will produce the greatest results?

THE SECOND COMING OF PUBLIC HEALTH

Recent studies appear to support the contention that the case for medicine, as it is conventionally conceived, has been grossly overstated. There is a growing body of evidence which suggests that there are limits to what medicine can be expected to accomplish, and that it is, in fact, quite possible that this society is on the threshold of such limits. Rick Carlson, a senior research associate to the Institute of Medicine, has noted:

Medicine has very little to do with health—it rarely has contributed to health, and today it may cause more ill health than cure disease. The major improvements in health have not been due to medicine, but to improvements in social, economic, and environmental conditions. Only early in this century through the impact of the decisive technologies of surgery and chemotherapy has medicine made a significant contribution. But the assaults of today are largely unamenable to the tools of modern medicine. We are becoming sicker and no longer can be cured by medicine.
  . . . We have constructed and we continuously elaborate a system of care that focuses on the elimination of disease—not on the generation of health—and the price we pay is twofold: extremely high costs and failing health. (1976, p. 6)

The major health problems facing this country today—heart disease, cancer, and stroke—are problems whose causes can best be dealt with outside the realm of medicine. It is widely acknowledged that obesity, insufficient physical exercise, smoking, hypertension, as well as carcinogens found in the air, water, food, chemicals, and other substances are primarily responsible for these three leading causes of death. Improvements in any of these factors will require significant changes in both personal life style habits and acceptable standards of environmental conditions.

Public health problems of a century ago matched the society's level of sophistication. Food contamination, for example, occurred until technology developed refrigeration and other appropriate methods for preserving food. Today, however, industrial society has reached a new level of sophistication—one which has brought with it pollution, carcinogenic substances, non-nutritional food products, life styles which breed stress, inactivity, excessive eating habits, and a host of other new forms of public health problems which sap the society of its health. To combat these new forms of public health hazards, this country needs a new, revitalized public health effort, one which is targeted at these highly sophisticated industrial, environmental, and social problems. In essence, a "second coming of public health" is in order.

The leap to this new plane will be no easy task. First, it will require an abandonment of the notion that medical intervention is the appropriate vehicle for solving all health problems. Second, it will require a reassessment of the resource allocation process and a recognition that, in the face of limited resources, priority must be given to those efforts which will benefit the greatest number of citizens. Finally, it will require individuals to accept greater responsibility for maintaining their own health—an activity which the mystique of modern medicine has virtually eliminated.

It is apparent that, if marked improvements in health status are to be achieved, a re-evaluation of our current approach to health care organization and delivery is necessary.

FORMULATING NATIONAL HEALTH POLICY

In any discussion of current health issues it is essential to evaluate the processes by which national health policies are determined. These processes include public and private sector efforts to identify needs, set priorities, develop alternatives, allocate resources, implement and evaluate programs, and, finally, although rarely, modify or terminate programs.

Although public debate over the cost, quality, and availability of medical services has highlighted these concerns as key national health issues, it is clear that decisions relating to these issues are not made in a rational and coordinated fashion. Instead, the current policy process frequently encourages judgments to be made in a fragmented manner, irrespective of the identification of priorities. Recently, in fact, individual legislative proposals, public programs, and private initiatives have often worked at cross-purposes with broadly identified national health goals.

There are several factors which contribute to this policy-making anomaly. Within the public sector, the responsibility for formulating health policies is held by a large number of groups, many of which have differing priorities and objectives. For example, there are currently six major committees in the Senate and House of Representatives with prime responsibility for health programs and issues, and thirty-five other important committees and subcommittees which have some jurisdiction over health matters. Almost every department in the Executive Branch—that branch of government responsible for administering federal programs—bears responsibility for some health-related activity. The largest concentration of these programs, of course, is found in the Department of Health, Education, and Welfare; but other programs which deal specifically with the provision of medical services can be found in the Defense Department, Veterans' Administration, and Agriculture Department. Programs which affect health in a broad sense, through such factors as housing, education, nutrition, and environment, are found in almost every department and agency. In addition to carrying out their legislative mandates, these agencies normally compete with private sector interests to lobby for their own point of view with the Congress.

At the state and local levels, health programs reflect the fragmentation and duplication of federal mandates. This is primarily because state and local agencies must adapt to federal guidelines to qualify for the funding available under federal programs. Thus, sensitivity to true regional and local needs and organizational requirements is ignored in the face of qualification requirements for federal funding.

The private sector—whose failure to self-regulate is largely to blame for increasing federal involvement—is equally as fragmented. Generally speaking, there are two levels of private sector input into the policy-making process. These include, on one level, the interest and lobby groups which represent health professionals, various components of the health industry, or a particular health or medical problem; the other level involves the purchasers of medical care.

The role of the interest groups in policy formulation can be characterized as follows: in addressing any given problem or issue, each group operates in a way designed to maximize its own goals and priorities. Essentially, this means that self-interest drives all activity; each group perceives its own specific set of goals to be more important than those of any other group. As a result of this independently motivated activity, the various competing groups are unable to agree on a broad unifying philosophy for identifying health priorities and appropriate solutions. Instead, each group expends its energy on attempts to maximize its individual position (or at least minimize its losses) irrespective of larger societal goals. There are numerous private sector groups which exert major influence in legislative and administrative policy development. Quite often, however, their influence is not enough to stop the legislative process or even to establish a prevalent point of view; these competing forces usually settle on compromises that, while mutually satisfactory, are ineffective in addressing specific problems.

The major purchasers of health benefits, such as business and labor, have their greatest impact on formulation of health policy by their choice of benefits. Since World War II, employers and unions have set most of the patterns by which health insurance benefits are structured and administered. These groups have had tremendous impact on the cost and performance of the health industry because of the amounts of money they spend for health insurance and the types of services they have chosen to purchase.

Because of a benign attitude toward their large investment in health care services, however, business and labor have had surprisingly little influence on the development of health policy. Thus, as a result of the health industry's promotion of the benefits of medical care, and employers' financing of health care benefits for workers, the consumer has developed the expectation that the access to medical care services is the key to better health. This widely accepted attitude toward the consumption of health care justifies the activities of the private sector.

The absence of coordination within both the public and private sectors, and between each of these sectors, has led to a fragmented approach to the development of health policy. Consequently, with the exception of the broad, overriding goal that all citizens should have access to high quality, reasonably priced medical care, there is little agreement as to more specific goals and priorities, and less agreement as to what means should be used to achieve these goals.

Until a consensus is reached regarding health priorities, and a more effective mechanism is developed which combines the best elements of the public and private sectors for the development of health policy initiatives, the outdated thrust of the existing patterns of medical care—which are growing increasingly unresponsive to the health needs of the nation—will continue to prevail. A restructuring of the health policy process to achieve a common concept of health appears necessary in order to refocus this country's efforts to develop any comprehensive national health care reforms or program.

REFERENCES

Carlson, R. J. "The End of Medicine." *Executive* 3, no. 1 (Fall 1976): 6.

Hanlon, J. J. *Public Health Administration and Practice* (6th ed.). St. Louis: C. V. Mosby, 1974.

National Leadership Conference. *Proceedings of the National Leadership Conference on America's Health Policy*. Washington, D.C.: National Journal, 1976.

Stevens, R. *American Medicine and the Public Interest*. New Haven, Conn.: Yale University Press, 1973.

U.S. Department of Health, Education, and Welfare. *Baselines for Setting Health Goals and Standards* (Publication no. HRA 76-640). Washington, D.C.: HEW, 1976a.

U.S. Department of Health, Education, and Welfare. *Health: United States, 1975* (Publication no. HRA 76-1232). Washington, D.C.: HEW, 1976b.

U.S. House of Representatives, Committee on Ways and Means. *National Health Insurance Resource Book*. Washington, D.C.: Government Printing Office, 1974.

U.S. Senate. "Hospital Cost Containment Act of 1977: Summary and Analysis of Consideration." Washington, D.C.: Government Printing Office, 1977.

Part I

The Changing Environment for Health Policy

1

Inconsistencies and Contradictions of Health Policy in the United States

Selection by Roger M. Battistella

Increases in the share of national wealth, as measured in terms of gross national product (GNP) allocated to health care in the United States, are progressing at a rate which, if allowed to continue unchecked, may lead to serious economic, social, and political disturbances in the form of lowered rates of economic growth, cutbacks in social spending in nonhealth areas, and higher levels of taxation. In contrast to the present figure of approximately 7 percent, it has been estimated that by 1980 the proportion of GNP going to health care may approach 10 percent (Rice and McGee, 1970). Clearly, the amount of money and manpower available for health services is not unlimited. In reality, health must compete with other demands for its share of national resources.

Though initially slow to materialize, recognition of the dilemma is becoming more widespread, to the point where government officials are beginning to engage in a systematic reexamination of basic institutional assumptions governing the structure and function of health services. This process of reexamination can be expected to lead to profound changes not only in the way in which health services are organized and delivered, but equally, if not more important, in the political control and social purpose of health care. The central proposition of this paper is that the pressures are not isolated to the United States but are, for the most part, characteristic of all highly developed countries. The dynamics are seen as an inherent property of the development or modernization process.

Reprinted by permission from "Rationalization of Health Services: Political and Social Assumptions," *International Journal of Health Services* 2, no. 3 (1972), pp. 331-48.

EVIDENCE OF CONVERGENCE

The results of cross-national comparisons by Anderson and Neuhauser (1969) suggest that rising costs may be an inherent problem in all advanced health care systems, because of common social, political, scientific, and techno-logical imperatives accompanying biomedical progress. Even though other post-industrial countries allocate a smaller share of GNP for health (under 5 percent) than does the United States, published sources reveal anxiety among government officials over the prospects of future increases. As is the case in the United States, there is a growing interest in the moulding of strategies for controlling costs by stimulating increased productivity and efficiency through the restruc-turing of existing organizational arrangements along more integrated, systematic, and unified lines (Owen, 1968; *Swedish Health Services System,* 1971; Ruder-man, 1969; Fry, 1969; Somers, 1971).

Most often discussed in the name of rationalization, the changes contem-plated represent a sharp break from past thinking and established ways of orga-nizing health services. With increasing pressure for changes, health care faces an uncertain future. By drawing upon recent experiences in the United States, this paper seeks to describe trends in the light of major public policy problems and to assess the probable future impact of any movement toward rationalization on selected political and social dimensions of health care organization. The implica-tions examined on the political side involve: (a) the size of expenditures and scope of substantive responsibilities falling within the boundaries of the health field; and (b) the role of health professionals in the formulation of health policy and program planning. Issues examined on the social side include: (a) the impact of organizational incentives in shaping the ethical-motivational orientation con-ditioning relationships at the point where services meet people; and (b) the rela-tionship of health to larger sociophilosophic ideals.

HEALTH POLICY OPTIONS IN THE UNITED STATES

The ferment and fluidity marking important transitions in policy com-pound the usual problems of description, understanding, and prediction. The movement toward rationalization is no exception. Though seldom overcome suc-cessfully, these difficulties may be lessened somewhat through the identification and assessment of major stress points and leading alternative points of view. By no means mutually exclusive, there are at least four major policy positions on the future of health services in the United States. While admittedly arbitrary, in the interest of convenience and to acquire perspective for a more detailed look at developments and trends later on, alternative positions have been classified into the following four groups of thought and opinion: (a) the traditionalist-expansionists, (b) the laissez-fairists, (c) the managerial-rationalists, and (d) the democratic-humanists. The respective views and positions of each of these groups may be described as follows.

The Traditionalist-Expansionists

There is a positive relationship between illness treatment services and health. Moreover, expenditures for health result in additional contributions to individual satisfaction and collective well-being. In a land of economic abundance, failure to increase share of GNP outlays for health is unforgiveable (Anderson, 1968).

The traditionalist-expansionist outlook is typical by and large of all parties engaged in the production and distribution of health services who have a stake in keeping things pretty much as they are. It also tends to characterize the leanings of governmental and nongovernmental agencies dominated by health professionals, if for no other reasons than the weight of conventional thinking in the professions and the effect of interlocking bureaucratic dependencies. Consumers and the general public, whether because of a general faith in the power of medicine, indoctrination in the doctor-patient relationship, or the rising standards of consumption which accompany affluence, also tend to subscribe to this point of view, although there is some reason to believe that things may be changing.

The Laissez-Fairists

Contrary to the understandable tendency of health providers and professionals to expound the benefits of what they do, the relationship between health status and health care is unclear. Health professionals and bureaucracies dominated by professionals act more in accordance with their self-interest than proclaimed public service ideals. The pull of self-interest leads them not only to oppose changes threatening to the status quo, but also to oversell services of dubious value and services which, in some cases, may actually harm patients. Given the uncertainty surrounding the benefits of many health services, innovation, progress, and the public interest may be better served by removing monopoly controls over practice currently held by professionals. Provided that the state acts appropriately to assure safety, market rationing and the provision of health care on a commodity basis may be an effective way of curbing governmental outlays. Paradoxically, market rationing may also promote health by making access to health services more difficult, and by stimulating greater individual responsibility for habits and behavior which are considered as threats to health, e.g., obesity, alcoholism, smoking, accidents. (One of the most cogent statements of the laissez-fairist position is provided by Friedman, 1962.) Acceptance of the conclusion that health care as a general class of goods falls short of meeting critical assumptions necessary for the successful operation of the competitive market has prevented this point of view from making much headway in policy-making circles in the past.

Previously confined in the main to academic debate, the market has surfaced recently within the ranks of policy makers as an ostensibly useful device for controlling costs and spurring innovation. Secretary of Health, Education, and Welfare Eliot Richardson (U.S. Congress, 1970, p. 62) put it plainly when in testimony before Congress he said, "One of our goals is to open the marketplace and provide opportunities for new delivery systems." Such laudatory references to market competition are misleading, however, in that public policy is aimed less at restoring the anarchistic features essential to the world of Adam Smith and the laissez-fairists, than in bringing about greater concentration and less of the uncontrolled competition which experience has found to be dysfunctional in the health field. What does appear to be receiving very serious attention, as we shall see, is the use of market-type incentives to stimulate and reward efficiency and economy among providers.

One portion of the laissez-fairist position has succeeded in acquiring a wide following among both the general public and policy makers, notably, that professionals act equally, if not more so, in accordance with their self-interest than with that of the public. This charge coincides with a growing reaction against professionals in the United States. The tough political questions necessitated by the growth in expenditures for human services, coupled with serious problems of recession and inflation in the general economy, have caused people to be more critical of budgets prepared by professionals and more sophisticated in demanding evidence, first, that stated goals are relevant, and secondly, that they will be met. The general defensiveness of professionals unaccustomed to having their expertise challenged has provoked disappointment and anger. To citizens worried about jobs and taxes, demands for higher income on the part of professionals and their organizations, no matter how justified, are easily interpreted as hypocrisy. Public opinion is supported by studies begun initially in the 1960s under the sponsorship of the Ford Foundation which pointed out that for a large number of complex structural, organizational, and personal reasons, service bureaucracies dominated by professionals tend to resist change and are not sensitive to the needs of clientele, particularly the lower classes and the poor. Whether consciously or unconsciously, professionals structure programs to suit their own needs and convenience, and select problems which appear most exciting from a standpoint of expertise. This finding led to the development of a number of significant experiments in consumer participation in decision making for health and related social services at community levels (Marris and Rein, 1967, pp. 33-55).

The Managerial-Rationalists

Because of the vagueness of health as a concept, it is difficult, if not impossible, to define and evaluate the output of the health services. There is, moreover, some tentative evidence to suggest that the health services may be manufacturing a considerable amount of illness (i.e., results of factors such as technological imperatives, latent consequences of complex therapeutics, categorization and lack of follow-up of treatment services, and unanticipated consequences of labeling and prolonged institutionalization of patients in mental hospitals and nursing homes). International comparisons suggest the possibility of an inverse correlation between health status and access to presymptomatic health care, number of physician contacts per capita, and volume of surgery per capita. Although persons in other developed countries receive less health care, they fare better than Americans. Given the degree of uncertainty, the burden of proof for justifying additional health outlays ought to be placed squarely on the shoulders of the health professionals, whose responsibility it is, through means of self-imposed ethics, to safeguard the public interest. There are other problems as well. In the absence of strong anti-inflationary controls, more health spending is futile. The extensive lead-times required for affecting the supply of services result in a fairly persistent situation of excess consumer demand. Further problems of inflation center on the labor intensiveness of health care and the difficulties of introducing mechanization and economies of scale without radically altering the present way in which services are organized.

The sources of the managerial-rationalist position are diverse but are drawn principally from economists such as Victor Fuchs (1968, 1969) who raise serious questions centering on the ambiguity of health as a concept and the paucity of data on the efficacy or benefits of health care. Additional criticism involves the bias toward economic expansion regarded as inherent in the socialization and careerism of professionals.

Dramatic evidence of the inflationary impact of unleashing new spending without first solving basic problems of productivity and efficiency is drawn from what happened following passage in 1965 of new federal programs for financing the cost of health care for the aged (Medicare) and poor persons on welfare rolls (Medicaid). In fiscal years 1966 through 1970, increases in expenditures totalled $11.5 billion for hospital care and $4.1 billion for physician services. Of these amounts, price increases accounted for three-fourths and seven-tenths, respectively (Rice and Cooper, 1971).

Improving efficiency and productivity will not be easy, however. It requires a major restructuring of the health field. As things now stand, too many small and independent parties are involved. An indication of the hopelessness of the present situation and the enormity of the change required is mirrored in the fact that over 7,000 hospitals, 1,700 voluntary health associations, 305,000 active physicians, and 1,600 insurance firms are engaged in the provision of health services and benefits. Among the hospitals, there are a total of 3,291 short-term, general nongovernmental, nonprofit institutions. These institutions, the so-called voluntaries, are known not only for their reputation as the mainstream of hospital care but for their autonomy and independence as well. Voluntary hospitals are also typically small in size—over 60 percent are under 200 beds —and are structured more for rural needs than a highly urban society. Of the total number of physicians, roughly 63 percent are in solo practice, in which the dominant form of payment is fee-for-service (*Hospitals,* 1971; U.S. Department of Health, Education, and Welfare, 1970, pp. 128-29; Wasserman and Wasserman, 1965; U.S. Congress, 1971, p. 79). Though some attempts have been made to encourage voluntary planning, there is little cooperation and coordination in practice, either within or among the various components of care. Against a background of fragmentation and noncoordination, greater planning, systematization, integration, and consolidation of producers into fewer and larger units loom as a logical, if not necessary solution.

The Democratic-Humanists

While the efficacy of illness treatment services may be dubious, the burden of proof ought to rest on the critics and skeptics. In recent years, the public has come to demand access to health care as an inviolable human right. Health services also play an important role in filling somewhat the emotional-spiritual void created in developed societies by the breakup of the extended family, the loss of primary community ties, and the diminution of organized religion. Mental health and family health services are particularly important in this regard. In an increasingly impersonal and materialistic world, health may be one of the few remaining outposts for the preservation of humanistic values of compassion, understanding, dignity, and self-worth. Furthermore, access to health care has become an important issue for the poor and minority groups aspiring to middle-class living standards. The middle classes for their part are more conscious of the instrumentality of health for achieving success in life, and more aware of the technical and psychological possibilities in medicine. Health has acquired considerable social as well as political importance. Health care may play a significant part in the maintenance of community integration and social order by alleviating unrest among the poor and relieving the anxieties of the middle classes. Regardless of one's interpretation of its larger function, there appears little doubt that health is becoming an important issue among the voters; as its electoral importance expands, no government, regardless of party, can afford to dismiss health care lightly (Pellegrino, 1963; Terris, 1968; Reissman, 1969, pp. 74-87; Fein, 1971).

The democratic-humanist outlook is commonly found among reformers who view health as an important symbol for improving the quality of life and a lever for more general social reforms. Pragmatists in this camp acknowledge the necessity for trade-offs between social ideals and managerial-economic exigencies. The question is largely one of balance and assurance that in the attempt to make better use of scarce resources, sight is not lost of the primary purpose of community life—the promotion of individual fulfillment and human welfare. In matters of policy formulation and program planning, democratic-humanism is distinguished by a frame of mind and general outlook born of an awareness of certain critical properties of health care and of the relationship between control of health services and governments structured on democratic principles. Democratic-humanism is anchored first of all in the conviction that health services are essentially ethical in nature. Secondly, the highly subjective and qualitative composition of health and health care compels restraint and caution in the application of quantitative measures derived from either market principles or scientific management, lest human values become distorted or lost. In addition, democratic-humanism takes the position that the claims of any society to democratic rule are meaningless unless public programs remain in the firm control of its citizens or their elected representatives.

TRANSITION IN HEALTH POLICY

Of the four points of view described above, the managerial-rationalist outlook is the most ascendant. It is indigenous to the systems analysis approach which emerged during national defense planning in World War II and carried over to large-scale organizations in contemporary business and industry. A strong appeal of managerial-rationalism is its disclaimer of ideology and values. The presumably greater scientific-objective nature of managerial-rationalism enables its proclaimers to raise questions and propose solutions ordinarily deemed heretical under other circumstances. While one of its major assets, the lulling of moral sensibilities also constitutes the greatest disadvantage and danger of this approach. The claim of superior ability to achieve superior performance in managerial efficiency, cost control, and technological innovation is a related attraction. As the pressure for efficiency intensifies, the influence of managerial-rationalism will no doubt grow. It will have to contend, however, with the rising concern for quality of life accompanying economic progress and development. The relationship of managerial-rationalism to democratic-humanism and the contest between them could be a milestone in the evolution of health affairs.

Much of health policy following the introduction of scientific medicine can be seen as a trial between traditional-expansionist and laissez-fairist schools of thought. On balance, the traditionalist-expansionists have had remarkable success. This success is reflected in the large and growing proportion of GNP going to health in all countries with advanced economies. Governments, whether from conviction or expediency, have not seriously challenged the assumption that money spent on health is a sound investment in future economic growth, despite the persistent objections of laissez-fairists who tend to look at the general category of health services as a form of consumption. Success is also reflected in favorable public opinion. More and more so, the public values progress in the power of medicine as an instrumentality for the achievement of the "good life." Rising consumer expectations for more and better services have served to transform the distribution of health care from a commodity provided on the basis of ability to pay and charity to a vital social service granted as a right of citizenship. In declaring it a merit good, the public has politicized health. The priority people give to health underlies its economic magnitude and supplies the dynamic for a bigger government role in the financing and distribution of services.

The very success of the health field in attracting resources creates conditions for criticism and sharper scrutiny of promises and results. With every addition, health expenditures impinge more heavily on the general economy, and invite comparison and conflict with competing demands. In the framework of the high rates of economic growth and better control of inflation to which developed countries appear to be committed, the investment function of health care may be found wanting. In the United States, economists have gone so far as to raise fears that expanding health employment and expenditures may depress economic growth because of productivity increases which are substantially smaller than those in other areas of the economy where employment is decreasing. Already the third largest industry in terms of employment, it is expected that the health field labor force will increase by two-thirds by 1980. Practical requirements for flexibility in management of the economy may facilitate attempts to depoliticize health in order to dampen consumer desires for more health services and amenities at odds with objectives of economic growth and control of inflation (Burck, 1970).

RATIONALIZATION: DEVELOPMENTS AND TRENDS

The spread of managerial-rationalism is manifested in the centrality of its concepts and techniques in the proposals recently introduced in the United States to deal with problems in the production and delivery of health services.

Following a historic hands-off policy, the federal government now appears committed to using its persuasive influence and the leverage of its purchasing power to restructure health care.

Health Maintenance Organizations

The chief element in the government's strategy to restructure health services is the replacement of solo fee-for-service as the predominate mode of physician practice by corporate groups referred to as Health Maintenance Organizations (HMOs). Together with an emphasis on consolidating physicians into fewer and more manageable groups, HMOs are designed to stimulate economy and efficiency through incentives for the substitution of ambulatory care in place of more expensive in-hospital care and the use of preventive services in place of illness treatment featuring high-powered, hospital-based specialists and costly technology. Reimbursement is seen as the key to lowering costs by controlling utilization. In place of prevailing modes of retrospective fee-for-service payment which tends to penalize more efficient and economy-minded providers, HMOs are based on principles of prospective capitation budgeting and provider sharing in any savings. That is to say, in return for an annual lump sum based on a capitation formula, physician groups would agree to provide a basic range of more comprehensive and coordinated services than typically found in solo fee-for-service situations and would be allowed to share in any difference between income and expenditures. Participation is open to profit-making as well as non-profit organizations. Among the groups expressing an interest thus far in the operation of HMOs are medical schools, private physicians, municipal and county hospital systems, voluntary nonprofit and commercial insurance carriers, and large private corporations active in such fields as aerospace, electronics, and pharmaceuticals. Among the persons most often cited as influencing government thinking on this subject is Paul M. Ellwood, Jr. (1971), a private consultant and chief architect of the HMO concept. For an official statement of the government's position on the subject, see U.S. Department of Health, Education, and Welfare (1971, pp. 31-40).

Although there are no published estimates on potential consolidation effects, a target reduction of 50 percent or more in the number of physicians in solo fee-for-service practice over the next decade seems a reasonable goal, provided that HMOs are given a serious enough push. (If there were a complete reconstitution of solo practitioners into three- or five-man groups, the decline in size would be 66 and 80 percent, respectively.)

A strong selling point of the HMOs is the potential provided for cutting costs through lowering hospital utilization. Control of hospital utilization is the key to any program of economy and savings, for the hospital stands at the center of the health care world. In the United States it commands the single largest share of expenditures for health care. If anything, the economic importance of the hospital is growing. In the eighteen-year period prior to 1969, hospital admissions increased by 63 percent and hospital days rose by 69 percent. Since 1966, the percentage of the personal health care dollar going to the hospital increased from 39 to 43 percent. If hospital care represents the main line in the struggle against illness, it is also the most costly and inflationary. While medical care prices have been rising twice as fast as consumer prices since 1965, hospital charges have been rising nearly five times as fast. The recent inflation in the general economy altered these relationships. In 1970 there was little difference in the growth rate for all prices (6 percent) compared with medical prices (6.4 percent). The rise in hospital outlays continued high, however—15 percent in 1969 (U.S. Social Security Administration, 1971). Expenses per patient for voluntary short-term general hospitals averaged about $81 in 1970, and among larger teaching hospitals and medical centers in cities like New York, expenses often run over $150 per day (*Hospitals,* 1971).

The experience of a number of prepaid group practice plans indicates that HMOs have the potential for reducing hospital utilization from one-fourth to one-third its present volume (Klarman, 1963; Donabedian, 1969). Provided that hospital and physician care is fully integrated and organized to exploit economies of scale and control of patient flow, businessmen who have studied the problem believe that total savings could reach up to 20 percent (*Nation's Health,* 1971).

Health Care Corporations

The most noticeable movement toward rationalization in the voluntary sector has come from the American Hospital Association. Perhaps because of fear of the implications of Health Maintenance Organizations for deemphasizing in-hospital care and the possible weakening of the hospital as the principal power in health care, the American Hospital Association has unveiled a plan (the Ameriplan) for transferring hospitals from narrow-focused, inward-looking, acute treatment institutions to broad-gauged corporate entities, called Health Care Corporations (HCCs). Each corporation would be responsible for the synthesis and delivery of a comprehensive array of health services to assigned geographic areas. The range of services to be provided comprises preventive health, primary care, secondary care, restorative care, and health-related custodial care (*Ameriplan,* 1970).

The Health Care Corporation is presented by the American Hospital Association as a vehicle better equipped than the Health Maintenance Organization to move the health services from what is often described as a "backward turn-of-the-century cottage industry" to a modern, coordinated, and comprehensive delivery system. Only the HCCs, it may be argued, have the scope and scale for economically integrating the various levels of mental and somatic skills and technologies embodied in the more inclusive and systematic approaches to personal health care widely recommended today. The HMOs, in comparison, would supply only a partial solution at best. While they may help improve the state of primary physician care, sizeable problems would remain in coordinating day-to-day family health care with more complex secondary and tertiary services, and in relating noninstitutionally based care to hospital and nursing home care. The HCC idea is grounded in assumptions of economies of scale, importance of management planning and program evaluation, and dysfunctionality of unorganized competition. In addition to fostering comprehensive care and lower unit costs, the assignment of geographic areas to single corporations would have the effect of promoting mergers and consolidations. The possibilities are enormous. In the course of a decade, the number of separate voluntary hospitals might well be diminished from over 3,000 to as few as one-half to one-third of this number. The average size of institutions could be reversed so that instead of the present situation (in which 43 percent of all voluntaries have under 100 beds, 68 percent under 200 beds, and only 9 percent as many as 400 beds or more) in the next decade few institutions would have under 200 beds and the majority would have the capacity for 400 or more beds (*Hospitals,* 1971). Should this occur it would still fall far short of the policy in Sweden by which all hospitals of under 300 beds are closed on grounds of economic nonviability. In England, the latest thinking appears attuned to larger minimum-sized units of 1,000 to 1,500 beds (Somers, 1971).

If adopted, the American Hospital Association plan would solidify and enlarge the position of the hospital in the health power structure. Hospitals may have their eye on raising their share of the personal health care dollar from the present level of 43 percent to a figure approximating that of hospitals in England and Sweden—between 50 and 60 percent (Somers, 1971). (Indeed, fear of this happening may be why the government is pushing the HMO idea. In the face of dubious efficacy, further centralization of patient care in specialist- and technology-dominated hospitals could be a prescription for more inflation and cost escalation.) Through various devices such as control of money flow to other providers through awarding of subcontracts and control of hospital-based technology essential to the modern practice of medicine, physicians would eventually be enticed to relinquish more of their autonomy to hospital corporations in return for greater security, more satisfying conditions of work, and a chance to participate in management. The political position of hospitals would be further assured by a system of state regulation operating through special five- to seven-man commissions subject to gubernatorial appointment. Working under the umbrella of broad guidelines set by a national commission, each state health commission would establish and assign geographic spheres of responsibility and approve rates of reimbursement. State regulation not only provides a measure of diversity and freedom consistent with regional cultural differences but, more importantly, because of hospital control of planning bodies, acts as a buffer against commercial penetration.

Proprietary Ownership and Unstructured Competition

Few developments have shaken the voluntary hospitals more than the swift rise of proprietary hospital and nursing home corporate chains designed to earn a profit for investor-owners. Some measure of the speed with which this development has occurred is provided by the fact that in a two-year period from 1968 to 1970, twenty-six investor-owned companies purchased or built more than 150 short-term general hospitals with more than 15,500 beds. These acquisitions comprised about 20 percent of the nation's proprietary hospitals and 32 percent of their beds. These twenty-six corporations have announced plans which, if implemented, will result in their obtaining control of nearly 230 facilities with more than 28,300 beds. All told, about fifty corporations now operate profit-making hospital chains and there are signs suggesting that many more—including nursing home operators—plan to enter the acute care field (Owens, 1970). This sudden turn from solo and small-scale patterns of ownership to large-scale corporate chains in the proprietary field is no doubt a reaction to the growth of health care as a major economic industry.

Extensively criticized by voluntary hospitals for selecting the best health care risks, avoiding patients unable to pay for the cost of care, and cutting out high-cost, low-volume services such as paramedical teaching programs and emergency and obstetrical services, proprietary spokesmen answer in defense that such charges are nothing more than envy over their demonstrated superior managerial ability, which makes it possible to simultaneously make money while charging patients less than voluntary hospitals, without any ostensible reduction in quality (Foster, 1969; Ferber, 1971). In the midst of such recriminations, and with little fanfare, the number of states requiring mandatory hospital planning and franchising based on proven community need has grown since 1968 from one to nine (*Hospital Week,* 1971). Proprietary hospital corporations look on this development as an infringement on the free movement of resources in response to competition and market opportunities. To the private sector, the proliferation of compulsory planning at the state level (most often with the overt support of hospitals which earlier viewed even less stringent voluntary planning as a threat to institutional autonomy and self-determination) appears suspiciously like a cabal to perpetuate voluntary hospital dominance and the status quo. The fact that voluntary hospital representatives and their allies dominate hospital and facilities planning bodies does nothing to assuage suspicion. Such charges can be expected to evoke sympathy and perhaps even transform the prevailing image of compulsory hospital planning from a constructive to an antisocial force.

Private Nationwide Corporations and Structured Competition

For persons interested in using private investment as a lever for expediting reorganization of hospital and health services (but worried about the possible social dysfunctionalities of intense market competition and "cream skimming" forms of profit taking which may relegate voluntary hospitals to the unhappy status of collection bins for non-money-making patients and services), the possibility of enlisting larger nationwide corporations, which by virtue of their size and complexity tend to stress planning, order, and stability in contrast to more tumultuous brands of competition, may be quite attractive.

The unusual combination in big corporations of easy access to the large amounts of capital necessary for financing today's costly health services, sophisticated approaches to problem solving, and outreach expansion capabilities of regional and national scope, provides an avenue for reorganizing hospital and health services quickly and unencumbered by deep-seated ideological suspicion and distrust of government power. Quite apart from the actual degree of involvement, the threat of private-sector encroachment may stimulate productivity by destabilizing relationships of accommodation and traditional practices in the health community which obstruct change and efficiency. Government officials may see another advantage—a chance to manipulate the health economy while simultaneously lowering the political risks of failure through the delegation of responsibility and clouding of accountability.

For their part, private corporations stand to benefit from the opportunity to expand security and growth needs through diversification of investments in an expanding market underwritten by governmental subsidies and guarantees. The annual value of medically related goods presently exceeds $6 billion and is growing at a compound rate of 10 to 15 percent a year (Meyers, 1970).

Interest in the private sector has been stimulated and encouraged by the ostensible success of the Kaiser Foundation Medical Care Program in lowering health care cost through the use of market incentives and managerial techniques structured to reward economy through the substitution whenever possible of less costly ambulatory and preventive care for in-hospital and acute care. An affiliate of Kaiser Industries (a large corporation specializing in steel manufacturing and heavy construction), the Kaiser Medical Care Program is characterized by an industrial-systems approach involving: (a) the introduction of large-scale, industrial-management capabilities into the health care system; (b) the separation of professional and administrative aspects of health care, with the former handled primarily by physicians and the latter by trained executives; (c) the provision of support services to both professional and nonprofessional activities; (d) the coordination of professional and nonprofessional manpower, hospitals and related facilities, and large amounts of consumable material to serve patients with needs for health care; and (e) conduct of the entire enterprise in an economically self-sustaining manner that generates enough income to permit amortization of large commercial loans, replacement of facilities, and an average growth of 10 percent per year. As a privately owned corporation with its own network of fifteen hospitals and twenty-nine clinics in the states of Washington, California, and Hawaii, and control over provider services through means of negotiated contracts with physician groups on a per capita, prepaid basis, Kaiser is the only medical program of its kind operating in the world. The potentially superior efficiency of involving big business in health delivery is indicated in Kaiser's claim to be able to provide family comprehensive in-hospital and ambulatory care on an annual per capita cost roughly one-third cheaper and at a quality equal to, and in many cases superior to, that offered elsewhere. Lower hospital utilization and higher rates of hospital occupancy are the secret. The advantages of a centrally managed system of hospital and physician care are striking. In relation to other comparable groups, Kaiser members use one-third fewer hospital days and require 40 percent fewer hospital beds (U.S. National Advisory Commission on Health Manpower, 1967, pp. 77-105).

POLITICAL IMPLICATIONS OF RATIONALIZATION

Despite the vaunted powers of modern medicine, health professionals are unable, for the most part, to demonstrate any clear relationship between services, e.g., somatic, mental, dental, and such end-result objectives as number of added years of socially meaningful life, degree of restoration of individual biologic and sociologic capabilities, and economic growth and productivity. There is a paucity of reliable benefit and trade-off information on alternative modes of treating illness conditions both within and between types of practice (medical, surgical, preventive, therapeutic, rehabilitative). In matters of outcome and cost-effectiveness, little is known about the value of treating many diagnoses medically or surgically, or the trade-offs between medical and nonmedical procedures compared with nonintervention. (For a review of conceptual and methodologic problems in measuring the benefits of health services, see Mushkin, 1962.)

Taking terminal cancer for an example, it could be that much of the surgery performed is questionable. Nonsurgical medical treatment may be not only equally effective in prolonging life but also more humane in alleviating unnecessary trauma to patients and unwarranted financial and emotional family strain. In cases where medicine cannot in fact accomplish much, it may be far better to rely upon nonscientific-humanistic means, traditionally better suited for handling emotional-supportive needs with compassion and dignity. Much of the surgery performed in questionable cases is probably due less to incentives for economic gain than the innate desire of highly trained individuals to want to apply their skills in the solution of problems. The recent wave of organ transplantations may be an illustration of the imperatives which drive specialists to employ their skills under even the most dubious circumstances.

Not only are the benefits of medical treatment often doubtful, but there is some reason to believe that, because of an irony of progress, medicine may be once again at the point where it does nearly as much harm as good to patients. Quite apart from obvious problems of human error and incompetence, the problem is largely one of the failure of health care organization to keep pace with changes in biomedical science and technology. The power and complexity of treatment processes today is such that up to one-third of all hospital admissions are estimated to be related to complications associated with chemotherapy (*Medical World News,* 1970; Cluff et al., 1964). Outmoded and restrictive state licensure laws often stand in the way of effective treatment by blocking the supply and distribution of skilled personnel and by perpetuating problems of manpower obsolescence. A haphazard scheme of financing health care provides incentives for unnecessary hospitalization and treatment. And the weight of habit and convention obstructs the abandonment of treatment procedures superseded by more effective methods in places such as mental hospitals and nursing homes where prolonged institutionalization and isolation from the community are known to be harmful. For a concise review of the literature on iatrogenic illness, see Freidson (1971, pp. 205-12).

Redefinition of Health Boundaries

Interest in economy and efficiency when coupled with doubt over safety and efficacy may provide a radical redefinition of illness and a sharply reduced sphere of authority and responsibility for the health field. In areas where jurisdictional claims are not backed up by evidence of demonstrably superior techniques and skills, the monopoly-hold of medicine may be broken and responsibilities reclassified and transferred to nonhealth authorities. For example, nonorganic mental illness may be considered a moral and behavioral problem more appropriately treated by the educational and legal systems. Similarly, responsibility for services dealing with mental subnormality, care of the elderly, preventive-health behavior, and social and environmental medicine might be transferred to authorities in education, housing, social services, and community and ecological planning. Arguments favoring such transfers have been advanced in the United States and abroad (Szasz, 1964; Seebohm Committee, 1968).

Reclassification and transfer of program responsibilities might be defended not solely on grounds of logic and functional specificity, but politically and economically as well. Transfer of operational responsibilities could better chances of achieving a more optimal allocation of national resources by placing competing needs on a more even footing in the politics of the budgetary process. Apart from the benefits of accounting legerdemain, some of the money savings could be real. Refusal to label nonorganically-based emotional and behavioral disturbances as mental illness (drug addiction, alcoholism, delinquency, sexual deviations, strained interpersonal relationships) could save large sums through cutbacks in expensive personnel and facilities, and by rechannelling such problems back into traditional treatment sources, such as the family and primary social groups, not reliant upon costly technology and training. Further gains would accrue through a reduction in the volume of illness resulting unintentionally from illness treatment procedures themselves. On this last point, if neither supply nor productivity of health services can be sufficiently increased to offset cost rises, then it may be worthwhile to think of tailoring the nature and amount of demand to meet the supply. Using cost-benefit analysis as a justification, a way to cut health costs and save money is to redefine illness and reduce the number of patients, especially in areas where the efficacy of treatment is questionable.

Control of Policy and Program Planning

From a managerial-rationalist standpoint, it may be concluded that health professionals are not well suited to deal with issues of policy and management. Their very training and vocational commitment is a liability. The twin processes of self-selection and socialization in preparation for entry into a career tend to place a higher premium on community service than on considerations of resource allocation and management know-how. Once committed to a career of service, the thought that one's actions are either ineffectual or harmful produces too much role conflict, with the result that such pressures are either rejected or altered in such a way as to constitute less of a threat. More often than not, professionals have an unassailable belief in the importance and value of what they do, and they are driven by a built-in impetus to expand service while simultaneously resisting evaluation of efficiency and effectiveness. An analysis of the social and psychological constraints affecting professionals in program administration and evaluation is provided by Freidson (1971, pp. 158-84).

Decisions are determined for the most part by the information that goes into them. To the extent that health professionals control the information systems and dominate important policy-making and advisory posts, their values and interests will understandably prevail. The solution is obvious: circumvent or downgrade the influence of professionals by giving persons not committed to health service values a more decisive if not controlling say in policy making and planning. The temptation to do so may be particularly strong in the health field. Because of their monopoly over healing, self-regulatory powers, and high status in the public eye, physicians are especially tough to control. Elected officials are most often at a loss over how to cope with physicians who in budgetary and planning negotiations raise implicitly or explicitly the possibility of life-threatening consequences should their recommendations go unheeded. Presented with the possibility of having to shoulder the normal and political responsibility for such terrible consequences, no matter how remote, elected officials invariably acquiesce. The problems elected officials have in coping with health professionals both within and outside the government bureaucracy are eloquently stated by former Minister of Health in England, J. Enoch Powell (1966).

In the view of public officials worried about having to meet total national needs within the constraints of fixed resources, experts conversant in the language of budgets but uncommitted to health care can appear as an effective buffer against the chauvinism, parochialism, and expansionist tendencies of career-minded health professionals and their bureaucracies. Consistent with this rationale, the center of gravity for decision-making in Washington has been quietly shifting from professionals based in the Department of Health, Education, and Welfare to a cadre of managerial and economic analysts working directly out of the President's Office in the increasingly prestigious and powerful Office of Management and the Budget.

SOCIAL IMPLICATIONS OF RATIONALIZATION

The social implications of rationalization are at least twofold: (1) a change in the ethical-motivational structure at the point of interface between patients and services, and (2) a change in the social purpose of health care.

Ethical-Motivational Orientation

Public service and commitment to humanitarian ideals has been the historic cornerstone of professionalism. The success of the doctor-patient relationship and much of healing depends upon an atmosphere of trust and faith on the part of the patient that his interests are foremost in the minds of those caring for him. While traditional values of empathy, understanding, and emotional support in health care may have declined due to the influence of science and technology in training programs, altruism and service remain a basic element in the socialization of professionals. It is a concern with client and community welfare, no matter how abstract and formal, that separates the professions from other occupations.

Although a weakening of service values might follow from any attempt to cut back the influence of professionals in health policy, use of market-type incentives to obtain efficiency and cost control is a potentially far greater hazard. In place of altruistic service ideals and incentives for advocacy of patient interests, rewards drawn from the market and industry are immersed in a tradition of egoism and self-interest and structured to place providers and patients in an adversary relationship. This danger is present in the incentives at the core of the corporate models proposed for reorganizing health care services in the United States. The crux of the idea is to stimulate efficiency and save money by allowing providers to keep a share of any difference between income and expenditures. Unlike fee-for-service systems whereby providers are encouraged to provide as much service as possible, the incentive here is to provide as little service as possible. It may be a reflection of the complexity of the politics of change that some well-known figures on the American health care scene reportedly feel that such a shift in incentives may be justified on the grounds that errors of overservicing and underservicing will tend to cancel one another (Greenberg and Rodburg, 1971). Without dwelling on the consequences of such logic, the situation seems tilted to place economics ahead of human service. Instead of acting too soon, physicians will now be encouraged to wait until it is too late.

It may be a sign of a desperate desire to control health care expenditures that top officials in Washington are openly urging an expansion of profit-making competition in the health field. Long held in check because of its widely acknowledged limitations, profit-making is now being refurbished as a socially constructive element for innovation and cost control. There is little reason to expect that the private sector has changed or that market principles are any more operable today than in the past. Indeed, leading pro-market theorists firmly insist on the incompatibility between social responsibility requirements and business goals, of acquisitiveness, profits, and capital accumulation (Friedman, 1970).

The role assigned to the private sector notwithstanding, the exaltation of management science and industrial systems techniques adversely affects democratic-humanist aspirations by their proclivity for defining health narrowly in statistically measurable terms rather than as a dynamic for personal and social well-being contained in the belief that health care is a right. The limitations stem from the not always clear predilection of management-industrial techniques for quantification and economic measures of performance which tend to deemphasize the importance of qualitative considerations and social goals. On balance, such methods are notoriously reductionistic and insensitive to the needs of people. In light of the essentially ethical and subjective nature of health care, it is illusory to think that the physically ill and the emotionally disturbed can be treated satisfactorily and humanely in ways that compare in efficiency and cost-effectiveness with the manufacture and sale of products in industry and business.

Relationship of Health to Social Goals

Rationalization and preoccupation with economic matters may also alter the mission of health services in society. Though the role of health services has always been broad, encompassing multiple diverse functions ranging from: (a) the mercantilistic accumulation of national wealth and power in which health is regarded as a resource of the state in the service of goals of defense, productivity, and economic growth; to (b) an instrument for social control in which health services act as a mechanism for the enforcement of a conformity of behavior for keeping existing institutions running smoothly; to (c) a vehicle for the attainment of social reform in such vast areas as civil rights, employment policies, income distribution, housing, and community relations; it has for the most part been perceived by the public as an expression of community adherence to the values of individual self-fulfillment and egalitarian sharing of precious life-support resources. The danger, of course, is that an overemphasis of economic and managerial values may change things so that, whether it is accurate or not, health services are viewed as an instrument for depersonalization and repression.

Any turn toward depersonalization and repressive controls would be grossly out of step with the general shift in values marking the movement from industrial to postindustrial society. In highly developed countries the constructs and values of early industrial development are believed to be in the process of giving way to a secular-humanistic outlook in which there is a greater recognition of: (a) community as opposed to individual ends; (b) egalitarianism and service ideals in contrast to principles of caveat emptor and egoism; (c) dignity and the intrinsic worth of the individual as opposed to impersonalization and dehumanization; (d) primacy of quality of life over objectives of economic efficiency and production of material goods; and (e) responsiveness and accountability of institutions to human needs as opposed to organizational and bureaucratic imperatives. (The increased importance of secular-humanism in the postindustrial society is described by Kahn and Werner, 1967.) It would be most ironic if values associated with health care were to march backward while social values in general moved forward. The creation of such a hiatus in health between democratic-humanist and managerial-rationalist values could sow the seeds for one of the more important controversies in the decade ahead and contribute significantly to the disintegration of individual and community life.

RESOLUTION

To the extent that service values have tended to dominate and overshadow managerial-economic values and have compounded problems of productivity, distribution, and effectiveness, then some redressing of the relationship between the two is desirable and necessary. However, in proceeding with such a realignment, caution is urged lest the pendulum be allowed to swing too far in the opposite direction. The challenge to policy makers is to work out an acceptable balance between these two value systems so that synergy replaces conflict.

It is apparent from experience that, although useful, the inculcation of humanist service values in the training of professionals is insufficient to guard against the forces of parochialism and insularity which lead individuals to interpret issues in a manner consistent with their specialized skills and personal convenience. Also evident is the effect of organizations on behavior. As pointed out by Freidson (1971, pp. 87-90), the organizational structure within which health care is produced and distributed exercises a profound influence and probably does more over time to shape behavior than does socialization and training in preparation for entry into health careers. In an era given to the accentuation of efficiency, it is essential that the attitudes of providers and the behavior-reward systems of organizations complement one another and reinforce acknowledgment of the paramountcy of man. Important as this union is, it does not go far enough. Since no one is a better judge of what is good and just than the persons most directly affected, vigorous consumer participation is required in every nonclinical (social, political, and economic) aspect of health decision making.

In defense of the managerial-rationalist principles contained in proposals for reorganizing health services, it is said that right things are often done for the wrong reasons. While this is true, it is no doubt also true that the chances of achieving right results are diminished by inconsistency and conflict of purpose. The inconsistency and conflict of purpose between professional values, organizational incentives, and social goals inherent in much of the discussion supportive of rationalization, is a formula best suited for confusion of objectives and obfuscation of public accountability. A more auspicious formula for minimizing the spread of alienation in contemporary life is based on the avoidance of any temptation to restructure health care from a social service to a purely economic and administrative activity, and adheres instead to a policy of building upon and strengthening (through appropriate reform in the structure of organizations and the education of physicians and related personnel) the already present altruistic service predilections of health professionals. While accountability and responsiveness cannot under any circumstances be guaranteed, the best assurance may well lie in a system of checks and balances, designed to stimulate, encourage, and reinforce socially desirable behavior.

SUMMARY AND CONCLUSIONS

Escalating costs and the rising proportion of gross national product going to health were examined from the standpoint of their significance for the future of health services. Rationalization driven mainly by pressures for efficiency and control of expenditures was viewed as posing a serious challenge to the continued leadership of professionals and the influence of service values in the field of health affairs. Although not excluding objectives of more and better care, the primary aims of rationalization were interpreted as more economic and managerial in nature: to foster productivity and efficiency in accordance with principles of economic self-gain and economies of scale; and to bring traditionally diffuse and autonomous health care elements under more effective central policy and planning control through consolidation and merger. The danger of too great a preoccupation with economics and management is that it may erode the traditionally humanistic-ethical foundations of health care, already weakened by the inroads of medical technology and specialization, and contribute further to the alienation of man arising from processes of material progress and depersonalization marking contemporary life.

Upon assessing the implications of rationalization, it was suggested that the inability to demonstrate a clear relationship between services and benefits might lead to a radical redefinition of health and transfer of program responsibilities to nonhealth areas based on less costly technologies. To counter the difficult-to-stop momentum for increases in health outlays rooted in consumer expectations and the career commitments of health professionals, government may turn increasingly for advice and leadership to experts uncommitted to service values and seek also to depoliticize health. The need to differentiate between means and ends was underscored and a system of checks and balances involving increased consumer participation was proposed for reconciling demands for efficiency with larger social and philosophic aims.

REFERENCES

Ameriplan—A Proposal for the Delivery and Financing of Health Services in the United States. Chicago: American Hospital Association, 1970.

Anderson, O. W. "Health Services in a Land of Plenty." *Environment and Policy: The Next Fifty Years,* edited by W. R. Ewald, Jr. Bloomington: Indiana University Press, 1968.

Anderson, O. W., and Neuhauser, D. "Rising Costs Are Inherent in Modern Health Care Systems." *Hospitals* 43, no. 4 (1969): 50-52.

Burck, G. "There'll Be Less Leisure Than You Think." *Fortune* 81 (March 1970): 87.

Cluff, L. E., et al. "Studies in the Epidemiology of Adverse Drug Reactions." *Journal of the American Medical Association* 188 (June 15, 1964): 976-83.

Donabedian, A. "An Evaluation of Prepaid Group Practice." *Inquiry* 6, no. 3 (1969): 3-27.

Ellwood, P. M., Jr. "Health Maintenance Organizations: Concept and Strategy." *Hospitals* 45, no. 6 (1971): 53-56.

Fein, R. "On Measuring Economic Benefits of Health Programmes." *Medical History and Medical Care,* edited by G. McLachlan and T. McKeown. London: Nuffield Provincial Hospitals Trust, 1971.

Ferber, B. "An Analysis of Chain Operated For-Profit Hospitals." *Health Services Research* 6, no. 1 (1971): 49-60.

Foster, J. T. "Proprietary Hospitals Go Public." *Modern Hospital* 112 (March 1969): 80-87.

Freidson, E. *Profession of Medicine.* New York: Dodd, Mead, 1971.

Friedman, M. *Capitalism and Freedom.* Chicago: Phoenix Books, 1962.

Friedman, M. "The Social Responsibility of Business Is To Increase Its Profits." *The New York Times Magazine* 33 (September 13, 1970).

Fry, J. *Medicine in Three Societies.* London: Billing & Sons, 1969.

Fuchs, V. R. "The Growing Demand for Medical Care." *New England Journal of Medicine* 279, no. 4 (1968): 190-95.

Fuchs, V. R. "What Kind of System for Health Care?" *Social Policy for Health Care.* New York: The New York Academy of Medicine, 1969.

Greenberg, I. G., and Rodburg, M. L. "The Role of Prepaid Group Practice in Relieving the Medical Care Crisis." *Harvard Law Review* 84 (February 1971): 926.

Hospital Week (May 7 and June 11, 1971).

Hospitals: Guide Issue 45, no. 15 (1971): part 2.

Kahn, H. C., and Werner, A. J. *The Year 2000: A Framework for Speculation on the Next Thirty-Three Years.* New York: Macmillan, 1967.

Klarman, H. E. "Effect of Prepaid Group Practice on Hospital Use." *Public Health Reports* 78, no. 11 (1963): 955-65.

Marris, P., and Rein, M. *Dilemmas of Social Reform: Poverty and Community Action in the United States.* New York: Atherton Press, 1967.

Medical World News 14-15. "Drug Experts Face Up" (November 13, 1970).

Meyers, H. B. "The Medical Industrial Complex." *Fortune* 81 (January 1970): 90.

Mushkin, S. J. "Health as an Investment." *Journal of Political Economy* 70, part II (October 1962): 129-57.

Nation's Health (June 1971): 10.

Owen, D. "Selectivity and the Health Service." *Social Services for All? Eleven Fabian Essays.* London: Pergamon Press, 1968.

Owens, A. "Can the Profit Motive Save Our Hospitals?" *Medical Economics* 76 (March 30, 1970).

Pellegrino, E. D. "Medicine, History, and the Idea of Man." *Medicine and Society. The Annals of the American Academy of Political and Social Science* 346 (March 1963): 9-20.

Powell, J. E. *Medicine and Politics.* London: Pitman Medical Publishing Co., 1966.

Reissman, F. *Strategies Against Poverty.* New York: Random House, 1969.

Rice, D., and Cooper, B. S. "National Health Expenditures, 1929-70." *Social Security Bulletin* 34, no. 1 (1971): 3-18.

Rice, D., and McGee, M. F. "Projections of National Health Expenditures, 1975 and 1980." *Research and Statistics Note no. 18.* Washington, D.C.: Office of Research and Statistics, Social Security Administration, 1970.

Ruderman, A. P. (ed.). "Canadian-American Conference on Hospital Programs." *Medical Care* 7, no. 6 supplement (1969): 1-90.

Seebohm Committee. *Report of the Committee on Local Authority and Allied Personal Social Services.* London: Her Majesty's Stationery Office, 1968.

Somers, A. "The Rationalization of Health Services: A Universal Priority." *Inquiry* 8 (1971): 48-60.

Swedish Health Services System. Lectures from the American College of Hospital Administrators Twenty-Second Fellows Seminar, Stockholm, Sweden, 1969. Chicago: American College of Hospital Administrators, 1971.

Szasz, T. S. *The Myth of Mental Illness.* New York: Harper & Row, 1964.

Terris, M. "A Social Policy for Health." *American Journal of Public Health* 58, no. 1 (1968): 5-12.

U.S. Congress, Senate Committee on Finance. *Hearings on the Social Security Amendments of 1970* (91st Congress, 2nd Session). Washington, D.C.: U.S. Government Printing Office, 1970.

U.S. Congress, Senate Committee on Finance. *Hearings on National Health Insurance* (92nd Congress, 1st Session). Washington, D.C.: U.S. Government Printing Office, 1971.

U.S. Department of Health, Education, and Welfare. National Center for Health Statistics. *Health Resources Statistics, 1969* (Public Health Service Publication no. 1509). Washington, D.C.: HEW, 1970.

U.S. Department of Health, Education, and Welfare. *Towards a Comprehensive Health Policy for the 1970s: A White Paper.* Washington, D.C.: HEW, 1971.

U.S. National Advisory Commission on Health Manpower. *Report* (vol. II). Washington, D.C.: Government Printing Office, 1967.

U.S. Social Security Administration. *The Size and Shape of the Medical Care Dollar: Chart Book, 1970.* Washington, D.C.: Government Printing Office, 1971.

Wasserman, C. S., and Wasserman, P. *Health Organizations of the U.S., Canada, and Internationally* (2nd ed.). Ithaca, N.Y.: Graduate School of Business and Public Administration, Cornell University, 1965.

2

Health Policy Developments in Other Highly Industrialized Nations

Selection by Roger M. Battistella

Health policy appears to be entering a new era within many advanced industrial nations, regardless of historic differences in culture and political systems and economic ideologies. In contrast to former confidence and optimism, the new outlooks are decidedly negative and modest. Instead of emphasizing the potential of scientific medicine, the inclination is to accentuate its limitations. The thrust of public policy is pitched to a lowering of public expectations.

This paper illustrates this new skepticism about the value of high technology medicine by examining three issues which are confronting policy makers here and in other countries. The issues are primary care, long-term institutional care, and the interface between health and social services. The paper draws upon a review of health system policies in the Soviet Union, Finland, Sweden, and the United Kingdom which the author visited in 1975 under a WHO fellowship (Battistella, 1977).

Except for the Soviet Union, where the function and organization of health services are noticeably different, the countries visited are in the process of levelling off spending for hospital services. In many instances, the process is well advanced. In the United Kingdom the entire hospital service is already midway

Reprinted from "Issues in Health Planning: An International Perspective," *Papers on the National Health Guidelines: Conditions for Change in the Health Care System* (Washington, D.C.: HEW, 1977). The section entitled "Trends in Health Policy: Revisionism and Convergence" appeared in "Study of Macrohealth Planning Developments in Finland, Sweden, Union of Soviet Socialist Republics, England and Northern Ireland," report submitted to John E. Fogarty Center for Advanced Study in the Health Sciences (National Institutes of Health, HEW, 1977).

through a planned ten-year reduction in which the hospitals' share of current and capital health service expenditures is scheduled to drop from 46 to 40.7 percent by 1980. In Finland a system of incentives was instituted in 1972 to stimulate the capital construction and professional staffing of community health centers; in Sweden, a moratorium has been placed on the construction of acute care beds in favor of long-term beds.

The justification for stabilizing and reducing budgets in acute hospital services is derived from the assumption that the saturation point has been reached in technological innovation and diffusion and in modernizing outmoded physical plants. These efforts, it is believed, have succeeded to the point where continuing high rates of increases in spending are inherently inflationary and counterproductive.

This is a plausible assumption being asserted with increasing trenchancy, but it presents some troublesome features. Closer inspection reveals a surprisingly low degree of definition among its proponents. It is questionable whether saturation is an easily recognizable phenomenon.

In practice, the assumption of saturation is used widely to conjure up a mixed bag of economic concepts, including economy, efficiency, productivity, and diminishing marginal benefit. Small wonder, then, that there is disagreement how one is to know whether saturation has been reached. A number of tests have been proposed; most of them are of the quick and dirty variety and many of them are easier to run in theory than in practice. They include, for example, the closing of a substantial number of beds (one-fifth or more) to see whether the same number of patients can be taken care of without a lengthening of waiting times and admissions delays. Presumably, if waiting lists are unaffected, then the saturation point has not been attained. Other approaches focus on bed occupancy, volume of procedures performed by doctors and other health personnel, and sharp changes in medical prices and costs. Many of the tests would be hard to implement because of the ability of doctors and other providers to exert control over the demand for their services, the rate of hospital admissions and lengths of stay, and the mix of technology and amenities they choose to use in diagnostic and treatment processes.

The saturation thesis is used also as a surrogate expression for the notion that it is costing more and more to accomplish less and less. But this notion may be overly simplistic, given that there is no agreement on the function of health services in highly developed societies, i.e., whether it is prevention and cure of disease, alleviation of suffering, human capital maintenance, or the promotion of social and political stability through achieving consumer satisfaction. There are also formidable methodological obstacles constraining the measurement of agreed-upon ends which is especially difficult in the health field because of the crossovers between such joint aims as teaching, research, and patient care and the effect of external factors on health status such as housing, nutrition, and the environment. The measurement problem is rooted in the chaos over the definition of health itself, that is, whether health represents long life expectancy, the absence of medically certified morbidity and disability, or advanced states of personally determined material and spiritual well-being—a range extending from the mundane to the metaphysical.

Until consensus has been formed at the fundamental level of definition, goals of health services will remain ambiguous. Saturation arguments against spending for high-technology services draped in the garb of ostensibly objective techniques for analysis should be viewed skeptically as a strategem, possibly for depoliticizing complex policy choices which can be defended ultimately only on political grounds.

PRIMARY CARE

Independent of the merit of the saturation hypothesis, there is widespread concern in many countries which have invested extensively in the development of high-technology health services that progress in this area has occurred at the expense of services for routine medical needs and/or the care of the long-term ill and permanently disabled. The growth in importance of the health problems of the aged and the chronically ill for which highly sophisticated and costly hospital services can do little are recognized increasingly as paradoxical reflections of improvements in the prevention and treatment of acute communicable illness and of improvements in standards of living.

Balanced development of the health sector has become a keystone of policy in advanced countries which are either committed to correcting imbalances due to one-sided development of acute hospital specialty services, or apprehensive about the economic consequences of unchecked expansion of technological innovation and forms of medical specialization which, sophistication notwithstanding, are extremely costly and of dubious efficacy. However, the momentum for the expansion of high-technology services will be difficult to arrest in an environment of faith entwined with political power. The public has been successfully proselytized to a belief in the benefits of medical technology and in the power of biomedical research and development to ultimately conquer disease and disability. Furthermore, there are many with political influence who are dependent upon continued investments in high technology.

Nevertheless, the concept of primary care is attaining symbolic significance as a panacea for correcting dislocations attributed to uncoordinated high-technology growth. To be sure, there are some developed countries which do not fall into this category, such as the Soviet Union, where there are opposite problems because of a historical bias favoring primary care, and England, which has been more careful to coordinate hospital services with general practitioner services so that the dislocations are less severe.

Defining Primary Care

While primary care is commonly invoked as a cure-all, there is not much agreement on what the concept means. It is used freely to represent constellations of services at levels of first- and last-contact medical care, which encompass such specific functions as: (1) disease prevention and health maintenance; (2) diagnosis and treatment of routine medical conditions; (3) palliation and care of the chronically ill and disabled; (4) certification of illness for sickness benefits; (5) control of referrals to assure optimal use of costly specialist and hospital services; and (6) emergency medical services.

The functions placed under the primary care umbrella tend, in practice, to be a reflection of the major gaps and problems arising from an overconcentration on high-technology services accorded a higher and more glamorous status by the value system of modern scientific medicine, which looks upon the subjective-qualitative component of medical practice as unscientific anathema.

In Sweden, a country where general practice was allowed to deteriorate to the point of near extinction, a major focus of the primary care renascence is to cut down on unnecessary use of hospital specialty and emergency room services by providing the population convenient access to modern, well-equipped health centers staffed by general practitioners working with interdisciplinary teams. Patients are free to go to hospital specialists directly.

In Finland, access to hospital specialists is by referral only. Under a 1972 mandate, primary care practitioners have also been granted control of low-technology beds in facilities set up for routine acute and chronic care. These facilities are said to average less than 60 beds in size. They are meant to achieve the cost-containment objective of reducing utilization of high-technology beds and also to improve the quality of care for nonambulatory chronic aged patients, since (in the opinion of critics in the medical profession) previously responsible social service authorities were performing unsatisfactorily. Granting such responsibility to primary care practitioners could backfire if the prestige and reward system of medicine is not modified to offset pressures to emulate high-technology colleagues through the technological enrichment of long-term beds.

Belief in the superiority of hospital-oriented specialty medicine dominates the medical establishment even in England, a country in which general practitioner services were never allowed to run down as badly as in many other developed Western countries and where they have been reasonably successful in screening access to acute hospital services. Patients in the United Kingdom cannot go to a specialist without first being referred by a general practitioner.

The decision taken in 1946 to remove general practice from the hospitals is currently being reconsidered as possibly shortsighted and unwise. Skeptics are troubled that the voicing of such sentiment by high-technology spokesmen may be a defensive reaction against the aim of the 1974 reorganization of the National Health Service to reallocate funds from the teaching and district hospitals to community care. The survival and aggrandizement of specialty interests may be served best by coopting general practice to preclude the formation of a powerful enough coalition in community care (involving general practice, public health, social work, and related human services) to challenge the hegemony of hospital services.

Inappropriate Hospitalization

In the countries mentioned above, it is generally accepted among policy makers that from 25 to 50 percent of the patients in hospitals could be taken care of elsewhere; in contrast, only about 5 percent of the hospital beds are said to be misused in the Soviet Union (mainly by aged awaiting home care and long-term care assignment). This is claimed to be one of the advantages of a highly organized system of primary care. Albeit the role of the doctor of first contact (the district doctor working out of a polyclinic who carries out the same functions as a general practitioner) has involved prophylaxis and referral mainly in the past, this is expected to change in the near future. Universal mass screening and computer applications are planned which will handle referrals automatically. When this is implemented, the district doctor will be free to spend more time in following up chronically ill patients in the home, whom he is required to visit once every ten days, and to do a better job on disease prevention and health maintenance.

In most of the countries visited, the depth of concern over the cost of hospital-based care is such that the main focus of primary care is on keeping the population out of hospitals and permitting the early discharge of hospitalized patients. For quality-of-care reasons as well as economy and cost containment, the emphasis in medical care is thus shifting from in-hospital care to disease prevention, ambulatory care, and home care. In assessing the stability and strength of this movement, it is prudent to keep in mind the pervasive opposing influences favoring the expansion of acute hospital services. There are, moreover, many resolved issues vital to the future development of primary care which require further reflection and study.

The Need for Research

The preoccupation of modern medicine with high-technology and acute intervention has retarded development of the objective base of primary care which is concerned with the natural history of disease during various stages of the life cycle, the efficacy of low-technology treatments, health maintenance, rehabilitation, and care of the incurably sick. The paucity of such essential knowledge is an obstacle to the proper staffing and organization of primary services. Except for the Soviet Union, where considerable and impressive research work has been done, Western countries have only begun to develop the necessary training and research capabilities for primary care. Thus, in the United Kingdom, Finland, Sweden, and the United States, medical schools are in the early stages of establishing full-time professorships and departments in primary care, under such headings as general practice, family medicine, community medicine, etc. Nevertheless, research in primary care continues to have a low priority.

The establishment of competent research as well as teaching is essential for the development of appropriate criteria and norms for guiding the future of primary care. All too often in the past, standards have been established by specialty and super-specialty interests which, in stressing academic or technological values, have been unrelated to the realities of primary care. In the light of the priorities in health policy for cost containment and community care, there is the danger that primary care may be subordinated to serving the economic security and professional self-esteem of high-technology interests. This is not to suggest that the assurance of the proper flow of patients to keep hospital beds and specialists sufficiently occupied to guard against underemployment and reduction of services is an unimportant function. The problem is how to assure a division of labor without a distortion of the mission and evolution of primary care which at the level of day-to-day reality does not have much in common with hospital-based specialty medicine.

It was with the specific intent of lowering the prospects for cooptation by high-technology interests that the Finnish government has financed the opening of two new medical schools with specially-designed curricula and staffing, in which the environment is skewed to favor primary care. Whether this approach will succeed remains to be seen, but it differs interestingly from the strategy followed in other Western countries and the United States in which incentives for primary care training are being introduced mainly in schools more clearly dominated by high-technology and super-specialty medicine.

Sharp differences of philosophy and practice characterize the organization of primary health services on the dimensions of technology and specialization. Americans may find that the conflict is articulated best in the debate in the United Kingdom on the future organization of primary care. Arrayed against proponents of low technology, common sense, and nonbureaucratic primary care represented by John Fry, is the medical education and teaching hospital establishment represented by highly respected spokesmen like John Brotherston, who believe firmly that the future of medicine belongs to technology and specialization, and who argue persuasively for restructuring general practice more closely in the image of hospital practice. (For a deeper understanding of these contrasting views, see Fry, 1966; Brotherston, 1969, 1971; Royal Commission of Medical Education, 1968; Department of Health and Social Security, 1971.) For this group the potential benefits of more highly scientific diagnosis and treatment far exceed the risk of depersonalization, lowered accessibility, bureaucratic complexity and the higher costs of medium-technology, interdisciplinary-staffed health centers, organized within the orbital influence of teaching and district hospitals.

Reduced to its simplest level, the debate in the United Kingdom can be represented as involving those who are conscious of the limitations of technology and the importance of the emotion-supportive aspects of healing and care and those who believe in the inevitability of scientific progress for the treatment and elimination of disease and disability. The consequences of how the conflict is to be resolved are not academic; at stake are issues which are enormously important, but hard to quantify, concerning the allocation of the gross national product, the doctor-patient relationship, the ethics of end-stage medicine, individual and family welfare, and sociopolitical stability. The question is whether the organization of primary care will be slated to respond to the roughly 90 percent of all complaints presented to general practitioners which are self-correcting in nature and susceptible to simple shotgun therapies, or to the roughly 10 percent or fewer conditions which authoritative medical opinion believes should be referred to specialists practicing in hospitals.

The future of general practice in the United Kingdom has not yet been determined. It could change vastly from its presently simple lines, in which approximately 85 percent of active practitioners continue to practice outside of interdisciplinary health centers in offices within a half-mile of where their patients live, with the barest amenities and diagnostic-treatment technology. Both public policy and the medical establishment favor restructuring general practice within multiprofessional, intermediate-technology health centers, in which from six to twelve general practitioners are assisted by clinical nurses, public health nurses, social workers, home visitors, domestic helpers, and secretarial help. Proponents of large-sized groups argue that small-scale organization militates against the close involvement of GPs with other health workers on a day-to-day basis.

Hospital Privileges

Whether general practitioners also will be routinely granted privileges in general acute hospitals or special small hospitals with beds for the care of routine acute problems and the care of the chronic aged as in Finland has not been resolved although sentiment for closer hospital ties is growing. As stated previously, the possible disadvantage of this approach is that primary care subjected to the influence of hospital medical specialty values can be more easily manipulated to thwart public policy by reinforcing the momentum for growth of high-technology services. A close relationship between generalist community medicine and hospital practice would make it easier for acute specialist interests at the top of the medical hierarchy to alter referral and treatment norms to assure full employment and expansion of high-technology services without adequate cost-benefit determination.

A rise in patient dissatisfaction can be expected from the increased travel time and the other inconveniences and the depersonalization resulting from centralization. It might also increase the costs of publicly financed health programs. In centralized health centers subject to the influence of hospital practice, practitioners have easier access to technology and the organizational values are tilted towards the substitution of complex and costly procedures for simple and inexpensive diagnoses and treatments. This could delay the adoption of universal coverage by countries which do not yet provide this while in other countries it could be an inducement to reduce benefits by mandating more restrictive eligibility requirements and use charges and would encourage them to redistribute financial responsibility from the central to local government. On the other hand, proponents of large, well-equipped interdisciplinary health centers tend to stress the potential benefits for both patients and doctors from a reduction in the need for diagnostic referrals to hospital outpatient departments—earlier treatment, greater patient through-put and a reduction in time lost in scheduling appointments and in awaiting the reporting of laboratory tests—which could help to contain costs and to facilitate an expansion in coverage.

The extent to which specialist services should be provided on an ambulatory basis in free-standing polyclinics or outpatient departments located within hospitals is another moot issue, as is the question of medical and nonmedical staffing. In none of the countries visited was there much sign of a preparedness to follow the Soviet model, in which primary care services are organized hierarchically in a system of multimedical specialties. This is in sharp distinction to the trend in the United States encompassing general practice, family medicine, internal medicine and pediatrics, which closely parallels the Soviet example.

In the United Kingdom, Finland, and Sweden, the preference clearly is for staffing by general practitioners, backed up by interdisciplinary teams. The major differences among these countries are the length of general practitioner training and the inclusion of social workers on the interdisciplinary team. Finland follows the Soviet example in omitting social service professionals, whereas Sweden appears to favor the English practice of including them. These differences may reflect differences in the importance assigned to cost consciousness and quality of care values. In both Finland and the Soviet Union there is a push to include economists in interdisciplinary treatment teams. Masters graduates in hospital and health services administration would be the U.S. counterparts.

Training of GPs

Though unofficial policy, the length of training of general practice in Finland has been cut in some schools to five years, the shortest in Europe. In the United Kingdom, Sweden, and the United States the movement is, of course, very much in the opposite direction—lengthening the period of training so that it more nearly matches that of hospital specialty practice.

The absence of consensus on productivity norms for first-contact practitioners also points to the need for controlled studies. The number of patients seen per hour in physician offices in the countries visited ranges from a high of six to seven in the United Kingdom and the Soviet Union to a low of two in some of the demonstration health centers in Sweden. Physician productivity is a controversial political issue both in Finland and Sweden. Doctors are upset over reforms for restricting hours of work and the number of patients who can be seen per hour, which have constrained their ability to supplement salaries with fee-for-service consultations, and over government efforts to get general practitioners to move from unilateral decision making in solo practice settings to interdisciplinary health center teams in which decision making becomes a collective responsibility.

Should general practitioner dissatisfaction escalate to the staging of work to rule actions, the government's attempt to rationalize primary care could be jeopardized. The idea of this happening is not farfetched. Some Swedish general practitioners new to health centers claim that the red tape and delays allow them to see only one-fourth of the patients they saw in solo practice, but admit that the length of the work week and the number of visits per hour previously may have been too high for quality care. Some of the changes are unpopular among consumers desiring quick and easy access to doctors.

Visits in Finland and Sweden are by appointment only and there is a high volume of complaint by the public over waiting times for nonurgent services, which can run an average of from three to four weeks. Open conflict over changes in primary care between general practitioners and government no doubt would be exacerbated by consumers who may themselves become dissatisfied with increased depersonalization and greater travel and waiting costs. The situation is precarious politically, especially if the frustrations associated with the changes should become translated among the public as a calculated strategy to control access of individuals to medical care rather than as a technical problem of adjusting the supply of manpower to meet growing needs for more and better primary care. A chronic shortage of physicians in a full employment economy led Sweden in particular and other Scandinavian countries to concentrate until recently on inpatient care as a means of optimizing productivity.

Queuing for primary care is not a problem in the United Kingdom and the Soviet Union, where the supply of primary care practitioners is much larger, nor is consumer dissatisfaction a problem. Public opinion polls in the United Kingdom consistently register a high degree of satisfaction with general practice. In the Soviet Union, patients are free to go to other first-contact physicians working in the polyclinic in their neighborhood, but over 85 percent are reported to go to their assigned physician. The Soviet polyclinic system provides patients with a system of airing complaints and the freedom to request second opinions and consultations.

The number of patients who can be cared for properly per primary care practitioner possibly has been underestimated. It has been demonstrated in the United Kingdom that two general practitioners sharing responsibility with a nurse trained to perform routine clinical tasks can care properly for a stable population up to 9,000 without impairing either the quality of care or consumer satisfaction (Fry, 1972).

INSTITUTIONAL CARE

Motivated, no doubt, by a combination of economic and humanitarian concerns, the long-delayed reaction against the conditions of overcrowding and neglect characterizing long-term hospital care has culminated in an explosion of demands for urgent reform.

General agreement on the need for action, however, is not matched by agreement on exactly what should be done. A variety of reforms are being undertaken, among them the following:

—Additional resources are provided to modernize facilities and alleviate overcrowding to allow more humane and efficacious medical and nursing care.

—The substitution of active treatment for purely maintenance services which, it is charged, reinforce dependence and promote physical and mental ill health regardless of how humane the intent and conditions are.

—The wholesale discharge of patients to family and community care on the assumption that (1) the long-term care sector is a mess that defies large-scale reform, so that any other form of care is preferable to the status quo, and (2) community care is both a cheaper and more effective way to restore individuals to normal living to the fullest extent permitted by their health and social status.

Commonly referred to as deinstitutionalization, this strategy has been established for at least a decade in the countries where it is being applied. In the United Kingdom and the United States, it has made considerable progress in meeting the goal of reducing the institutionalized population in mental hospitals and hospitals for the mentally handicapped by as much as 50 percent. It is now being expanded to include the chronically ill aged in long-stay hospitals and/or nursing homes.

Questions of Deinstitutionalization

There is considerable dissension on the general merits as well as specific details of each of the broad strategies being followed, so that policy in the entire long-term care field is not only fluid but somewhat confused. Important policies like deinstitutionalization are often chosen without benefit of careful comprehensive study and analysis of short- and long-run implications. Among the unexamined questions are the impacts on other health services such as general practice, public health, and community nursing services; the impacts on nonhealth services such as housing, income maintenance, and social services financed by local government; and the impacts upon the family.

The pell-mell rush to substitute action for inaction is an invitation to overreaction. In the United Kingdom, for example, data have been compiled which show that many previously hospitalized long-term-stay patients (mainly mentally ill and mentally handicapped) receive less care following discharge to the community than when they were in the hospital previously. The Government underestimated the speed with which the deinstitutionalization policy would be implemented and overestimated the willingness or ability of local government to finance and administer support services such as social work, halfway houses, foster care, and sheltered workshops. Other problems were the obstacles and disincentives to coordination and continuity between health and social services because of separate administration, contradictory-inconsistent economic incentives, professional rivalries, and the preference of social service professionals to work with patients who respond quickly and positively to intervention rather than with the hard-core chronically ill. Newspaper accounts of comparable problems with the deinstitutionalization movement in this country suggest a need for more careful screening of community care and the importance of postdischarge planning to optimize effective follow-up treatment through coordination of community health and social services (see Schumach, 1974).

Care of the Aged in Sweden

The number of aged in Sweden is one of the largest in the developed world, close to 14 percent of the total population. The need for health and social support for them has been intensified by the paradoxical effects of improvements in the standard of living. These have increased life expectancy and at the same time have resulted in a greater unwillingness on the part of adult offspring to care for aged parents living in their households. The percentage of aged persons living with their children a decade ago was approximately 10 in Sweden (3 in Stockholm), contrasted with 20 in Denmark, 30 in the United States, 40 in England, 70 in Poland, and 90 in the USSR.

Sweden's policy of placing a moratorium on the construction of new acute beds in favor of long-term beds has foundered because of the discovery that, if done right, care in a long-stay facility, while less costly than an acute facility, may still be prohibitively expensive. The staff-bed ratio requirements for the chronic aged are higher than for acute patients, especially with respect to nursing and rehabilitation personnel.

Payroll is the single most important budgetary component in all branches of the hospital service, accounting for over 60 percent of total costs. Payroll expenditures have grown sizably as the result of advancing standards of industrial justice which challenge the validity of the historic idea that health workers other than medical practitioners should work for lower wages than persons doing comparable work elsewhere in the economy because of the eleemosynary and humanitarian ethic of patient care. The effects of the progress of women in securing greater parity with men in income and employment opportunities are especially notable in the health field where women, who comprise roughly three-fourths of the labor force, have been concentrated disproportionately in low-paying and low-status jobs.

In nearly all highly developed countries recently the policy has been to bring the wages of low income hospital workers into line with those in industry and manufacturing, in order to improve recruiting and reduce costly rates of labor turnover. Even so, the conditions of employment are unattractive and staffing remains a problem, especially during off hours, weekends, and summers when persons prefer to be with their families or off on vacation. The magnitude of these problems is greater in long-stay than in short-stay facilities, because of the differences in prestige and responsiveness of patients to intervention. Problems such as these have prevented the attainment of staffing norms and precipitated cutbacks in less immediately essential programs like library and hairdressing services and organized day care activities. In Finland and Sweden the difficulty of getting married women employees to work during periods traditionally set aside for family vacations makes it necessary during summer to shut down as many as one-fifth of the available beds. Low wages and high taxes also contribute to this situation.

Although the number of long-term beds per thousand persons in Sweden aged 70 and over went up from 4.5 in 1955 to 5.5 in 1972, medical experts believe that the number should go up to 6.5 by 1980 (an increase of 20 percent) if present long waiting lists are to be shortened. In 1972 close to 20 percent of all hospital spending went to long-term care. The priority for long-term care is reflected also in other data. The number of beds expanded from 4,000 in 1942 to 40,000 in 1975, and the number of medical doctors specializing in long-term care shot up from 25 in 1965 to 325 in 1975. It is questionable, however, whether the 1980 target will be reached, not just because of the money pinch, but because doubts have arisen about the benefit of medical and nursing treatment modalities.

Improvement in Outcomes

Paradoxically, the cutbacks in long-term care spending in Sweden may have contributed to an improvement in treatment outcomes. The requirements for economy reasons that patients take on maximum responsibility for their own care has lessened dependency and fostered rehabilitation. A similar principle of self-care applies to the treatment of the mentally retarded and the aged. In addition to the patient care benefits, significant economies can be obtained, demonstrating that the two objectives are not necessarily incompatible.

To cite one example, as reported by the medical director of a large-sized long-term care facility, it has been found that, in the case of the aged over 80, multiple patient rooms are better than single patient rooms. Older and mentally disoriented patients are much quieter when they have roommates and, because of the tendency of people to help one another, they require less staff time. The amount of staff time per day for each patient is directly correlated with the number of beds in the room, decreasing from 217 minutes for single rooms to 99 minutes for four-bed rooms. With these advantages in mind, many new long-term hospitals for the psychogeriatrics of advanced age are being designed for four to five beds per room, with smaller-sized rooms reserved for younger patients who have a greater need for privacy. Self-help activities are, however, planned and supervised to match individual needs and abilities. The reaction to resource scarcity has resulted in unexpected contributions to patient welfare and is facilitating a reexamination of conventional treatment models and a more favorable climate for experimentation with alternatives.

The Stockholm County Council is conducting a controlled experiment to determine whether discharge rates and quality of survival both within and outside the hospital can be improved by greater use of physical and occupational therapy in place of traditional medical and nursing services for the long-term aged patients. Patients admitted to long-stay hospitals are said to have an average life expectancy of five years. The hope is that the need for hospitalization can be reduced, thereby lowering governmental expenditures for care while simultaneously enriching the lives of the chronically ill aged.

Two diagnostic groups responsible for 15 percent of all hospital utilization and 30 percent of long-term utilization were selected, i.e., senile patients and patients with broken bones. The experimental group showed dramatic progress, despite an advanced average age of 77. In contrast to the prediction of a panel of medical experts that 70 percent of the study population would go into long-term care, 2 percent to day care, and 28 percent to home care, it was found after less than five months that 34 percent were admitted to a long-stay care, 8 percent to day care, and 58 percent to home care. In less than eight months' time, the figures were 22 percent, 11 percent, and 67 percent, respectively. In summary, about 80 percent of patients in the study are believed to have benefited from the treatment, omitting 25 percent of the sample who died. Only 20 percent of the survivors showed no improvement after one month of intensive treatment and were reassigned to conventional care.

There were benefits to the staff, as well. Professionals previously eschewing long-term care as unchallenging work showed greater motivation and interest. The method by which these results were achieved was to limit stay in the acute hospital from five to ten days prior to transfer to a specially equipped and staffed unit of a long-stay hospital, where intensive rehabilitation therapy was applied every day of the week for as long as patients could stand until the rehabilitation was completed.

Although the findings are tentative and final results must await the completion of follow-up studies and studies which will examine what happens to people after they are returned to the community, several provocative conclusions have emerged from the research done in Sweden on the efficacy of alternative treatment modalities for the institutionalized long-term ill. It has been shown that doctors and nurses know little about rehabilitation and the potential of social care and that occupational and physical therapy are the key components to an early hospital discharge program. A big unanswered question is how lasting are the results? In any event, the research questions the value of designing and staffing long-term facilities too closely in the image of the acute hospital medical and nursing model. Paradigms stressing social, recreational, and rehabilitative dimensions, e.g., physical, occupational, and speech therapies, will likely be more efficacious. It also casts doubt on the wisdom of cost containment measures in government-funded long-term care programs in the United States (Medicare and Medicaid) which place social work and occupational and physical therapy among the first services to be eliminated.

Hospital vs. Community Costs

Another important unanswered question is whether community care is cheaper than hospital care when economic and social costs are totaled broadly. Because of the dispersal of patients in large numbers of small-sized units in wide geographic areas, the productivity of professionals is lower in community care. Travel time and the lack of critical mass in the concentration of patients mean that fewer patients can be seen hourly than in highly organized settings like hospitals and physicians' offices. For these reasons, it is also much more difficult economically and administratively to monitor the quality of services provided in community care. In periods of economic recession and reduced budgeting for health services, such as many highly developed Western countries are presently experiencing, the expense of staffing community services with costly professionals can be prohibitive. More study should be given to how much authority can be delegated to nonprofessionals without adversely affecting outcomes, not only in medical terms but from the standpoint of consumer and provider satisfaction. Moreover, the accounting of costs should not fail to consider both short- and long-term transfer burdens to nonhealth institutions such as social work and the family, and how these transfers might eventually affect gross national product formation and the viability of the sociological as distinct from the administrative community.

The justification for the trend toward medical specialization in the treatment of the aged sick also should be reexamined. Whereas the United Kingdom and Sweden appear convinced of the value of geriatric specialization, the United States seems indecisive and the Soviets openly skeptical. The potential limitations of specialization need to be considered carefully. Among these are fragmentation of care; segregation of the elderly; designation of long-term care as a medical backwater because of low status and inability to compete successfully for scarce resources with more prestigious medical subsectors; and weakening of family structure with resultant greater social disorganizations and pressures to expand welfare state services.

In Sweden, the combination of weakened family structure and high taxes have contributed to the attitude among middle-aged and young adults in metropolitan areas, where traditional family ties are weakest, that it is the responsibility of the state to care for the aged totally. Some medical directors of understaffed long-stay hospitals deplore the fact that when asked to help out by taking parents for walks and outings, relatives become sneering and indignant. In an attempt to slow down the trend toward costly institutional care, the Swedish Government has, since 1960, provided families and relatives with modest cash payments (typically about $125 per month, but in certain exceptions monthly payments could go as high as $375 to $400), to care for aged sick in the home. In light of the pressures for a major expansion of the long-term sector, the success of this program seems marginal, at best.

Finally, the deep-seated bias in modern medical education for technology and acute intervention with the promise of quick and favorable results is cause to wonder what maintenance and palliative services may be like in the future. The status of services for the aged, the mentally ill, and the mentally handicapped is ambiguous in countries where the imperatives of medicine favor the curative services. If, on the one hand, the momentum for science and technology leads inevitably to the neglect of maintenance services as an unpleasant reminder of medicine's recent entry from the primitive stages of religion, magic, folklore and tender loving care, the medical establishment is, on the other hand, reluctant to sever its ties with low-prestige services, if for no other reason than the size of the cash flow and the opportunities to capture overhead support for low-volume high-cost services and high-technology development. This is especially true now that the specter of spending reductions is materializing.

Thought should be given to the question of whether maintenance services should be transferred from the health sector to other sectors which have the know-how and willingness to assume unequivocally the responsibility for the care of the incurably sick and the reintegration into the community of those who can be rehabilitated. In this context, controlled risk-benefit studies should be performed to ascertain whether, for example, it is either cheaper or more efficacious to assign the educable and trainable mentally handicapped to educational authorities; the terminally ill to social workers, the family, and volunteers; and the mentally ill to social workers, the legal-penal system, and indigenous community influences. Barring some major breakthrough in medical research, the interest and welfare of those needing long-term care might be served better outside of the medical field than within it.

INTERFACE BETWEEN HEALTH AND SOCIAL SERVICES

The human tragedy resulting from skimming and dumping practices prevalent in the classification and referral of patients in deinstitutionalization and demedicalization programs has been described earlier. It is a consequence of the uncoordinated administration and antagonistic financial and professional objectives between separate and competing health and social services.

The attempts of central government in the United Kingdom and the United States to contain unacceptably high rates of inflation in the general economy and to stimulate employment recovery in the private sector by cutting back on public spending for social services and other domestic spending further jeopardize the short-term future of community care. Higher-level government cutbacks invariably place greater pressures on already heavily burdened local governments to raise politically unpopular taxes to support community services. Illustrating the dilemma encountered by local governments are the current attempts of many of the larger local governments in New York State to impose a ceiling on the amount of tax revenues which can go to support community programs for the mentally retarded. As of July 1976, such major centers of population as New

York City, Syracuse, and Buffalo had imposed or were considering ceilings which would, if allowed to stand, cut spending for mental health services by as much as 20 to 25 percent below 1975-76 levels (Greenhouse, 1976). This is occurring despite increases in fifty-fifty matching funds in the state's budget. Many local politicians are fearful of the political backlash of raising taxes in order to take advantage of matching funds and others openly doubt whether the state government can be trusted to continue subsidizing community care, once the objective of halving the inpatient population in state institutions is achieved. This would force local taxpayers to assume total responsibility for financing a program of unknown, but costly, dimension.

The realpolitik of resource allocation in times of recession typically works against newly established and politically weak programs. When push comes to shove, longer established, more highly organized and politically stronger programs suffer less in real terms than their weaker competitors. The depth and length of the present economic decline in most Western countries can be expected, therefore, to impair the implementation of community care, together with other new priorities for disease prevention and health maintenance.

Less obvious in the context of short-run crisis management objectives are the long-run monetary losses such as the undoing of costly hospital intervention because of poor follow-up care in the community, and the expenses of income maintenance and dependency due to improper rehabilitation. The United Kingdom and Sweden are attempting as a compromise arrangement to provide for the joint planning and the joint occupation of health centers so as to alleviate gaps resulting from the separation of health and social services financing and administration.

Success in the Soviet Union

In contemplating the significance for the United States of foreign experience with the intergovernmental coordination of nonunified health and social services, one is impressed favorably by the apparent success of the Soviet Union. Notwithstanding a separation of administration and financing, and the difficulties of coordinating multiple levels of government, the Soviets claim to have achieved a high degree of success in coordinating health and social services. The explanation that cooperation between naturally competitive professions is a measure of the coercive power of the Soviet system may appeal to Westerners whose thinking has been conditioned by Cold War rivalries, but this may be too reductionistic. Possibly more important are differences in philosophy and practice concerning the role of social services. While maintaining a comparably strong service-ethic orientation, social services in the Soviet Union are not as highly professionalized as in the West. That is to say, full-time graduate training is not a requirement for entry and Freudian-oriented behavioral theory, with its emphasis on the subconscious, is rejected as contrary to party ideology, which stresses the importance of free will for shaping the character and morality of Soviet Man.

Social work in the Soviet Union concentrates pretty much on the provision of economic security against the hazards of life (old age, sickness, disability, and premature death of the breadwinner), and care in sheltered environments of invalids who can no longer benefit from active treatment and rehabilitation, for whom the society has a duty to provide humane and compassionate care in accord with common sense principles of socialist humanism. Therefore, the competition between health and social services for jurisdiction in the treatment of behavioral and sociomedical problems (mental illness, alcoholism, drug addiction, etc.) common in Western countries, is not found in the Soviet Union. The absence of competition for control of patients makes it easier to get cooperation when necessary. Thus, for example, doctors sit together with social services personnel on panels for determining the eligibility of workers for sickness and disability benefits. The medical and nursing supervision of institutionalized invalids is provided by doctors and nurses, who are employed by social service authorities but receive their graduate and continuing education training from medical school faculty. Invalids requiring prostheses are attended by specially trained experts employed in the health sector.

The decision of whether to classify a problem as medical or social is made at the top, the most important criterion being the efficacy of medical intervention relative to alternative forms of treatment in restoring individuals to the community. For example, acute mental illness is treated as a medical problem with treatment provided in special psychiatric hospitals, but the chronic mentally ill are the responsibility of social services, which stress work therapy. Educable and trainable mentally handicapped are the responsibility of the schools, whereas the nontrainables are a social service responsibility. There is no discernible pressure or interest on either side for the joint staffing of health centers.

The relationship between health and social services in the USSR raises an interesting possibility regarding cross-national approaches to the evaluation of quality of medical care. Ironically, the exigencies of industrial development and corollary higher value assigned to labor because of capital scarcities in the Soviet Union favor an environment in which quality of care is viewed in outcome terms, rather than from the standpoint of inputs and processes which is more prevalent in the more affluent Western countries not experiencing shortage of capital. The emergence in the West of unaccustomed resource scarcities may be a powerful stimulus for the development of outcome measures.

Question of Status

Conditions in Finland closely approximate the Soviet situation in terms of a clear division of labor between health and social services and the exclusion of social workers in the staffing of health centers. However, some pressure is developing from the social services side for closer cooperation in the form of joint planning and staffing. This pressure may reflect the greater exposure of social service workers in Finland to the Freudian-oriented professional social work model prevalent in England and the United States, which leads them to believe that they can either contribute to, or do a better job in, the treatment of the mentally ill presently classified as medical problems. The competition for jurisdiction over patients between the two professions was revealed by the proud boast of several health officials interviewed that average length of stay in long-term facilities for the aged went down 60 percent (from 100 to 49 days) following the transfer of responsibility in 1972 from social services to community health centers. Social services officials complained, on the other hand, about what a terrible job the health services do in rehabilitating the mentally ill, and claim to be able to do better.

Since the profession of social work in many Western countries, including the United States, is in a difficult period of transition due to the reaction against the vagaries of Freudian theory, and since the future of schools of social work is very much in doubt, the time may be right for reconsidering the relationship with the health sector before any irrevocable decisions are taken in the restructuring of primary care.

One can expect that the status relationships between medical practitioners and social workers will become a manifest source of tension in the future. In the United Kingdom, even at the highest decision-making levels, the tension is obvious to the outside observor. In interdisciplinary decision making the social service representative emerges as the lesser of equals, and a sort of second-class citizen. Policy and planning discussions are dominated by medical practitioners and other health professionals. There is a tendency for them to pull rank, even when the subject deals with social services. Social service representatives, for their part, are conspicuously deferential to medical colleagues. It will take considerable time before the two can interact as equals. Serious thought may have to be given to revamping social services curricula and the possibility of joint training at the postgraduate level, if not in programs of full-time degree instruction.

TRENDS IN HEALTH POLICY: REVISIONISM AND CONVERGENCE

When looked at from a distance, the observations and impressions of the countries discussed here form a pattern which suggest that many orthodox assumptions of macrohealth policy have been reexamined and are in the process of being replaced by a new generation of assumptions. The confusion invariably accompanying momentous shifts of policy is exacerbated by the crisis atmosphere in the financing of health services which has been hastened, if not caused directly, by the twin problems of unemployment and inflation bedevilling many national economies. The psychology and politics of crisis management is conducive to suboptimization in decision making, which often produces inconsistent and contradictory short-term policies and programs which are hard to follow, let alone grasp, because of the resultant contradictions and inconsistencies.

The consequences of crisis management are especially severe in the United

States, where, unlike the countries visited, a logically coherent centralized policy has not materialized because of the power of traditional free market values. The role of government has been subordinated to private interests and confined mainly to the provision of subsidies on the assumption that the forces of efficiency intrinsic to free enterprise health services will reassert themselves, if primed periodically. Structural intervention to compensate for deficiencies in the private structure of medicine, consequently, has been constrained, reluctant, and ad hoc. The absence of a clear, uniform, and consistently applied national policy not only has obscured vision, but fostered a cultural penchant for reducing complex issues of policy to simplistic dimensions, which is expressed frequently in a search for scapegoats and the attribution of blame for failure to petty motives. In contrast to other developed countries with a clear and consistent national health policy, the underlying assumptions of policy actions tend to be hidden more and harder to follow in the United States.

Americans grown accustomed to scientfic progress, economic affluence, and high standards of private consumption, not only are less sensitive to waste, but less knowledgeable than Europeans about the effects since World War II of the enormous growth in public confidence in medicine and the proliferation of technology and specialization arising from increased public investments in biomedical research and hospital services—i.e., fragmentation of patient care, imbalances in the relationship between primary, secondary, and tertiary care levels, and the strains on obsolescent systems of financing and organization developed in the 1920s and 1930s, when medicine was simpler and far less costly.

It is not commonly recognized in the United States that until as recently as World War II many people continued to look on the hospital as the place where one went to die. If earlier advances in asepsis and anaesthesia made hospitals safe and surgery less hazardous, and if the development of nursing as a profession contributed to more humane patient care, there still was little that medicine could do to alter the course of disease. With the exception of advances in public health and sanitary engineering, which contributed substantially to the control of communicable diseases, the medical profession in the U.S. was preoccupied after World War I with implementing the Flexner-inspired reforms for combating earlier ethical excesses stemming from the riotous commercialism of medical education, and with establishing the scientific base for modern medical research and teaching. Most of the progress in successful intervention has occurred in the past thirty years (antibiotics, chemotherapy, tranquilizers) and, as recently as a decade ago, few hospitals had intensive care units and coronary care units or were equipped to perform organ transplant surgery.

Assumptions Underlying Postwar Expansion of Health Services

The rate of technological innovation and diffusion has been especially rapid in the past several decades and, together with rising public expectations and the transformation of medical care from a semi-market good to a merit good (provided freely as a right), accounts disproportionately for the stresses responsible for the reexamination of the following assumptions. These assumptions provided the justification for the enormous growth in public expenditures for the capitalization of health services.

First: Concentrated and massive investments in biomedical research and development will lead to vast gains in life expectancy and reductions in disability. The investment program in the health sector was influenced greatly by the successful wartime crash programs to develop radar, the atomic bomb, and other military innovations. It is manifested especially in the growth of target-specific categorical research centers in the National Institutes of Health. The faith prevalent in the scientific community in the superior advantages of serendipity, such as that experienced in the discovery of penicillin, when coupled with the solo fee-for-service traditions of American medicine, mitigated against the introduction of parallel management controls.

Second: The best place to provide patient care is in the hospital, where the proper technology and skilled staff are concentrated. This assumption, of course, contributed vitally to expansion of the bed supply and acceptance of the minimum norm of roughly 4.5 acute beds and 5 long-term beds per 1,000 population, which was exceeded by a wide margin in countries like Sweden and the Soviet Union for reasons of low population density, medical manpower shortages, an aged population, low housing standards, or an even greater faith in the value of hospitalization.

Third: Medical specialization is both necessary and desirable. The glamour, income, and superior working conditions which stimulated the growth of specialty practice, not only produced a sharp decline in the percentage of medical graduates going into general practice, but provided broad support for the attitude in the medical field that a generalist is nothing more than a failed specialist. From 1950 to 1970 the supply of active physicians in general practice in the U.S. declined from roughly 60 percent to 25 percent. The decline was even greater in other countries. Even in England, where the supply of general practitioners was kept at higher levels (through use of controls over approved residencies similar to those now being proposed in the U.S.), there was a sharp deterioration of morale and productivity which made it necessary to raise the status of general practice through increases in income, liberalization of conditions of practice, and reforms in medical training. The nascent attempts to establish family practice in the U.S. are a manifestation of this reform movement.

Fourth: Spending for health services is finite. There was widespread belief in the assertion by Lord Beveridge who reportedly said (in arguing the case for the British National Health Service over the objections of critics who protested it would break the Treasury and economic theorists who insisted that medical care was a private good) that public expenditures would rise steeply in the short run, but would level off once the backlog of unmet needs was provided for. It was also believed that expenditures would decline, once the benefits of more systematic and comprehensive disease prevention and early detection programs were felt.

Fifth: The role of government in the health sector should be limited mainly to the provision of consumer purchasing power to eliminate financial barriers to early diagnosis and treatment to guard against the threat of unpredictable and costly illness to the economic security of the family. Subsidies to providers, in the form of support of medical research, hospital construction, medical education, and the guaranteeing of minimal incomes to practitioners, were also widely endorsed. This "buying in" philosophy was grounded in the corollary assumption that the established structure of health services was performing well and there should be as little interference with the status quo as possible. The prevalence of this philosophy possibly accounts for why doctors and hospitals in England were allowed considerable freedom from outside interference following the nationalization of hospitals and their reorganization into regional systems. In the National Health Service the major professional groupings pretty much do what they want and individual clinicians are left alone to do what they believe is best for the patient, once the central government sets the ceiling on aggregate expenditures for the fiscal year.

Grounds for Revisionism

The expansionary policy of the past quarter century has been surprisingly successful. Most of the objectives have been met and, indeed, surpassed in many instances. Understandably, the feeling has developed among policy makers that the time has come to focus on new areas of investment. Sentiment for a change of direction of public spending gains support, of course, from the recognition of resource scarcity in even the wealthiest nations. The decline of the general economy has put pressure on governments to better manage budgets, with a sharper eye on the relationship between consumption and investment spending best suited for generating savings for financing economic growth which, in turn, can provide the surplus to support additional health and related welfare state services required by an aging population, the weakening of the family-support structure, and rising public expectations.

It is perhaps wishful thinking for proponents of the status quo in health services to expect that things will return to normal once the performance of the general economy improves, since even political parties historically committed to health and other welfare state programs are showing a recognition of the need to better balance consumption and investment spending in the future (e.g., the Labor Party in England and the positions taken in the 1974 presidential campaign by President Carter following his winning of the nomination of the Democratic Party).

While justifiably proud of the accomplishments of increased public spending for health care in the promotion of technological progress and social justice, a growing number of government officials and politicians have also become disillusioned by the failures of conventional health policy in terms of the inflation and waste in the health sector, the dubious effects of health services on health status, and the unresponsiveness of health services to new disease and treatment priorities. More and more, the critics of publicly financed health care appear convinced that the problems cannot be solved by more spending or by a mere change of direction in investments, but require, instead, a thorough overhaul and reworking of fundamental assumptions.

An important cause of the disillusionment with conventional assumptions is the persistently high rate of inflation and rates of increase in spending for publicly financed health services which have consistently exceeded by a wide margin rates of increase in other sectors of the economy. Financial experts, previously dismissed as misanthropes, have succeeded in alerting politicians to the dangers of voting increasingly larger sums of money for one of the fastest growing components of the government's budget, when for every dollar allocated the return in new services is worth only fifty cents or less in constant values.

Additional disillusionment stems from evidence which questions the existence of a strong positive relationship between health spending and health status, and the mounting awareness that nonhealth services in the form of nutrition, housing, income, life style, occupational safety, and environmental protection achieve better results.

The fact that all of the new spending intended to increase the supply of medical personnel has not done much to correct problems of maldistribution in isolated and low-income rural areas also has produced a shock effect, particularly among policy makers believing in the workings of the market and the laws of supply and demand. Equally or more upsetting is the realization that subsidies for medical education unwittingly have exacerbated problems in manpower supply and distribution by specialty, and that the oversupply of surgical and other hospital-based specialists is a key factor, not just to inflation and overlap and duplication, but to a rising volume of medically questionable and unnecessary procedures. The growth in consumer complaints about the unavailability of medical practitioners to care for routine medical complaints and the costly substitution of the emergency room for general practitioner services contributes further to the climate of disillusionment.

Finally, whether motivated by disillusionment with the shortcomings of past policy or concern over future demands on public financing, many policy makers are troubled by the increasing numbers of population groups whose need for health care and related social services is high—the aged, the mentally ill, the mentally handicapped, and the physically disabled. It is a paradox of medical progress that it makes it possible for more and more people to survive who require as a condition of survival disproportionately large health and social support services. Even on the chance that high technology and acute and long-term hospital services are prepared to respond to these needs, it is doubtful whether they are properly equipped and oriented from a cost-benefit standpoint. In England, for example, these population groups account for two-thirds of all health services, but receive only one-third of the resources. Without additional substantial amounts of new money, the resources to provide for the chronically ill and handicapped can be obtained only at the expense of acute high-technology services, thereby contributing to tensions and divisions within the health sector generally.

In light of the prevailing climate of disillusionment with current programs and the concern over the financing of future needs, the central issue in health policy today is how much more money is the government prepared to spend for health services at the expense of other needs during a time of growing doubt about the contributions of increased spending for health services to health status.

Convergence of Policy

In all of the countries visited, and including the U.S., the old policy assumptions are in the process of being replaced by a new generation of assumptions. The new assumptions radiate a greater skepticism toward the value of high-technology medicine and place higher priorities on social equity and economy in the allocation of health resources. They signal a stronger interventionist role for government, a weakening of the influence of the medical profession, and more systematic controls for the planning, monitoring, and evaluation of health services.

Diminishing returns of high-technology services

Foremost among the new assumptions is the belief that spending for high-technology medicine has entered the stage of diminishing marginal social benefit, i.e., it is costing more and more to do less and less. There is, therefore, more interest in the possibilities provided by low and medium technologies. Interest in lower cost alternatives extends also to the application of common sense in shaping life styles conducive to good health. The argument against high technology is attractive. Whereas costly high-technology eradication of the three leading causes of death (heart disease, cancer, and stroke) would lengthen life expectancy from birth by an average of six to seven years, and at age sixty-five by one to two years, adherence to six inexpensive and simple rules for good living would add eleven years to life expectancy from birth—three meals a day, moderate exercise, seven to eight hours sleep nightly, no smoking, moderate weight, and moderate use of alcohol. A study by Belloc and Breslow (1972) has shown the physical status of persons aged sixty-five following all six rules is equivalent to that of persons aged thirty-four to forty-four who follow only three of the rules.

Spending for health services is limitless

There also has occurred considerable growth in the belief that spending for health services is endless because of insatiable consumer wants and the monopoly of the medical profession in standard setting. Especially important to proponents of this view is the autonomy of individual clinicians to do what they believe is best in treatment and utilization decisions for, more than any other single factor, it is responsible for the condition whereby supply creates its own demand. Retrospective fee-for-service payment of physicians and other economic disincentives contribute managerially to a situation in which all of the imperatives and controls favor technological enrichment, modernization of amenities, and high rates of growth in overall spending. These expansionary forces are hard to check, even in systems with centralized financing and budgetary controls, like England.

Importance of first-contact medicine

The restoration of the generalist function in medicine is perceived increasingly as a worthwhile means for facilitating the treatment of routine problems and chronic illness in low-cost community settings and for better rationing, through a system of organized referral, of costly hospital and specialty services by assuring that resources are fully employed and the right patient is in the right place at the right time. It is recognizably shortsighted, to say the least, to have an elaborate hierarchical pyramidal structure of specialty medicine without an accompanying broad and solid base in general practice.

This convergence on the need to revive general practice is not free of contradiction and conflict, however. The major disagreements on the role of the first-contact practitioner center on length of training, access to bed privileges, and whether medically led interdisciplinary treatment teams should include social workers. Medical educators, in the main, display a preference for modeling general practice training after the preparation of specialists in terms of emphasizing the application of advanced techniques circumscribed by anatomical, disease, and population foci. A counterview which is very much in the minority stresses the role of elementary technology and common sense, in accord with the constraints imposed on medical intervention by the natural history of disease and the aging of populations in developed countries. Within this framework the general practitioner is seen as a composite of roles, including health educator, diagnostician, gatekeeper to high-technology services and illness benefits, counselor for the provision of continuous care for routine illness and medical complaints, and social worker to assure that patients receive the proper follow-up services (income maintenance, housing, rehabilitation, job retraining, etc.) to optimize the chances for recovery and independence. A parallel goal centers on the restoration of humanist values in medicine as a check on the narrow efficiency values of science and management, and as a means for coping with the rise in consumer dissatisfaction over the depersonalizations of treatment which threatens to erode the political base of medicine.

Given the validity of such assumptions as the technological imperative, the creation of demand by supply, and the diminishing marginal benefit of technologically intensive modes of medical treatment, the implications of which course governments choose finally for the development of general practice are certain to be profound.

Iatrogenic hazards of modern medicine

Recognition is mounting that hospitals are dangerous to patient welfare because of the problems of coordination and control due to the diseconomies of scale in the organization of hospital services and the vastly increased power of therapeutics to do harm as well as good. For example, in the U.S. it has been reported that as many as 10 percent of hospitalized patients suffer compensable injuries during their confinement, that 50 percent of the surgery performed annually is done by noncertified surgeons, and that as much as 20 percent of all the surgery performed may be medically unnecessary. It is, moreover, commonly recognized in all countries that long-term hospitals for the chronic aged, mentally ill, and mentally handicapped often do more to perpetuate and manufacture dependency and illness than to restore patients to normal living. Awareness of these limitations complements the cost containment objectives behind the movement toward community care, and efficiency and quality-of-care aims are decreasingly regarded as being mutually exclusive.

Oversupply of beds

Accompanying the above changes in beliefs is the conviction that there are too many beds and that in rough terms the proportion of acute beds could be reduced by as much as one-fourth or more without any deleterious effects. The experience of the privately owned Kaiser Foundation Health Plan in the United States is particularly impressive to policy makers, for it appears to have demonstrated that it is possible to get by with as few as two acute beds per 1,000 population, if the leverage of financing is used to provide physicians with economic incentives to organize in groups and to weigh the economic implications of patient-treatment decisions.

Too many doctors

Closely related to the belief that there are too many acute beds is the belief that, except for certain specialties, there are, or soon will be, too many doctors. In following up on this assertion, many governments have begun to restrict the entry of foreign medical graduates and to make plans to level off and possibly cut back on medical school enrollments. Widely disseminated data from Canada which indicate that each graduated doctor generates throughout his working life costs of $225,000 annually as the result of clinical decisions, has translated into understandably concrete terms the implications of the theory that supply creates its own demand.

Health spending impedes economic growth

It is no longer accepted uncritically that health spending has an important investment function in contributing to economic growth. Health spending is seen, instead, as a form of consumption, largely because of doubt about the existence of a positive relationship between health spending and health status on the one hand, and the demand, on the other hand, for health services resulting from a rapidly growing retired population. This thinking gives rise also to the assumption that spending for high-technology services has reached the saturation point.

Breakdown of self-regulation and free enterprise

Finally, the philosophy of "buying in," or passive intervention, in the provision of publicly supported health services is being rejected in favor of a more active interventionist role. In this role, government is believed to be justified, if not compelled, to use the leverage provided by its purchasing power in a manner conducive to comprehensive planning and managerial monitoring of delivery. In other words, government must attempt to assure accountability, economy, and efficiency in the delivery of publicly financed services.

Priorities for the Next Decade

The ongoing reexamination of policy assumptions provides the framework within which the priorities for the next decade will be formed. If one accepts the proposition that programs typically will follow rather than lead policy, an understanding of the reformulation of underlying assumptions can prove useful for predicting, at least in the time frame of a decade or so, the form and thrust of new priorities. Some of the new priorities have been declared already in important government publications in the West, such as the Department of Health, Education, and Welfare's Five Year Forward Plan for Health in the U.S., the Consultative Document in England dealing with Priorities for Health and Social Services, the Seven Kroner Reform in Sweden, and the 1972 reforms of primary health care services in Finland. These priorities include:

First, construction of an infrastructure for comprehensive-integrated health planning and systematic flow from the bottom up of five- to ten-year rolling plans in accord with broad guidelines responsive to the realities of national economic and social development. Progress in this area inevitably spells the end for neo-market supply and demand strategies in cost containment and social equity goals.

Second, revitalization of general practice in the context of bureaucratic models of primary care for purposes of promoting more effective programs of disease prevention and health maintenance and the rationing of high-technology services.

Third, modest increases in investments in rehabilitative and other services for the long-term ill and physically and mentally disabled.

Fourth, experimentation and demonstrations of means for improving coordination between health and social services without alteration of presently separate systems of administration and finance.

Fifth, expansion of preventive health services geared to changing harmful life styles and the promotion of occupational safety, automobile safety, and environmental protection.

Sixth, resocialization of the public to become more knowledgeable about the limitations of modern medicine and to accept a greater personal responsibility for health maintenance and routine treatment.

Seventh, reductions in rates of annual increase in spending for hospital services from presently high levels of 15 percent or more to a more modest 5 to 10 percent range, in order to generate savings to finance expansion of first-contact medical services and services for the chronically ill and permanently disabled.

Eighth, substitution of contract target arrangements for loosely supervised grant funding of biomedical research and development, with a greater emphasis on applied problems, rather than basic studies, and the subjecting of new technology to rigorous analysis for safety, efficacy, and costs prior to controlled diffusion guided by principles of economies of scale and equitable geographic distribution.

Ninth, imposition of ceilings on central government financing of health services through the termination of open-ended funding provisions and the sharing of responsibility with the private sector, with lower levels of government, and with consumers. In accord with this priority, the prospects for comprehensive universal national health insurance financed from general revenues is bleak in the United States. Countries already possessing comprehensive schemes of national health insurance can be expected to attempt, whenever politically possible, to substitute the principle of selectivity for universalism in benefit coverage and to impose charges at the point of consumption, especially for less essential services. It is instructive in this regard to note that, in announcing in July 1976 public spending plan for 1977, England's ruling Labor Party has increased patient charges for medication, eyeglasses, and dental services for adults; increased social security payroll taxes for industry; and cut back on grants and subsidies to local government for support of personal social services. While the pressures will lessen, once world and domestic economic activity returns to normal, the basic trend of tighter controls over central government spending will continue, because of the powerful role of government in the modern economy and the expansion of its responsibility to include national economic planning. In this context, compulsory uniform and comprehensive national health insurance with services provided free at time of use may be an idea whose time has gone. More pragmatic alternatives can be anticipated in which government seeks to fulfill rising standards for territorial and social justice in the distribution and consumption of services while limiting the claims on budgetary allocations. This could be accomplished through a policy of entitlement to a minimum floor of benefits stratified by age and employment status and a system of pluralistic financing with the mandated participation of business and industry and lower levels of government, and liberal provisions for individuals and families to supplement basic levels of coverage.

Summary

A pattern of increasing governmental intervention in the health sector discloses the obsolescence of financial and organizational arrangements formulated at a time earlier in this century when medical specialization and technology was less highly developed. Recognition of the inflationary effects of promoting the capital development of hospital-based services through increased public spending, without coming to grips with an outdated structure, is tangible in the strengthening of machinery for compulsory regional planning, and the movement toward prospective reimbursement. Recognition of the gaps between resources and needs, which result when the training and supply of health manpower are not harmonized with changes in the organization of health services and illness treatment priorities, is tangible in the movement toward formal manpower planning and in the attempts, by a combination of controls and incentives, to improve the supply and distribution of practitioners by specialty. And recognition of the exorbitant costs and risks to quality care, which result when consumers and practitioners have too much freedom of access to costly and complex therapies, is tangible in the growth of interest in primary care and in the role of controls and incentives for rationing utilization of health services.

The potential advantages of described changes in policy are substantial: Services more responsive to changing disease patterns and the needs of aging populations; greater equity of access to health services by geography and social class; coordination and balance in the relationship among primary, secondary, and tertiary levels of care; earliest feasible restoration of the ill and disabled to work and conditions of normal living; and resource allocation attuned to the realities of scarcity, population needs, and feasibility of delivery and follow-through.

The degree to which these goals can be attained and the pace of change will be conditioned by the politics of competition for scarce resources and the psychology of crisis management which may lead decision makers to focus disproportionately on immediate results without sufficient regard for secondary and tertiary externalities over longer periods of time. More specifically, the dangers include: Resistance to new health priorities by vested interest groups fearful of change; subordination of human service and social justice values to depersonalized and narrow criteria of managerial-economic efficiency and cost containment; and an over-reaction to the limitations of modern medicine which could jeopardize the stability of fragile capabilities in high technology requiring prolonged lead times, impede the health sector's ability to recruit its fair share of competent young men and women, and create an overall milieu of cynicism and nihilism inimical to technological innovation and quality patient care.

Striking the right balance between high- and low-technology medical services and between health and social services will not be easy but it is the key to the provision of services which are more responsive and compassionate in relation to the needs of the population and which are, moreover, attuned to the realities of resource scarcity and the interdependence of hospital and ambulatory services geared to health maintenance and the fullest reintegration possible of the sick to normal social functioning.

REFERENCES

Battistella, R. M. "Study of Macrohealth Planning Developments in Finland, Sweden, Union of Soviet Socialist Republics, England and Northern Ireland." Report submitted to John E. Fogarty International Center for Advanced Studies in the Health Sciences, 1977.

Belloc, N. B., and Breslow, L. "The Relation of Physical Health Status and Health Practices." *Preventive Medicine* (August 1972): 409-21.

Brotherston, J. "Change and the National Health Services." *Scottish Medical Journal* 14 (1969): 130.

Brotherston, J. "Evolution of Medical Practice." *Medical History and Medical Care,* edited by G. McLachlan and T. McKeown. London: Nuffield Provincial Hospitals Trust, 1971.

Department of Health and Social Security, Welsh Office. *The Organization of Group Practice.* London: Her Majesty's Stationery Office, 1971.

Fry, J. *Profiles of Disease.* London: E. & S. Livingstone, 1966.

Fry, J. "21 Years of General Practice: Changing Patterns." *Journal of the Royal College of General Practice* 22 (1972): 521.

Greenhouse, L. "Cuts Proposed in Mental Aid." *New York Times* (August 8, 1976): 41.

Royal Commission of Medical Education. *Common Paper 3569.* London: Her Majesty's Stationery Office, 1968.

Schumach, M. "Shift in Mental-Hospital Theory." *New York Times* (August 20, 1974): 23.

3

New Directions for Health Policy

Selection by William R. Roy

Shattuck Lectures have always been timely.

One can trace the history of modern medicine reasonably well by review-ing the titles of the lectures.

The lectures have been primarily clinical and scientific in nature, following the precedent of Dr. George Brune Shattuck's first presentation in 1890 on the subject of influenza. The greatest accomplishments of medicine after Koch and Lister have been revealed and reviewed here by the men who were, or are, the miracle workers of modern medicine. During the span of their work, medical care has contributed greatly to the doubling of the life expectancy of the citi-zens of the industrialized nations.

We, the modern physicians, can do more than care; we can oftentimes cure. Over the six generations since Dr. George Cheyne Shattuck's legacy for the establishment of this lectureship was announced in 1854, medicine has by any imaginable yardstick been successful.

Yet, honored by success, we find ourselves also beset by even closer scru-tiny and evermore frequent criticism from all segments of our society.

As a result, there has been a dramatic change in the subject matter of the Shattuck Lectures. My talk today will be the eighth of the last eleven Shattuck Lectures to deal with matters social, economic, and political. Only two lectures on medical education and Dr. Nevin S. Scrimshaw's learned lecture of last year

Reprinted by permission from "Shattuck Lecture—An Agenda for Physicians and Legislators, 1976," *New England Journal of Medicine* 295, no. 11 (September 9, 1976), pp. 589-96.

have interrupted this steady tattoo of the consideration of the relation of medical care—usually expanded to health care—to the balance of American society.

In this, our Bicentennial Year, 200 years of solutions have not left us without serious problems, challenges, and opportunities.

As the locus for health decisions has switched from the meeting halls of organized medicine to the capitol of our nation, we physicians are asking, "What is happening and why?" and, "Can we participate and how?"

In an attempt to address these questions I will be presumptuously global in approach, because I believe that the indispensable prerequisites for physician participation in health decision making are an understanding of the forces that determine the current health scene, a recognition of the truly critical decision areas, and a knowledge of the tradeoffs that exist among the limited choices available to us.

I shall first present my perspective about the current health scene, derived from fifteen years of private practice, from working within organized medicine at the state level, from four years of congressional health legislative activism, and from a series of unusual opportunities to visit intimately with health professionals, politicians, and many social scientists.

After an analysis of the current health scene, I will present an agenda of decisions that must be made and that I believe can best be made affirmatively rather than left without definition to happenstance and other societal forces. In spite of my title, this is an agenda for all citizens of this nation and not only for the hierarchy of physicians and legislators. However, the identifiable actors on the stage will certainly include legislators, and, I believe, if we are to achieve the best possible result, it should also include those whom I classify as enlightened physicians.

THE CURRENT HEALTH SCENE

Over the past decade, there has occurred the sequential recognition and definition of several forces that are determining our nation's current health problems and must be dealt with directly and intelligently if we are to change the American health system for the better. Some of these forces, such as economic laws, are immutable. Others are deeply embedded in the traditions, history, and culture of our nation and of the practice of medicine, and therefore, for practical reasons, probably must be dealt with as if they were immutable.

Three medical facts of life emerge: that we cannot do everything that is scientifically possible for everyone everywhere; that if we cannot do everything for everyone everywhere, we must decide what we are going to do for whom where; and that personal health care is only one of the determinants of health.

All these conclusions, I believe, are undeniable. In private conversations nearly all physicians agree, and many of you may say that these conclusions are so obvious that they require neither listing nor explanation.

However, I do not find that we physicians as a group behave in ways that indicate both an understanding and an acceptance of these medical facts of life.

Because these facts dictate our agenda for decision, permit me to review these conclusions, and the associated forces, with you.

We Cannot Do Everything That Is Scientifically Possible for
Everyone Everywhere

We, as a society, have long accepted this economic reality about nearly every service and product except health care.

Fuchs (1974) has put the basic economic laws simply and succinctly. "The first is that resources are scarce relative to human wants; second, is [that] resources have alternative uses; and third, that people have different wants to which they attach varying degrees of importance."

Reinhardt (1976), speaking at the recent "National Leadership Conference on Health Policy," looked at the furor about expenditures for health and the measurement of the expenditures as a percentage of the gross national product (GNP) and asked in effect, what is all the excitement about? People simply place a high value on health wants—we should be receptive or perhaps pleased that the people of our nation spend as much or nearly as much for physicians' services as they spend for alcohol or tobacco. He contends that people must be left free to make this choice in a market economy. To say the least, this point of view has a great appeal to most of us, and it found great favor among the 600 representatives of the health industry who were present.

Expenditures for health increased from $38.9 billion in 1965 to $118.5 billion in 1975, a 300 percent increase over a ten-year period. The portion of the GNP spent for health increased from 5.9 percent in 1965 to 8.3 percent in 1975.

One of the forces at work is undeniably the value that people place on health, and the high expectations that people have about personal health services. The presence of this force is best illustrated by the majority acceptance that "Health care is a basic human right." This concept of a right is a subjective force, and, as such, it may be changed, but it now appears so generally accepted that it must be dealt with when modifying the American health system.

The single, greatest force responsible for increased health expenditures is the fact that we live in a time of scientific and technologic revolution. Medical knowledge, it is said, has a half-life of four to seven years. Likewise, medical technology has a similarly short half-life, and this brief span propels constant and expensive changes.

Hiatt (1975) amply documents the impact of new medical technologies on health costs in an article in which he analogizes the finite resources available in our economy for health services with a limited commons available to herdsmen for the grazing of their cattle.

A commons is not a marketplace. All members of the society are entitled to use a commons. Overutilization and ruin of the commons is the inevitable result because each individual rushes to use the commons in his or her own self-interest.

We have established a health services' commons for most Americans by the adoption of private health insurance for many people and government payment for services for some people. The adoption of mandatory and universal national health insurance would entitle everyone to use the medical commons.

Combining with third-party payment is the force of provider determination of services. We physicians are trained to use every available resource of possible benefit to treat our individual patients—regardless of cost. To my knowledge this has always been so, and it has been my expectation that it must always be so.

In sum, four prominent forces have caused the medical system to be characterized as a vast vacuum cleaner that will suck up all dollars made available to it: (1) the expectations of patients, (2) the scientific and technologic revolution, (3) open-ended third-party payment, and (4) a physician ethic to provide all health care for each patient.

Some of these forces are modifiable; others are not.

Under any circumstances, few or none within our society will contend that it is mathematically or politically possible to continue indefinitely present trends in increased expenditures for health, or that it is possible even in wealthy, modern America to do everything that is medically and scientifically possible for everyone everywhere.

We Must Decide What We Are Going To Do for Whom Where

This conclusion is a corollary of the recognition of limited resources for health.

In any society, when there is not enough of something to go around, there are ways, formal or informal, organized or unorganized, of determining who gets what.

Schwartz (1975) has written that any national-health-insurance law will be a method of rationing health care. I agree. But it is also my contention that we are now rationing health care by several mechanisms, including the barrier of cost for some people, the unavailability of services for others, and for others the inability to find a point of entry into a complex health care delivery system. For others, it is a matter of the chance utilization of already limited resources—for example, which victim of aplastic anemia gets into the sterile cocoon first.

In the poor nations of the world, the rationing of health care has been a long-time thing. Most inhabitants of poor nations only aspire to modern health care as we know it.

The extent of the health care rationing problem for poor nations is dramatized by the fact that over half the world's people have annual incomes of less than $500, the amount that each of us Americans spends each year for health care alone.

Most of the world's wealthy nations, the industrialized nations, have been attempting to provide equal access to all health services for every citizen. Each of these nations is now impaled on the dilemma of expenditures for health rising much more rapidly than nearly any other classified group of expenditures.

As a result, nearly all the world's wealthy nations are today attempting to withdraw their open-ended promise for all health care for each citizen and to ration services equally for all. Where there is equality of access to existing services, there has until this time been little social or political strife.

The fact that our task of rationing health care is one that we have in common with others does not lessen the formidable nature of the task. Our difficulty is increased by the absence of a tradition of equality of access to health services for all citizens.

In sum, it is a matter of the first magnitude of importance that we recognize and articulate that our deliberations and actions are directed toward the rationing of personal health services.

Personal health care is only one determinant of health

If our goal is individual and national health, we cannot afford to consider medical care or health care separate from other determinants of health.

Greatly increased expenditures for health have been made primarily for personal health services. Simultaneously, there has been little improvement in the gross indicators of health. From this one can conclude that more personal health services alone can provide only marginal improvements in health.

Once we have established equal access to personal health services by the financing and organization of the personal health care system, then what?

The Canadians, as most of you know, have reasonably well accomplished equal access to personal health services, and have asked this question and have attempted to answer it in the Lalonde Report, "A New Perspective on the Health of Canadians."

His categorization of health determinants into four areas is extremely helpful to us in our considerations. The four areas are (1) human biology, (2) environment, (3) life style, and (4) health care financing and organization. The report lays out in seventy-six readable pages the conflicts, considerations, and possible solutions that are derived from this "health-field" concept.

I believe the Lalonde Report has great relevance to us not only because of the similarities of our two nations, but also because the Canadians established universal hospital insurance in 1958 and universal physician insurance in 1968. (Incidentally, their rate of increase of expenditures over the past ten years under their government financing mechanism is nearly identical to ours, indicating, I believe, that our current financing mechanism is about as open-ended as it can be; also, it should be noted that the Canadians are now initiating limitations on federal government expenditures for health.)

The health-field concept should be considered by us in two contexts. The first is the need for the assessment of outcomes and cost benefits for personal health services, and for all other expenditures for health.

If we are going to ration personal health services, we need to know the cost benefits of such services. Likewise, if we choose to expend more resources in an attempt to intervene in the areas of human biology, environment, and life style, we had better also determine the cost benefits of these efforts. For example, it is conceivable that we can spend hundreds of millions of dollars on health education without substantially changing American life style in ways that improve health. Current measurements of cost benefits are equally soft for personal health services and for other expenditures for health.

Secondly, I believe the Lalonde Report should be read by citizens of this nation with the full recognition that expenditures in the health field other than those for personal health services are traditionally expenditures from state and federal funds. Money for public health, education, research, planning, data gathering, and similar purposes does not come directly from private sources. It comes through the public treasury.

Public funds for other health initiatives are now being greatly reduced because of the impact of expenditures for personal health services on governmental budgets. If the Lalonde Report concepts have validity, many of our actions in this country at present are directly opposed to modifying the causes of discomfort, disability, and death, and thereby are futile or counterproductive in improving the health of Americans.

The explanation of this apparently irrational governmental behavior is rational. The cost to the federal government of Medicare and Medicaid—i.e., personal health services—is increasing at a rate of nearly five billion dollars annually and is dictated by laws entitling Medicare patients to personal health services and entitling states to matching funds. The President and the Congress can justify only so much money for health. Therefore, most available money is spent where by law it must be spent, and money for all other federal health initiatives, which is currently about five billion dollars for research, education, new delivery systems, data gathering, planning, and direct health services to identified populations (migrants, Indians) is systematically cut back in presidential and congressional budgets.

In sum, rapidly increasing expenditures for personal health services and the absence of gross indications of substantially improved health have led us inevitably to the re-examination of other determinants of health and to ask how these determinants can be modified. Conversely, we are spending relatively less each year for these other health initiatives.

If this is a reasonably accurate description of current forces and current health system problems, what, then, is our agenda?

DECISIONS THAT MUST BE MADE

It is difficult enough to have to deal with decisions and change. It is even more difficult to have to decide among alternatives all of which are in one way or another unacceptable. And this is the situation that occurs when there are limitations on resources for anything so highly valued as health services.

How Shall We Determine Total National Expenditures for Health?

The method of payment for personal health services, in combination with government regulation, will determine the total national expenditures for personal health services.

I believe alternative mechanisms should be measured by at least two criteria. First, the nation's total expenditures for health should reflect the importance that the people of this nation place on health; and, second, total expenditures should assure adequate resources to provide for a healthy nation commensurate with the state of the art and science of health care, and commensurate with our abilities to modify other health determinants.

The first criterion preserves our respect for individual values and needs, and the second criterion indicates a recognition of societal and national values and needs. The harmony of these two often conflicting values is ultimately reconciled by the government, which determines the combination of market forces and regulation in the health industry at any given time.

Consideration of alternatives will focus on expenditures for personal health services because such expenditures account for over 80 percent of all expenditures for health, and because it is assumed that public money will continue to be the primary source of financing for expenditures to modify other determinants of health.

Some alternatives are:

The present system. Our present system, which combines private health insurance, government payment for the indigent, and out-of-pocket payment for uncovered services and for people without insurance or government payment, is unsatisfactory, and change is inevitable.

The advantage of the present system is that it makes unlimited funds available for health services and, therefore, there is great latitude for innovation and the adoption of new services. As a result, it makes the world's finest health care available to many Americans.

The disadvantage is that costs are increasing to the point of unaffordability of services. Also, we have two classes of medical care—one provided for full-pay patients, and the other provided for government part-pay patients and the poor.

A return to market forces. Total national expenditures for health would then equal the sum of hundreds of millions of individual decisions made annually and based on the laws of supply and demand and the specific importance that the individual places on health services. This very effective means of allocating resources would require a law prohibiting private health insurance. A return to market forces would also require either some kind of guaranteed annual income for each citizen, so that each citizen could realistically make his or her own choice to spend or not to spend for health, or a continuation of government payment of health services for the poor.

A return to market forces would also require modifications on the supply side, including antitrust actions and provisions for increased freedom of access of providers of services to the market.

A return to a free market for health is exceedingly unlikely because of the obvious value the American people place on health, the size of present-day health care bills, the present reliance on health insurance, and the demand for equity in health care.

Present system plus catastrophic health insurance. This system would leave in place present open-ended funding for ordinary services and would put in place either private or government-funded insurance for catastrophic care.

Total third-party payment for catastrophic care would very quickly result in a further explosion of health care costs. Most of the expensive new technologies do not cure but only temporarily relieve disabilities and marginally prolong life.

If catastrophic care were paid for by the government, strong federal regulation would be necessary to contain costs. Possibilities include a limitation of total annual expenditures for catastrophic care, preauthorization of services, and a federal Food and Drug Administration-type regulatory agency to approve the implementation of only the new procedures that are found by pretesting to be adequately effective to justify their costs.

Continuation of the present system for ordinary care would perpetuate the nonchoice of individuals to pay what is asked in premiums and taxes for total health expenditures. Catastrophic insurance would remove the barrier of cost and thereby provide greater equity for those with large expenditures for health services, but current inequities for noncatastrophic care would continue.

National health insurance (NHI): total federal payment. This system would greatly limit total resources for personal health services because the government would decide the precise number of dollars to be spent for personal health services, and this expenditure would be determined in relation to all other federal spending, including defense, welfare, and transportation.

Such a system, absent a black market or substantial additional private health insurance, greatly diminishes direct individual choice of expenditures for health care. It relies on a governmentally determined limitation (a "cap") on total expenditures for health. It requires central or regional planning to allocate limited services.

The advantages are equity and affordability. The disadvantages are the risk of inadequate funding and the dangers of central planning and regulation.

NHI: government payment—private insurance. This system is likely to resemble the West German system or a more comprehensive Nixon Administration Comprehensive Health Insurance Program (CHIP). Its primary advantage is that it permits nongovernmental determination of total resources for health services and thereby guarantees less arbitrarily determined total expenditures.

The degree of equity will be determined by whether or not the government purchases insurance coverage for the poor identical to that owned by other citizens and whom the government classifies as poor.

In the absence of new government regulation, this system would have the other advantages and disadvantages of the present system.

In sum, we will adopt universal mandatory national health insurance. We will eventually adopt first-dollar, comprehensive coverage.

How much money is enough money for personal health services? If we look to the federal government to pay for all health services, Congress will decide—and the decision will reflect other national priorities and the fact that people always want more services and less taxes.

For this reason, there are strong arguments for the retention of a private-sector component in the financing of personal health services in the form of private health insurance. Only in this way can we, the American people, be assured that there will be enough money available to provide the personal health services that are known to be effective.

For reasons of equity, everyone must own the same "ticket"—i.e., have the same insurance. This means that the government will have to buy health insurance for the people in our society who cannot afford it.

But because national health insurance will finish off even the charade of a marketplace for health services, extensive government regulation will be necessary and important.

How Can We Assure Adequate Money for Other Health Initiatives?

The evidence is undeniable that personal health care is only one of the determinants of health.

If we are to modify appreciably other determinants of health, substantial and consistent amounts of money must be made available. Moreover, such funds probably must come from government or governmentally determined sources because research, health education, data gathering, planning, preventive services, rehabilitative services, and organization modifications, as I have noted before, are only to a small (although important) degree underwritten by private sources. Paradoxically, the more government spends for personal health services, the less government spends for other health initiatives.

The method or methods of assuring adequate money for other health initiatives will be related to and probably will be dependent upon how we are paying for personal health services at any given time.

Two modifications can be used to increase funding for other health initiatives without changing present payment mechanisms. One is a form of entitlement whereby an amount proportionate to government expenditures for personal health services would be stipulated for other health initiatives.

A second is a tax on private health insurance premiums with the establishment of a fund for other health initiatives.

Each of these methods consists of placing a taproot into the broad mainstream of health money, that spent for personal health services, and each is adaptable to all other payment mechanisms, which include large government or private insurance payments for personal health services.

One or both of these mechanisms, or similarly effective mechanisms, for assuring adequate money for other health initiatives should be made an integral part of any national health insurance program.

How Shall We Ration Health Services?

To this point, I have discussed possible payment mechanisms and how each would be likely to affect the total funds available for personal health services. I have also stressed the importance of assuring adequate money for other health initiatives, and I have indicated two ways of assuring that money.

This brings us to the critical question of how we decide who gets what where, the rationing question.

Let me first discuss the physicians' specific roles in rationing health services.

It is increasingly necessary for physicians to measure the outcome of health services on the basis of cost benefits. In addition, physicians are expected to play a major part in deciding who will provide services and where services can be most effectively and economically and humanely provided.

Can the physician be expected to consider "not only the medical but the financial aspects" of the care of his or her own individual patient? I have always thought not, but there is evidence to the contrary in a remarkable resolution adopted by the 1959 House of Delegates of the American Medical Association (1971).

It reads: "Medical Profession Responsibility: (1) The individual physician and the medical profession as a group must also be concerned with maintaining *a proper balance between adequate medical care for the welfare patient and economical use of public funds.* (2) The individual physician, as the key person in the care of the welfare patient, must, therefore, take into consideration *not only the medical but the financial aspects* of various acceptable modes of treatment" [emphasis mine].

It follows, of course, that if the physician can balance costs and care for his individual welfare patients, he can do this for all his patients.

Furthermore, on May 11 of this year, J. Alexander McMahon, president of the American Hospital Association, speaking at the annual meeting of the American College of Obstetricians and Gynecologists in Dallas, Texas, stated: "As efforts to regulate hospitals continue, the physician will have to balance benefits with cost, recognizing his responsibility not only to the individual patient but to the hospital and all its patients."

Thus, we find the American Medical Association as long ago as 1959, and the American Hospital Association as recently as May, saying that the individual physician must balance benefits with cost for his or her individual patient.

It follows that if every physician knew the cost benefits of his services, and if every physician were equally able to implement the "proper balance between adequate medical care . . . and economical use of . . . funds," we would need no further rationing system. But I believe we know that this cannot be done.

While we physicians have special responsibilities for the rationing of health care, the entirety of our society must deal with the moral and ethical implications of who shall get what services, when everyone cannot have all services. Although we cannot expect our society to arrive at unanimous or definitive answers on such questions as when to discontinue a life-support system or how many resources are to be used to maintain life for a badly damaged one-pound baby (or the even more subtle questions of resource use—e.g., what laboratory tests), we can expect concern, debate, guidelines, and the understanding of these omnipresent questions.

I have already pointed out the mechanisms now operating that determine our present rationing system for health services. On balance, these mechanisms as now used are totally ineffective in limiting the utilization of resources, and consequently total costs, but for some people in our society, they are very real deterrents to adequate or even minimal personal health services.

Many of the mechanisms now being used for health services rationing—namely, costs, government-imposed limitations on expenditures, and other regulation by government—will also be the mechanisms for future health services rationing. The amount and mix of these levers will be varied in an attempt to gain maximum equity and effectiveness while limiting total resources for health.

Costs. In the area of costs, we have found the worst of both worlds. The absence of marketplace considerations is blowing the lid on health services' expenditures. Conversely, the absence of universal, mandatory, comprehensive, first-dollar health insurance is rationing services for a small number of Americans.

There is one other problem. Reimbursement or nonreimbursement is determining what services will be provided where, as well as for whom. Legislators and insurors are effectively making medical decisions when they decide that one service is reimbursable and another is not. And they also prejudice the site of service when they decide to pay for a service in a hospital, but not in a physician's office or a nursing home.

As physicians we know that the disincentives built into health services' benefit packages often make health care more expensive, of lower quality, and less convenient and acceptable for the patient and family.

For reasons of equity and because of the tradition of health insurance, most services will continue to be reimbursable. There are strong arguments that in the near future all health services should be totally reimbursable.

If personal health services are reimbursable, there must be some other rationing mechanism. The only other alternative is government regulation.

Regulation. Arbitrary payment limitations for government-funded programs. This rationing mechanism is now being partially implemented. There are "caps" on Medicaid expenditures, and the President and the Congress are asking for caps on total expenditures for Medicare.

The results are (1) a widening of our dual system of one level of health care for the indigent, aged, and disabled and another level of health care for all others; (2) unpredictable and oftentimes irrational curtailment of services; (3) a shifting of institutional costs to others; (4) the withdrawal of services from the poor by physicians and other health professionals; and (5) oftentimes greater costs than if services were fully reimbursable in a variety of settings. For example, some patients are forced to receive services in teaching-hospital outpatient departments at a much higher cost than if the same services were received in a private physician's office.

If we adopt NHI with total federal payment for health services, the inequity problem is eliminated, but the other undesirable and unpredictable results of government-determined payment limitations would occur. These results can be modified or eliminated, however, by the implementation of other regulatory mechanisms.

Utilization review and professional standard review organizations (PSRO). The health care system is presently highly but ineffectively regulated by government. Efforts to contain costs have prompted the formation of utilization review committees, and professional standard review organizations, which are asked to control utilization on a case-by-case and day-by-day basis and are also asked to fit the individual patient into the most effective and economic treatment site regardless of the patient's insurance provisions.

Patients, physicians, and institutions frequently do not perceive utilization and PSRO activities to be in their own best interest. For example, it is not perceived by the patient to be in his or her best interest to be moved from a site where care is paid for by insurance to a site where care is not paid for by insurance. It is often not perceived by the physician to be in his best interest to take the time necessary for such efforts or to try to supersede his judgment for a colleague's judgment. And it is not perceived by a hospital that is half empty and running in the red to be in its best interest to send patients out of the hospital at the earliest possible moment.

Because even the government cannot expect individuals or institutions to do the things that they believe are not in their best interest, these regulatory efforts have a doubtful future as effective cost-containment mechanisms. However, PSRO, properly implemented, will improve quality of care and, equally importantly, will provide a data base for outcomes assessment and the measurement of cost benefits. Both are indispensable information for health care system planning and development.

Because current cost-containment efforts are ineffective, there will be greatly increased government regulation of health. Further regulation is made more certain because of the great improbability of the reinstatement of substantial free market forces, and the likelihood of mandatory, universal, and comprehensive national health insurance, with an increase in the government-payment component.

Wage-price controls. Wage-price controls are a favored regulatory mechanism when there are runaway costs, and wage-price controls for the health industry are under continuous consideration by the Administration and Congress. This form of regulation has all the problems of arbitrary government caps on expenditures, which I have already listed, with the additional problem of the virtual impossibility of long-term success unless there are wage and price controls on all related industries.

In addition, most increased health expenditures are the result of the provision of more services and more expensive new services rather than the inflation of costs for existing services.

Input regulation. The regulation of "inputs," which would eventually determine the function and size of the health care system, is the newest regulatory mechanism being implemented, and further considered by Congress.

The major component of input regulation is the planning of the health system instead of leaving its size and function just to happen as a result of reimbursement and other forces.

Other components are the development of approved plans, and sanctions to prohibit unplanned development.

One major group of inputs for providing personal health services is facilities, including hospitals, skilled nursing homes, and, to a lesser extent, physicians' offices. Specific inputs, such as the equipment necessary to establish cardiac-surgery units, renal-dialysis services, and radiation-therapy departments, further refine the nature and functions of the hospital.

Each physical improvement requires the expenditure of capital. The Health Planning and Resources Development Act, which requires each state to issue a certificate of need for each hospital capital improvement, is a capital-expenditure regulation law.

The other major input for personal health services is manpower, the educated, trained, skilled people who provide services by using the facilities and special equipment that are available.

Proposed federal health-manpower legislation, which would reapportion residency positions among the various specialties, is a manpower input regulation bill, and passage of such a law would eventually determine the kinds of physicians we have available to provide care.

At any one time the facilities and manpower available will determine total health services available. And all or nearly all services available are likely to be used to capacity if the services are paid for by private insurance or the government.

In sum, in the absence of a marketplace, there are only two alternatives for effectively limiting total health-services expenditures. One is an arbitrary government cap on payment, which to be effective requires government payment for all or nearly all services. The other is limitation of the size of the health care system by control of inputs.

If we cannot do everything for everyone everywhere—and we cannot—the least acceptable alternative is for us to decide what personal health services we need and want and are willing to pay for. And for us then to make certain that the facilities and skilled people are available to provide these services on an equitable basis to all citizens of our nation.

The new planning law looks to the people in over 200 geographic areas throughout the nation to decide for themselves what health care facilities they want. The law provides the structure and process for planning, but it leaves the final planning to local and state determination, and the implementation of plans mainly to the private sector, which today provides 80 percent of all health services.

Input regulation either can substitute for government determination of total expenditures for health services, or it can be used to minimize the adverse effects of an arbitrary government cap on health care expenditures.

However, only with successful input regulation and the resulting limitation of the size of the health care system can private health insurance be continued as a substantial component of the total health funding mechanism. Otherwise, the open-endedness of private health insurance payment will eventually bankrupt the system by perpetuating the present trend of uncontrolled increases in health expenditures.

One disadvantage of input regulation is that planning, even decentralized planning, can lead to mistakes that we must live with for a long time. But formal planning on a local basis is not likely to be more wasteful or inefficient than present duplication and obsolescence.

Another disadvantage of input regulation is that it establishes local monopolies, which in turn require rate setting and quality control—i.e., more regulation.

However, input regulation has the following substantial advantages.

It does not require changing the organization, ownership, or legal structure of health care institutions. It does limit their size and determine their function.

Input regulation does not make necessary any change in the nature or organization of medical practice. It does not limit choice of physician. It does not favor fee-for-service or capitation payment.

If we are willing to pay for planned services, we should be able to avoid payment of less than costs with its resulting starvation of institutions and services with the associated risk of the lowering of quality of services.

Finally, input regulation does not preclude innovation and change, but encourages planned change.

Government ownership and operation of health services institutions. This is the ultimate rationing mechanism, and it is being increasingly used by governments throughout the world. In this system the government owns the health facilities and hires the personnel.

THE PRIMARY CAVEAT

This point has been alluded to but bears special attention.

It is essential that we maintain the ability to innovate and change.

The history of national health insurance in other nations too often is a history of the freezing of the health system of the respective nations as of the date of passage of NHI. To avoid this freezing, I believe most of our laws should provide structure and process for local, regional, or state decision making rather than attempt to provide final answers and rather than look only to the federal government for central planning and regulation of the health system. Even more importantly, there must be a private component of total expenditures for health.

Just as illness is dynamic, and science and technology are dynamic, the health system must be dynamic. The total funding, the organizational form, and services available must remain open to change.

So the primary caveat is that we must retain flexibility in the American health care system.

CONCERNING THE ROLES OF PHYSICIANS

At times I considered addressing my entire presentation to the role of medicine in a time of change. I have demurred because I have no idea how we can make organized medicine (the state medical societies and associations and the American Medical Association) an instrument for constructive change. This is not to say that organized medicine cannot continue to do some important things well.

However, I will comment briefly because perhaps my perspective about organized medicine needs to be heard, and also because I want to take this opportunity to recognize the many physicians who individually and in settings other than organized medicine are making selfless and invaluable contributions to society and government.

I have carefully read and reread the 1970 and 1971 Shattuck Lectures given by Dr. C. Rollins Hanlon (1971) and Dr. George Himler (1971). Both men dealt extensively with the role of organized medicine. Dr. Hanlon expressed optimism for a positive role for the then newly organized Institute of Medicine of the National Academy of Sciences.

Dr. Himler came to the lectureship after having reported to the American Medical Association the recommendations of its committee on planning and development which he chaired. He stated: "Some of the opinions expressed in it aroused . . . a surprising degree of hostility." Dr. Himler then recommended the establishment of statewide institutes to do health planning, data collecting, negotiation, and other functions that he saw organized medicine being unable to do.

These observations, as well as my own, lead me to conclude with regret that organized medicine is organically incapable of playing a constructive political and planning role in the change of the health system.

What then can you and I do? I can see two good ways of providing positive input. One is through our specialty societies and many medical organizations other than state societies and the A.M.A. For example, committees of the American Academy of Pediatrics and the American College of Obstetrics and Gynecology are doing yeoman work in establishing regionalization of obstetric and newborn care. The roles of the American Academy of Family Physicians and the American Group Practice Association have been consistently constructive and helpful. The Study on Surgical Services for the United States sponsored jointly by the American College of Surgeons and the American Surgical Association is a major contribution. Public officials are extremely receptive to these efforts by physicians working in concert.

A second role can be played individually. The American political process is remarkably open. We can play the role of advisers to the decision makers or we can become one of the decision makers.

Personal action requires time, effort, and sacrifice, and I realize that someone must stay home and practice medicine, which I believe is one of mankind's highest callings.

But I also deeply believe that each of us should do all he can to assure health, in the broadest sense, for ourselves, our families, our nation, and our fellow human beings.

The tradition of high public service by physicians was established for us 200 years ago by Dr. Josiah Bartlett, of New Hampshire, Dr. Lyman Hall, of Georgia, Dr. Benjamin Rush, of Pennsylvania, Dr. Matthew Thornton, of New Hampshire, and Dr. Oliver Wolcott, of Connecticut, signers of the Declaration of Independence—and by Dr. Joseph Warren, patriot and martyr, who was mortally wounded commanding troops on Breed's Hill not far from where we are now in the City of Boston.

Our tasks today may not be so hazardous as theirs, but we should approach them just as fervently and selflessly. And if we do, I am convinced not only that we as physicians will make equal contributions to our nation's third century, but also that the practice of medicine will continue to be one of life's most rewarding and satisfying professions, even in a period of ever accelerating change.

REFERENCES

American Medical Association. *1959-1968 Digest of Official Actions of the American Medical Association* (vol. 2). Chicago: AMA, 1971.

Fuchs, V. R. *Who Shall Live?* New York: Basic Books, 1974.

Hanlon, C. R. "Shattuck Lecture: The Physician and Organized Medicine." *New England Journal of Medicine* 284 (1971): 1131-34.

Hiatt, H. H. "Protecting the Medical Commons: Who Is Responsible?" *New England Journal of Medicine* 293 (1975): 235-41.

Himler, G. "Shattuck Lecture: The Anatomy of Our Melancholy." *New England Journal of Medicine* 284 (1971): 1406-13.

Reinhardt, E. Presentation before the National Leadership Conference on Health Policy, Washington, D.C. (April 1976).

Schwartz, H. "Rationing Medical Care." *New York Times* (September 16, 1975).

Part II

Underlying Forces for Change

4

New Patterns of Mortality, Morbidity, and Disability

Selection by Ernest M. Gruenberg

I would like to begin by taking you back to the years preceding the Second World War, because the problem I wish to discuss must be seen as a historical process if it is to be understood. I am going to talk about a particular chapter in the history of disease, a chapter characterized by the surprising fact that the net effect of successful technical innovations used in disease control has been to raise the prevalence of certain diseases and disabilities by prolonging their average duration. The beginning of this historical period coincided with the introduction of the systematic clinical trial and of the sulfonamides in 1937 and 1938.

The health situation regarding modern man's chronic diseases and disabilities immediately before that period was well described by Osler in 1904 in his famous textbook, *The Principles and Practice of Medicine*, and the same description was still present in the 1935 edition revised by McCrae (Osler, 1935): "There is truth in the paradoxical statement that persons rarely die of the disease with which they suffer. Secondary *terminal* infections carry off many patients with incurable disease." Osler could not have anticipated the coming successes in curing the terminal infections associated with these incurable, or chronic, diseases that were to be introduced by a new era of medical research—the era of the clinical trial. What happened was that at the beginning of the era, in 1936, on a very small grant from the Rockefeller Foundation, a group of investigators searching for a cure for puerperal fever revealed to the world the antibacterial powers of sulfanilamide. The impact that sulfa drugs were to have on

Reprinted by permission from "The Failures of Success," *Milbank Memorial Fund Quarterly: Health and Society* 55, no. 1 (Winter 1977), pp. 3-24.

pneumonia, the most frequent of the terminal infectious diseases at that time, was as dramatic as it was serendipitous. Figure 4.1 shows the steep decline in death from pneumonia after 1936, following the introduction of sulfa drugs.

FIGURE 4.1

CURVE OF THE MORTALITY RATE PER 100,000
FROM PNEUMONIA BETWEEN 1930 AND 1950 (as prepared by
the Metropolitan Life Insurance Company)

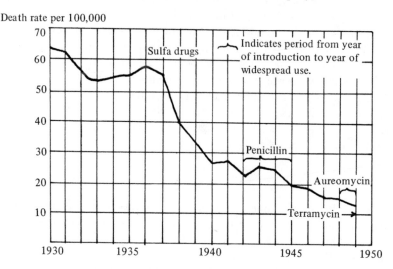

Source: Hobart A. Reimann, *Pneumonia* (Springfield, Ill.: Charles C Thomas, 1954).

Coincidental to the discovery of the sulfonamides was the invention of the clinical trial, the seeds of which had been developing for many years. In 1937 Professor A. Bradford Hill gave researchers a means for comparing a new treatment with an old one on a carefully selected population, and getting a definitive answer, usually within a few months. Quite by accident, the first new treatment that was tested adequately by the clinical trial was sulfanilamide. The clinical trial was then used to examine the efficacy of treatments whose effects, while not so apparent as those of the sulfa drugs, represented major clinical successes.

The rate at which new, effective remedies were discovered accelerated suddenly. The most important of these turned away impending death by simple techniques. The once fatal disease or injury might be in an otherwise healthy or vigorous person. As it turned out, these successful life-saving measures were disproportionately needed in people suffering from an incurable disease or disability. But these new techniques did not cure the chronic diseases, nor did they prevent them in the next patient.

If we assume no change in the age-specific annual incidence of the diseases formerly terminated early by now curable infections, and that, in fact, the anti-infectious drugs have been postponing death, then the average duration of these conditions has presumably been increasing. Therefore at the same time that persons suffering from chronic diseases are getting an extension of life, they are also getting an extension of disease and disability.

It is obvious that, with increasing duration, we would expect the proportion of the population in any given age group suffering from these conditions to rise. And, in fact, as the result of advances in medical care, we are seeing a rising prevalence of certain chronic conditions which previously led to early terminal infections, but whose victims now suffer from them for a longer period. The goal of medical research work is to "diminish disease and enrich life" (Gregg, 1941), but it produced tools which prolong diseased, diminished lives and so increase the proportion of people who have a disabling or chronic disease.

That is a major but unintended effect of many technical improvements stemming from health research. These increasingly common chronic conditions represent the failures of success. Their growing prevalence and longer duration are a product of progress in health technology.

MONGOLISM

How much does the elimination of fatal complications increase the proportion of the population with a specific chronic condition? That depends on how much the duration is increasing.* The increased duration has been measured best for mongolism (Down's syndrome).

Mongolism has long been known to be associated with a high susceptibility to respiratory infections (Record and Smith, 1955; Penrose, 1932). Children born with Down's syndrome rarely reached maturity until the 1940 birth cohort started to age. Persons in that cohort are now passing their thirty-sixth birthdays. However, their predecessors who managed to survive the first few years of life have also experienced an increased life expectancy—a much larger increase than that of the general population. For the first time in human history we are seeing seventy-year-old mongoloids. Spain's excellent pathology text (1963) on diseases resulting from medical advances does not describe the consequences of this new type of extended disease process in adults which the pathologist sees at the autopsy table. According to the director of the new Institute on Aging, Robert Butler, the geriatrics program will have to include plans for mongoloids, a situation that would have been unimaginable forty years ago!

Several sets of life tables for mongolism have been prepared, but none allows us to measure with precision how the life expectancy has changed and

---

*The duration of each person's illness extends from the time he becomes ill until he no longer is ill. A person with an incurable chronic illness will remain ill until he dies.

how much the prevalence rates have been rising since 1939. However, Carter (1958) makes what I think is a reasonable set of estimates of the prevalence rate of mongolism at age ten years. The rate doubled between 1929 and 1949, and doubled again in the following decade, reaching a level of more than one per thousand by 1958.

If we look at prevalence data from Victoria, Australia, in 1961 (Collmann and Stoller, 1963) and Salford, England, in 1974 (Fryers, 1975), we see that this trend is continuing. The overall prevalence rate increased by about 150 percent between 1961 and 1974. For children aged five to fourteen years, the prevalence rate per 1,000 was 1.3 in 1974, or almost twice the 1961 rate of .70.

Prevalence rates for mongolism would have risen dramatically even if nothing had been added to medical technology beyond antimicrobial drugs. Cardiac complications, which today are the most common cause of mortality among mongoloids (Deaton, 1973), usually do not occur until the teens or twenties, whereas previously most mongoloid children died of pneumonia before the age of six years. The most dangerous period of life for mongoloids is still the first year, but gains in survivorship have also been the most dramatic in this early period.

Of the mongoloid children who survive to age five years today, 50 percent live on into their fifties (Øster et al., 1975). Even this situation is changing. As more and more cardiac and gastrointestinal lesions are being surgically corrected, and patients with leukemia and other cancers are receiving life-prolonging treatments, we can expect to see an even greater rise in the prevalence of Down's syndrome.

Yet, no large-scale searches for preventable causes of mongolism are underway. Such inquiry seems to represent no one's priority. Even the door to new studies, which opened dramatically in 1959 when mongolism was shown to be due to trisomy, has given us no new insight into how to keep this condition from beginning. Fetal diagnosis of the trisomic condition followed by elective abortion does indeed represent an attempt to reduce the incidence of live-born mongoloid infants. At best it is a method for recognition of the condition early enough in fetal development so that women willing to do so can arrange for an early termination of the pregnancy. But this is merely a method of precipitating death, not an attempt to find preventable causes of the condition itself.

If this phenomenon of rising prevalence had occurred only in mongolism, the situation would be disturbing, for mongoloids now represent one-fourth of the severely retarded population (Kushlick, 1966). But because the prevalence rate of the severely retarded has been growing in general, it becomes alarming. The lives of youngsters with other causes of severe mental retardation are also being extended more rapidly than those of the general population due to the falling neonatal, infant, and childhood mortality rates associated with these conditions. The best data on the subject of rising prevalence rates come from Salford, the industrial suburb of Manchester, England (Fryers, 1975). There the school-age prevalence rates of the severely mentally retarded more than doubled between 1961 and 1974. We do not have much information on the diagnostic groups represented, but if I interpret correctly the criteria for severe retardation, many young people are going to live handicapped lives of unpredictable duration.

SENILE BRAIN DISEASE (SBD)

Another example of the failures of our successes occurs at the other end of life. We have long known that the age-specific prevalence of serious mental disorders rises rapidly in the last decades of life (Figure 4.2). We also know that the general population is aging.

With the exponentially rising age-specific prevalence rates of mental illness with age, and with an increasing number of aged in the population, it is clear

FIGURE 4.2
"SERIOUS" MENTAL DISORDER

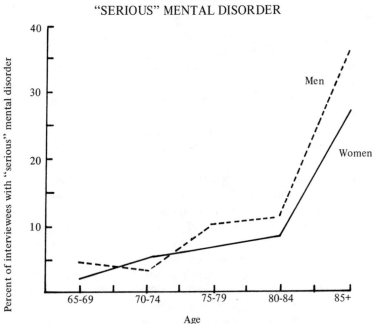

Note: "Serious" in this study meant with enough evidence of dangers to self or others, or, more commonly, inability to care for self that an involuntary mental hospital certificate could have been properly signed by a physician *if* those in the individual's home situation stopped being able and willing to provide care.

Source: Staff of the Mental Research Unit, New York State Department of Mental Hygiene, "A Mental Health Survey of Older People," *Psychiatric Quarterly* (supplement) 34, no. 1 (1960), pp. 34-75.

that we are headed for a great increase in serious mental disorder associated with aging. I can see no reason to think that the incidence of senile brain disease might be falling, nor do I think there is evidence that it is rising. I suspect that psychosis with cerebral arteriosclerosis may be getting more common, because coronary artery disease is getting more common, but I know of no assembled facts on this issue.

However, since senile brain disease was probably the condition which led Osler to think of pneumonia as the old man's friend, we may properly ask whether the large-scale conquest of pneumonia has reduced the usefulness of this friend, stretching out the course of senile brain disease, which produces the mental manifestations of "senile dementia."

We have some facts from a small (approximately 2,500), south Swedish population which was carefully screened for psychiatric illness in 1947 by Essen-Möller (1956), and rescreened in 1957 by Hagnell. Gruenberg and Hagnell (1976) selected two diagnoses believed to be dominated by cases of senile brain disease, although the classification might be slightly contaminated by cerebral arteriosclerosis and depressive states. (The silent cases of senile brain disease which occur will, of course, be missed by the type of clinical screen used.)

There were twenty-four people over the age of sixty with senile dementia in 1947, and there were forty-eight over the age of sixty in 1957. All twenty-four of the people found to have senile dementia in 1947 died by 1953, but of the forty-eight cases prevailing in 1957, five were still alive in 1967. The average duration of the episodes had at least doubled in a decade. The data suggest no concentration of this doubling in either sex or in any age group, but the number of cases is too small to examine this issue with confidence.

From 1947 to 1957, the prevalence rate of senile dementia in women over sixty years old rose from 3.2 percent to 5.7 percent, and in men from 2.3 percent to 4.9 percent.

Survivorship of the cases prevailing in 1957 closely resembled that of the general population, whereas cases prevailing in 1947 died off faster than the general population. The evidence suggests that this process did not end in 1957, but probably still continues today.

WHO ELSE WAS KILLED BY PNEUMONIA?

The chronic disabilities I have discussed so far—Down's syndrome and senile brain disease—are only two examples of the failures of success. What other conditions have been extended because of the elimination of fatal complications? First let us ask what other conditions have risen in prevalence due to the advent of antimicrobial drugs. Collins and Lehmann (1953) examined the excess death rates caused by conditions other than pneumonia during local influenza and pneumonia epidemics in the 1920s and 1930s. From this material, they were able to provide us with evidence regarding those diseases which were frequently

terminated by these respiratory infections in the days when the treatment resources against them were limited. From their data, we can infer what those conditions were (table 4.1).

TABLE 4.1

CONDITIONS SHOWING EXCESS DEATH RATES
DURING EPIDEMICS OF INFLUENZA AND PNEUMONIA

Heart Disease
Tuberculosis (especially before 1921)
Intracranial vascular lesions
Nephritis (especially before 1929)
Diabetes
Puerperal diseases
Cancer
Chronic bronchitis

Source: Collins and Lehmann (1953).

If no other causes of death had been conquered by modern medicine except those which respond to the sulfa drugs and antibiotics, we would be
justified in suspecting that the durations of these conditions were being prolonged. They are conditions which do not recover spontaneously. They are also
diseases for which no cures have been developed, and for which no preventions
have been found.

But there have been other major advances against the killing complications
of chronic diseases, some of which I will mention to illustrate the fact that the
rising prevalence of chronic diseases and disability is not merely the result of a
decreased case fatality rate in pneumonia.

SOME OTHER CONDITIONS

In Table 4.2 are listed some of the conditions which should be looked at
from the same point of view—diseases made more prevalent by medical progress.
I have listed them approximately in their rank order in terms of prevalence rates,
regardless of which age group experiences the highest prevalence rate. In doing
this I have taken the unusual step of eliminating discrimination by age.

Arteriosclerosis

Most cases of arteriosclerosis cannot be recognized by clinical examination. We have no good estimate of the prevalence of subclinical cases, but we do
know that arteriosclerosis represents the most important single cause of chronic
brain disease interfering with mental functioning, as well as the largest cause of

TABLE 4.2
CONDITIONS SHOWING INCREASED PREVALENCE
IN THE LAST THIRTY YEARS

Condition	Highest prevalence*	Next steps in research
Senile brain disease†	300/1,000 (80 years)	Case-control; autopsies; laboratory diagnosis
Arteriosclerotic‡		
Heart disease	140/1,000 (65-74 years)	Case-control
Brain disease	100/1,000 (65-74 years)	Case-control
Hypertension‡	150/1,000 (over 65 years)	Case-control
Schizophrenia‡	12/1,000 (35-44 years)	Penetrance factors
Diabetes†	9,1,000 (65-74 years)	Case-control on individuals with similar indices for metabolism of glucose
Severe mental retardation†	4.7/1,000 (5-15 years)	Nutritional preventive trials
Spina bifida†	2.5/1,000 (birth)	?
Down's syndrome†	1.3/1,000 (birth)	Is increased incidence in older women due to more trisomic mutations or decreased lethal effects of trisomy?

*Author's best estimate, based on available data
†Pretty certain
‡Inferred

chronic heart disease in this country. Chronic kidney disease and hypertension are also closely related to this condition. Previously, cases of arteriosclerosis were terminated by a number of complications: pneumonia, coronary occlusion, and ruptured arteries in the brain (stroke) and aorta. In the last forty years, medical research workers have developed a variety of means for outmaneuvering each of these fatal complications.

Hypertension

The prevention of fatal complications by moderating the level of hypertension with diuretics seems to be working. Most hypertensive patients lead almost normal lives and experience only a low level of disability. We have discovered an ideal way to control this disease, but we have yet to learn how to prevent it from occurring.

Schizophrenia

This is a common enough condition to worry about and a damaging one. While the highest point prevalence rates run only a little over 1 percent (Kramer, 1976), the proportion of the population who will at some time in life get clinical treatment for a schizophrenic episode is close to 5 percent. Its prevalence may be rising because in the recent past schizophrenic patients in mental hospitals had much higher mortality rates from many conditions than the general population (Malzberg, 1934). Yolles and Kramer (1969) have shown that since then this high mortality rate has declined. The pattern of community care has reduced the implications of these institutional death rates radically. But the frequency of schizophrenic diagnoses has also risen with the expansion of outpatient treatment and the broadening of diagnostic criteria. Balancing these two forces which affect the available data, I estimate that the life expectancy of schizophrenics has been increasing faster than that of the general population.

Diabetes

The discovery of insulin in 1922 dramatically changed the life expectancy of diabetics. While formerly the majority died of fatal complications (in conformity with Osler's paradox) over 40 percent died in diabetic coma. This figure rapidly dropped to a tiny fraction. Pneumonia continued to account for over 10 percent of the deaths until approximately 1944. By the 1960s over three-fourths of the diabetic deaths were due to vascular complications (Marble, 1972) which must be occurring at older ages.

Spina Bifida

In 1963, a British surgeon developed a marvelous operation to save newborn babies with extreme spina bifida, a congenital anomaly of the spine. Over half those who survived this surgery were severely or very severely disabled (Laurence, 1974; Hunt, 1973). They were doubly incontinent, immobile, and often retarded and incoherent. Ford (1970) estimated that this surgery would add 358 children with severe mental and physical handicaps to the British population each year. Routine use of this surgery in the United States would result in about 1,700 families each year being "blessed" with totally crippled children (Eisenberg, 1975). No one yet knows how many years these children will survive because this is a new "advance." Previously they would have died in the newborn nursery; now they will be saved to live crippled lives.

Other advances have had similar effects. The fatal complications of pernicious anemia have been thwarted, since this condition can now be suppressed with medication. Cases of Huntington's chorea have been prolonged by successfully treating terminal pneumonia. Hemophiliacs can now be treated so that they less often die of hemorrhages. The thoughtful reader will undoubtedly be able to list numerous other examples.

DISCUSSION

Why are we preventing death in the presence of illness and disability? Why these successes which produce these failures? Is it because the scientific period of modern medicine and public health continues to gain its drama from the idea

of a life and death struggle against the causes of death? Public health departments once routinely put falling death rate curves on the outside cover of their
annual reports. This was their index of success. They only gave up using crude
death rates as a selling point when their successes in lowering childhood deaths
increased the proportion of old people in the population, which resulted in a rise
in the crude death rate. In fact, many health officers no longer know what the
death;ates in their jurisdictions are or how they compare with those of the country as a whole.

I, among others, predicted that morbidity would become the priority of
public health once the giant killers had been conquered and the average age of
the population rose. Events have refuted my hopeful expectation. Yet our research programs continue to put primary emphasis on causes of death rather
than on causes of nonkilling chronic diseases. More and more of the health dollar
is being used to provide services to the chronically ill and disabled. A recent
estimate (R. Morris, 1976) of the health and medical care and transfer expenditures for the chronically disabled was around $83 billion—almost as much as the
hotly debated defense budget.

The major advances in medical science have in fact been against killing diseases. It is noteworthy that the sulfonamides emerged out of the fight against
maternal mortality in a search for a treatment of puerperal sepsis. The other
effects of the sulfa drugs were all serendipitous to that goal.

NEXT STEPS IN RESEARCH

It seems obvious that the rising prevalence rates of serious conditions
should lead to new priorities for research. We should focus on furthering our
understanding of the forces which determine the patterns of occurrence of these
conditions, and thus try to identify some modifiable causal factors. Intensive
searches for preventive measures are at least as important for bettering the people's health today as were the searches to gain control over plague, smallpox,
cholera, diphtheria, tuberculosis, pellagra, and lung cancer a generation or so ago.
In principle there is no reason to think that different types of epidemiological
forces are at work in the causation of these diseases. Infections, poisons, genes,
physical agents, and nutritional deficiencies are the classes of agents we have
come to worry about, and we should continue to worry about them. The epidemiologists of the future must seek out such modifiable agents in the causal
chains which lead to these newly stretched out diseases of medical progress.

In order to indicate that this precept is not just empty rhetoric, I have
undertaken to suggest a next step in epidemiological research for each of these
conditions (table 4.2). In selecting a next step I have tried to keep in mind Sir
Peter Medawar's excellent dictum: "If politics is the art of the possible, science
is the art of the soluble" (Medawar, 1967). Selecting the next issue to investigate
is not a science but an art—it is a matter of judging what problem is soluble

today with today's understanding and research techniques. "Any fool can ask a question, the trick is to ask a question which can be answered" (Lemkau and Pasamanick, 1957).

Trisomy 21

We have known for some time that mongolism (Down's syndrome) is the most common of the human trisomic disorders. I will confine my suggestions to those cases caused by nondisjunction, the failure of the chromosomal material to divide properly when the ovum is being formed in the mother's ovary.* The obvious approach to this problem is to look for the causes of nondisjunction and to look at its epidemiology. The nondisjunctions which occur in the various trisomic conditions (for example, mongolism, Turner's syndrome) may be caused by different agents or they may have a single underlying cause. If all nondisjunctions have similar causes and result only in different patterns of trisomy because they affect different chromosomes, we should then turn our attention to all the nondisjunctions including those which do not cause human disease. Most trisomic patterns are likely to be lethal to the embryo, so the obvious research step is to compare fetuses which spontaneously abort with those that do not. We would then be able to tell whether trisomy of chromosome 21 (which produces mongolism) is the most common human trisomy, or only the most common one which survives the fetal period and produces disease.

I suspect that trisomies are fairly common and that quality control occurs by weeding out the "misfits" during fetal development. One way to pursue that hypothesis is to determine whether the much higher rate of mongoloids born to older women is associated with a higher rate of trisomic conceptions or with a decreased ability for discriminating weeding through resorption, abortion, and miscarriage. There is abundant evidence that the mortality rate in mongoloid fetuses is enormous. How does it compare in women of different ages? That, I think, is a soluble problem.

Senile Brain Disease

Clinical diagnosis of senile dementia is not terribly difficult but this does not identify the frequent asymptomatic silent cases of it. So we need autopsy surveys on clinically surveyed populations. Case control studies cannot yet be done because we know too little about the age of risk. There is some evidence in Hagnell's data that incidence rates, which soar between age 70 and age 80, begin to fall off after age 80. Perhaps everyone who is going to develop this condition does so by age 85 or 90. If so, we know that our case control studies should be

*The normal human cell has twenty-three pairs of chromosomes, one of each pair coming from the father's sperm and one from the mother's ovum. The ovum and sperm each have only twenty-three chromosomes. Nondisjunction in oogenesis results in an egg having twenty-four chromosomes because one pair failed to split. When fertilized such an egg has three chromosomes where a pair normally exists, hence the name "trisomy."

done on people who have passed their ninetieth birthday. All of the important questions about the epidemiology of senile brain disease would become rapidly answerable if we had a reliable, valid means of knowing whether senile plaques were present during life. The new evidence about aluminum deposits in the senile plaques suggests the possibility that some clever biophysicist might develop a noninvasive device for ascertaining the presence of such deposits.

Arteriosclerosis

We need a means of identifying people in the early presymptomatic stages of this group of diseases. These early stages can be detected at autopsy, and autopsy surveys for this purpose can be done on young people who die of other conditions, particularly accidents. This would provide an opportunity to compare the characteristics of cases and noncases—a simple case-control study.

Schizophrenia

The next fruitful step in elucidating the pathogenesis of schizophrenic conditions may be reached by identifying populations with high levels of familial aggregation of the condition and comparing these families with the families of schizophrenics in which the concentration of secondary cases among first degree relatives is low. This is based on the general notion that there are two types of factors which must interact to produce clinical schizophrenic syndromes: factors associated with the family of origin (polygenic mechanisms, dominant gene with low penetrance?) and external environmental factors. Comparing the environments and living habits of these two sets of families would be an attempt, through a type of case-control study, to identify risk factors other than the familial tendency to develop schizophrenia. That is a long shot, but it attracts me. I have used the single word "penetrance" in table 4.2 to signify this line of reasoning.

Diabetes

The individual's inability to metabolize glucose, which was earlier thought to be the hallmark of the diabetic condition, is no longer an adequate criterion for case identification. Survey findings have revealed that the indices which measure the ability to metabolize glucose fall with age in the general population, whether diabetes is present or not. This has made the task of the epidemiologist more difficult, as has the fact that these falling indices are accompanied by greater variations in value for older age groups. A next worthwhile step for research would be to compare diabetic and nondiabetic individuals who have low index values with respect to factors associated with clinical diabetes (overweight, familial aggregation, and so on).

Severe Mental Retardation

Epidemiology cannot help us to find causes for this group of conditions when approached collectively. Some forms of retardation are associated with genes. Some are caused by the trisomic conditions discussed above. But there is a large group which is not familial and is probably associated with brain damage early in fetal development. The "continuum of fetal damage" concept introduced by Lilienfeld and Parkhurst (1951) and elaborated by Pasamanick and Knobloch (1961) has not been picked up and elaborated sufficiently in more concrete investigations. Causative agents often interact with suboptimal nutrition to produce disease, and many women who become pregnant are in a suboptimal nutritional state. Preventive trials in which nutritious food is supplied to pregnant women would seem to be the logical next step in research.

There have been so many examples in the last forty years of how our health technology too often advances by postponing death and thus increases the duration of chronic conditions, that one might conclude that this trend is inevitable. But there is one great victory during the same period which went just the other way. It may not be as impressive as the conquest of smallpox, but as a consequence of the discovery that a very large proportion of tooth decay was due to a correctable deficiency of the trace element fluorine, millions of persons who would have lost their teeth in early adulthood have been able to keep them. The final link in the chain of evidence came from the great preventive trial which compared the incidence of caries in Newburgh and Kingston (New York) after one of the towns had flouridated its water supply. Our techniques for treating dental decay have improved only slightly, but we have made great strides in reducing the incidence of decay. The fact that more dentists are making more money than ever should relieve any anxiety that the medical fraternity might have about successful disease control programs.

ENVOI

In assessing the effect of our technical advances in the past four decades, I have attempted to demonstrate that the net contribution of our successes has actually been to worsen the people's health. The prevalence of chronic diseases and disabilities depends on both the frequency with which they occur and their average duration. It is true that we have lowered the occurrence of certain chronic conditions through preventive measures; the prevalence of dental decay and lost teeth has diminished, and the prevalence rate of paralytic poliomyelitis has fallen. However, these few reductions in the occurrence of chronic conditions have been more than offset by the increased average duration of a wide range of conditions whose fatal complications we have learned to postpone.

You will recall that Semmelweis was led to connect puerperal sepsis with contamination from the autopsy room after a close friend of his, a pathologist, had died with tissue changes similar to those seen in puerperal sepsis after he had been pricked with a knife during an autopsy on an infected person. I can give you no such dramatic episode which forced me to the conclusions outlined in this paper, but I do have enough recollection of transient ideas and insights to know that I was extremely resistant to the generalizations laid out here. I now recognize that we should have predicted by 1940 that some chronic diseases and disabilities would become more common because we had better techniques for thwarting killers which had been weeding out the chronically ill.

I tell you about this resistance within myself to let you know that if you find alien the whole idea that the techniques we have to improve life expectation perpetuate sick lives more than they do healthy lives, I was recently of your company. I know that part of my resistance and caution stemmed from a feeling that colleagues would also be resistant and that I would have to be able to defend myself against much methodological quarreling. But after looking at the issue from many angles, and examining multiple sources of information, I am convinced that this unpleasant proposition is true.

The paradoxical fact about death is that it is at once the great leveler and the great discriminator. It is the greatest of all equalizers because it is everyone's ultimate end, and the lowliest beggar can be no more dead than the most eminent monarch. But it is also a great discriminator because it comes later for those more privileged than for those less privileged. As Sir Thomas Browne (1642, 1889 ed.) said so elegantly in *Religio Medici,* "There is little difference between one man's death and another's except in the time and the manner of dying."

While the universal fear of the great plagues might leave us with the impression that they were no respecters of persons, in fact, all the great killers have discriminated, more readily taking those who were half dead or half grown than those who were healthy and in their prime. There are a few examples of killers which discriminate in the opposite direction. The generals have always wanted the flower of our youth for cannon fodder. Paralytic poliomyelitis selected people of strong athletic build who were more vigorous than the average person (Draper, 1917). In this instance, it was later discovered that higher social status was associated with a lower chance of having a subclinical immunizing attack of poliomyelitis in early childhood. But the few real exceptions only underline the general rule that the large-scale killers are cowardly and select those least able to defend themselves. That greatest of all iatrogenic killers, puerperal sepsis, was concentrated in women of childbearing age, but from all the records I can find, showed special favoritism for the weakest of them.

But now our technological successes defy death's claim on the sick and the weak. We are proud of these successes, and perhaps it is partly our pride which prevents us from seeing that the successes result in the prolongation of sick lives.

Surely another reason why it has been so difficult to see the effects of our medical successes is that we have been suffering from that terrible ailment of modern technological man, his fragmented specializations. I did not see, for example, the way that chronic brain syndromes are made more common in the population by the systematic application of new health technologies until I stopped thinking of mental disorder epidemiology as somehow isolated from general epidemiology. It seems obvious to me now that general epidemiology also needs to be capable of dealing with the mental conditions which are manifestations of brain disease or of cerebrovascular disease. But our thought processes have been suffering from excessive hardening of the categories.

It is easy to see, in such cases as Karen Ann Quinlin's, that maintaining the vital systems artificially is not maintaining an intact person. And it is easy to see that there are profound ethical, professional, and legal questions involved. But my concern is not these small gains in extending life at the last moment before death. Such cases, which Jerry Morris (1975) has aptly called "snatch victories," make up only a minute part of the paradoxical effect of medical progress which I am trying to make more visible to you. The vast bulk of the increases in prevalence rates consists of only slightly impaired lives: memory loss in elderly people who are continuing to get and give pleasure in their lives, generally well-controlled cases of diabetes, or early hypertension. I am myself a handicapped person who survives by courtesy of modern medical care at its best. The extensive antishock and reconstructive surgery procedures I had following an automobile accident saved my life. The same injury would have been fatal a few years earlier.

So the successes I have been referring to are real successes representing real advances. But the increase in disease and disability which ensues is also real and must be faced. What then are the proper lessons to learn from these failures? Not the silly notion that we should give up our efforts to overcome the killers. Not that we should go backward to a pre-enlightenment stage of society in which we throw away the umbrellas and say, "If God meant you to stay dry, he wouldn't have made it rain." Nor should we conclude that the cheapest solution to chronic disease is the best solution. Hitler knew that the cheapest "solution" to cases of chronic illness was death. If our technology has blunted the edge of the grim reaper's scythe, that's exactly what it was meant to do and we should rejoice. We cannot avoid the successes. We must learn to overcome the ensuing failures.

As a first step, we must come to recognize that the socially organized application of health technology is one of the greatest epidemiological forces in the world. We have seen how the provision of medical care, while it has served as an important means of postponing death, has done so, to a great extent, by defeating the fatal complications that used to terminate the diseases people were suffering from, thus making those diseases more common in the population.

Today's socially organized campaigns to prevent killing diseases can have a similar effect; that was the object of the swine flu vaccination program. The eradication of smallpox from the earth—perhaps public health's greatest single victory—may have a similar effect. Smallpox must have been weeding out some individuals with chronic conditions. Who had it been killing? I admit to feeling foolish in raising this question only after the campaign has been completed. If we had posed the question before the campaign got started, we would now be in a position to state what conditions will become more common as a result of the eradication of smallpox. If we are to be more sensible in our efforts to improve the people's health we must have the foresight to look for these failure as soon as we recognize the possibility for advance.

The increase in chronic illness and disability which results from our advances makes finding ways to prevent these chronic conditions a matter of top priority for research programs. We are now over thirty years late in recognizing the failures that are bound to follow such successes. We should not waste time crying because we are so tardy, but rather hasten to see how quickly we can catch up.

I have indicated in the last column of table 4.2 a few ideas which I think are worth pursuing. To my eye, what is dramatic about these conditions is the paucity of existing epidemiological data. We don't even have good case-control data for many of them. We haven't failed in our efforts to find preventable causes of these conditions—we have hardly made any effort at all! There are whole sequences of investigations which are obvious even when we have no clues. But even in cases where we do get a clue, I think that we are unduly passive in our approaches to preventing chronic diseases.

Preventive trials are interventions based upon an accumulated body of experience. Their great value lies in their ability to prove or disprove seemingly credible hypotheses. If preventive trials were done often enough, most would yield negative results, and we could rid ourselves of a number of erroneous "common sense" ideas. But preventive trials are not used to the extent that they should be. Most often, they are thought to be too expensive. Frequently they are viewed as "manipulations" which raise social and ethical problems, even though in most applications (like improved maternal nutrition) they are innocuous and involve interventions known to be desirable. Frequently, preventive trials are not done because they call for stable research teams which cannot be organized under the present project grant system.

Our weakness today in finding preventive measures for chronic illnesses in contrast to our strength in finding curative measures for fatal complications is due largely to the way health research money is organized. I think the time has come to examine afresh the administrative mechanisms by which research is supported. Can't we find new ways to encourage research which will emphasize chronic disease *prevention*? If we don't, research which produces means for thwarting fatal complications—research which, when applied, increases the frequency of postmature deaths—will continue to advance more rapidly.

I have always been mortified by public health's preoccupation with death. We have always known that there are fates worse than death. But epidemiology and biostatistics have never sufficiently weaned themselves from John Graunt's great bills of mortality studies and William Farr's brilliant use of birth and death records. I have long been sick and tired of this morbid preoccupation with the first and last months of life. But it doesn't matter that this backwardness in public health made *me* sick. Now that we know that instead of enhancing the people's health this kind of deathly thinking has been increasing the people's sickness and disability, it is time to call for a change.

Now that we recognize that our life-saving technology of the past four decades has outstripped our health-preserving technology and that the net effect has been to worsen the people's health, we must begin the search for preventable causes of the chronic illnesses which we have been extending. Epidemiologists must play a key role in finding these causes, but without the application of social pressures in that direction, few will take up the opportunity. For a period, at least, health saving must take precedence over life saving. And we will not move forward in enhancing health until we make the prevention of nonfatal chronic illness our top research priority.

REFERENCES

Brown, T. *Religio Medici*, 1642. Reprinted in *Religio Medici, A Letter to a Friend, Christian Morals, Urn-Burial and Other Papers*. Boston: Roberts Brothers, 1889.

Carter, C. O. "A Life-Table for Mongols with the Causes of Death." *Journal of Mental Deficiency Research* 2 (1958): 64-74.

Collins, S. D., and Lehmann, J. "Excess Deaths from Influenza and Pneumonia and from Important Chronic Diseases During Epidemic Periods, 1918-51." *Public Health Monograph* no. 10. Washington, D.C.: Government Printing Office, 1953.

Collmann, R. D., and Stoller, A. "Data on Mongolism in Victoria, Australia: Prevalence and Life Expectation." *Journal of Mental Deficiency Research* 7 (1963): 60-68.

Deaton, J. G. "The Mortality Rate and Causes of Death Among Institutionalized Mongols in Texas." *Journal of Mental Deficiency Research* 17 (1973): 117-22.

Draper, G. *Acute Poliomyelitis*. Philadelphia: P. Blakiston's Son, 1917.

Eisenberg, L. "The Ethics of Intervention: Acting Amidst Ambiguity." *Journal of Child Psychology and Psychiatry* 16 (1975): 93-104.

Essen-Möller, E.; Larsson, H.; Uddenberg, C. E.; and White, G. "Individual Traits and Morbidity in a Swedish Population." *Acta Psychiatrica et Neurologica Scandinavica*. Supplementum 100 (1956).

Ford, A. B. "Casualties of Our Time." *Science* 167 (1970): 256-63.

Fryers, T. "Life Expectancy and Causes of Death in the Mentally Retarded." *British Journal of Preventive and Social Medicine* 29 (1975): 61.

Gregg, A. *The Furtherance of Medical Research*. New Haven: Yale University Press, 1941.

Gruenberg, E. M., and Hagnell, O., with the assistance of L. Ojesso and M. Mittleman. "The Rising Prevalence of Chronic Brain Syndrome in the Elderly." Symposium: Society, Stress and Disease: Aging and Old Age. Stockholm (June 14-19, 1976).

Hunt, G. M. "Implications of the Treatment of Myelomeningocele for the Child and His Family." *Lancet* I (1973): 1308-10.

Kramer, M. "Population Changes and Schizophrenia, 1970-1985." Paper presented at the Second Rochester International Conference on Schizophrenia. Rochester, N.Y. (May 1976).

Kushlick, A. "A Community Service for the Mentally Subnormal." *Social Psychiatry* 1, no. 2 (1966): 73-82.

Laurence, K. M. "Effect of Early Surgery for Spina Bifida on Survival and Quality of Life." *Lancet* I (1974): 301-04.

Lemkau, P. V., and Pasamanick, B. "Problems in Evaluation of Mental Health Programs." *American Journal of Orthopsychiatry* 27, no. 1 (1957): 55-58.

Lilienfeld, A. M., and Parkhurst, E. "A Study of the Association of Factors of Pregnancy and Parturition with the Development of Cerebral Palsy: Preliminary Report." *American Journal of Hygiene* 53 (1951): 262-82.

Malzberg, B. *Mortality Among Patients with Mental Disease.* Utica, N.Y.: State Hospitals Press, 1934.

Marble, A. "Insulin—Clinical Aspects: The First Fifty Years." *Diabetes* 21 (Supplement), no. 2 (1972): 632-36.

Medawar, P. *The Art of the Soluble.* London: Methuen, 1967.

Morris, J. N. *Uses of Epidemiology* (3rd ed.). London: Churchill Livingstone, 1975.

Morris, R. "Alternative Forms of Care for the Disabled: Developing Community Services." *Developmental Disabilities: Psychologic and Social Implications,* edited by D. Bergsma and A. E. Pulver. New York: Alan Liss, 1976.

Osler, W. O. *The Principles and Practice of Medicine* (12th ed., revised by T. McCrae). New York: D. Appleton-Century Company, 1935.

Øster, J.; Mikkelsen, M.; and Nielsen, A. "Mortality and Life-Table in Down's Syndrome." *Acta Paediatrica Scandinavica* 64 (1975): 322-26.

Pasamanick, B., and Knobloch, H. "Epidemiologic Studies on the Complications of Pregnancy and the Birth Process." *Prevention of Mental Disorders in Children,* edited by G. Caplan. New York: Basic Books, 1961.

Penrose, L. S. "On the Interaction of Heredity and Environment in the Study of Human Genetics (with Special Reference to Mongolian Imbecility)." *Journal of Genetics* 25 (1932): 407-22.

Record, R. G., and Smith, A. "Incidence, Mortality and Sex Distribution of Mongoloid Defectives." *British Journal of Preventive and Social Medicine* 9 (1955): 10-15.

Spain, D. M. *The Complications of Modern Medical Practice: A Treatise on Iatrogenic Diseases.* New York: Grune & Stratton, 1963.

Yolles, S. F., and Kramer, M. "Vital Statistics." *The Schizophrenic Syndrome,* edited by L. Bellak and L. Loeb. New York: Grune & Stratton, 1969.

5

Changes in Population Structure

Selection by U.S. Department of Health, Education, and Welfare

GROWTH RATE

The rate of population growth in the United States is slowing down. Between 1960 and 1970 the total resident population of the United States grew 13 percent, reaching 204 million in 1970. This is significantly lower than the 18 percent increase registered between 1950 and 1960. Bureau of the Census estimates for 1980 indicate that the increase over 1970 may be as low as 8 percent (U.S. Department of Commerce, 1974).*

The rate of population growth varies considerably from region to region in the United States. While the U.S. population as a whole grew 13 percent between 1960 and 1970, the population in the West grew 24 percent, the population in the South grew 14 percent, and the population in the Northeast and in the North Central regions grew less than 10 percent (see figure 5.1).

Thus, although the total United States population continues to increase, the rate of increase is declining appreciably, particularly in the Northeast and the North Central sections of the country.

The slowdown in population growth should cause health care facilities to be more cautious about expanding than they were during the years of sizeable

*The 1970-1980 growth rate would be as low as 8 percent only if the average number of births per 1,000 women upon completion of childbearing is as low as 1,800.

Reprinted from "Changes in the Environment Affecting the Health Care System," *Health Planning Information Series no. 1, Trends Affecting the U.S. Health Care System* (Washington, D.C.: HEW, 1976).

FIGURE 5.1
UNITED STATES POPULATION GROWTH, BY REGION: 1920-1990

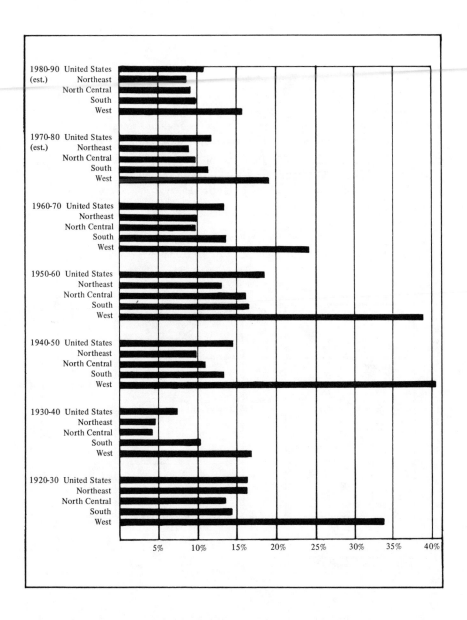

Source: U.S. Department of Commerce (1974). The 1980 and 1990 population projection is the Census Bureau's projection under Series I-E, which assumes 2,100 births per 1,000 women upon completion of childbearing and continuation of 1960-1970 migration patterns.

population increases. Population projections for a facility's service area should be carefully studied before embarking on an expansion program.

BIRTH RATE

The principal reason for the slowdown in population growth is the dramatic drop in the birth rate since 1957. In 1957 the number of births per 1,000 population was 25.2; by 1973 the birth rate had fallen to 14.9.

The fertility rate has plummeted even faster than the birth rate. In 1957 there were 122.9 births per 1,000 women of childbearing age (age 15-44); by 1973 the fertility rate had fallen to 69.3, a drop of nearly 50 percent (see figure 5.2). Women today are having only 1.9 children per completed family—less than the population replacement rate of 2.1 children (*New York Times,* 1974).

FIGURE 5.2

UNITED STATES BIRTH RATE AND FERTILITY RATE: 1935-1973

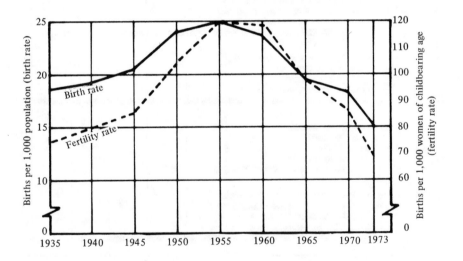

Source: U.S. Department of Commerce (1974).

The baby boom in the 1940s and early 1950s, however, is currently creating a spurt in the number of women of childbearing age: By 1980 the number of women in the high fertility ages of 20 to 29 will jump 14 percent over the 1974 figure (*New York Times,* 1975). Therefore, even though these women are having smaller families, the birth rate—births per 1,000 population—may rise for a time. However, the fertility rate—births per 1,000 women of childbearing age—seems likely to continue its downward trend, unless there are unforeseen changes in life styles and values. Among the many reasons for the falling fertility rate are the following:

—Better contraceptive methods are now available.

—Abortion laws are less restrictive.

—Family planning services are increasingly available to the poor as well as the middle class. As a consequence, the fertility rate among the poor has fallen considerably faster than the rate among other segments of the population. The fertility rate among women in the poverty level classification fell from 153 in 1960-1965 to 121 in 1966-1970, a 21 percent decrease. In contrast, the fertility rate among women in the nonpoverty level classification fell from 98 in the early 1960s to 81 in the later 1960s, a decline of 17 percent (Jaffe, 1972). Thus, the fertility rate of the poor was 56 percent higher than that of others in the early 1960s but only 49 percent higher in the later period. If the analysis could be extended up to 1973, the statistics would presumably be even more striking.

—The escalation in college tuitions and other costs may make people more concerned about restricting the size of their families.

—More women are working and therefore concerned about limiting the number of children they must care for.

—With women's liberation, exuberant motherhood is less fashionable than it once was.

—Religion is no longer having such an impact on family planning. For example, the birth expectations of Catholic women aged 20 to 24 declined more than twice as much as those of non-Catholic women (Gold, 1973).

The declining fertility rate will affect the health care system in many ways, although the temporary rise in the birth rate in the next few years may mitigate some of these effects for a time.

—Those hospital obstetric units already suffering from low occupancy levels may be under increasing pressure to close. There may also be less demand for the services of obstetricians, though abortions may keep some obstetricians and some hospital OB units busy.

—The demand for hospital pediatric units will also decline, in part because of the lower fertility rate and in part because of medical advances which are reducing the need for hospitalization of sick children. For example, the polio vaccines have dramatically reduced the incidence of this disease, and antibiotics have reduced the need to hospitalize children with pneumonia.

—Better contraception and greater ease in obtaining abortions may reduce neonatal mortality, for mortality rates tend to be higher among illegitimate babies, among babies born of older mothers, and among babies born to mothers with a large number of children (Chase, 1974; Barnett, 1974). Mortality rates tend to be higher also for babies born into poor families (U.S. Department of

Health, Education, and Welfare, 1972a), and it is in these socioeconomic classes that the fertility rate is falling the fastest.

—Differences in fertility rates among various population segments seem to be diminishing. Therefore, health facilities serving population groups that in the past had particularly high fertility rates may face a steeper drop in the demand for their services than facilities serving population groups whose fertility rates were always comparatively low.

—With smaller families, there may be less migration to the suburbs. The population served by inner city health facilities may cease,to fall, and the population served by suburban health facilities may not grow so rapidly as in the past. This trend will, of course, be accentuated if gasoline shortages or very high gas prices increase the difficulty of commuting from the suburbs.

AGE DISTRIBUTION

The population of the United States is growing older. Fewer babies are being born, and people are living to more advanced ages. In 1920 life expectancy at birth was 54.1 years; in 1950 it was 68.2 years; today it is over 71. The advancing life expectancy in the United States can be ascribed to a number of factors including a higher standard of living, new medical discoveries, better and more sophisticated health care, and improved public health programs.

One major reason for the greater life expectancy, however, is not the improved health of adults, but the steep decline in infant mortality. A male baby born in 1971 has 5.5 more years life expectancy than a male baby born in 1939-41, but a twenty-year-old male in 1971 has only 2.7 more years life expectancy than his equivalent in 1939-41. The drop in maternal mortality is one reason life expectancy has risen far faster for women than for men. Life expectancy for female babies rose 8.3 years between 1939-41 and 1971, and for twenty-year-old females it rose nearly 6 years (U.S. Department of Commerce, 1974).

Although life expectancy continues to creep upward, particularly for women, the death rate has not fallen appreciably since 1950. Many diseases have been conquered by modern medicine—and modern public health practices—but the U.S. health care system has been less successful in combating the debilitating effects of old age that have become a greater health problem now that people are no longer dying of typhoid or diphtheria. And changes in our life style are creating new health problems: increasing pollution, greater use of drugs and alcohol, heavier smoking, greater incidence of overweight, less exercise, greater tension and pressure are creating medical problems that can not be successfully tackled by improved medical care alone.

Advancing life expectancy is greatly increasing the percentage of the U.S. population that is over sixty-five years old. In 1930 only 5.4 percent of the total population was sixty-five or older; in 1973 the older segment of our population had grown to over 10 percent. The percentage of older people is expected to continue to increase during the 1980s and 1990s (see figure 5.3).

FIGURE 5.3
PERCENTAGE OF UNITED STATES POPULATION AGED SIXTY-FIVE
AND OLDER: 1950-1990

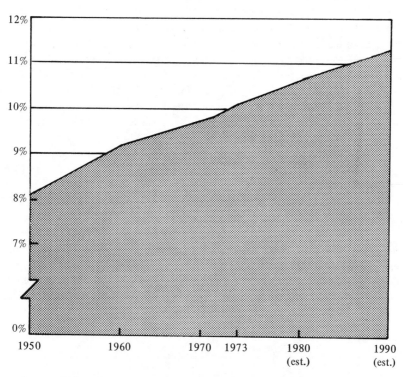

Source: U.S. Department of Commerce (1974). The 1980 and 1990 population projection is the Census Bureau's Projection under Series I-E, which assumes 2,100 births per 1,000 women upon completion of childbearing and continuation of 1960-1970 migration patterns.

The percentage of the population that is over sixty-five varies considerably from state to state. Variations from town to town can be even greater. As a consequence, the size and the nature of the demand for health care can differ markedly from one area to the next.

The trend toward an older population, which is hitting some areas more than others, affects the demand for health care in innumerable ways:

—Older people, on a per capita basis, suffer from more health deficiencies than do younger people and therefore require more medical attention at all levels of care.

—Physician visits per person per year increase considerably with age. On the average, persons over seventy-five years of age visit physicians 7.4 times a year, while younger people—for example, those between the ages of seventeen and twenty-four—see a physician less than 5 times a year (U.S. Department of Health, Education, and Welfare, 1973a, p. 26).

—Hospital admission rates are also higher for older people. In 1972, nearly 17 percent of the population over age sixty-five were hospitalized (in short-stay hospitals) at least once during the year, compared to only about 12 percent of those in the seventeen to twenty-four age group (U.S. Department of Health, Education, and Welfare, 1973a, p. 21). Age has been determined to be one of the most important factors affecting the demand for hospital facilities, and even small changes in the age distribution of the population greatly affect hospital utilization rates. In one study (Anderson, 1973), age represented the third most important influence on the use of short-term general hospitals; age was surpassed in importance only by economic factors (i.e., hospital insurance status and coverage, family income) and by a variable reflecting sex and marital status (see table 5.1).

—When hospitalized, older people tend to require a longer hospital stay than do younger patients with the same illness, thus increasing the demand for hospital beds. For example, patients over sixty-five years of age hospitalized for fractures stay an average of 27.5 days in short-term hospitals, while those under seventeen leave after about 5.4 days. Older patients with malignant neoplasms require an average of almost 17 hospital days; those between the ages of seventeen and forty-four stay only about 10 days (U.S. Department of Health, Educa-

TABLE 5.1
AGE DIFFERENTIALS IN HOSPITAL UTILIZATION:
1965, 1970, 1972

Age group	Discharges from short-stay hospitals per 1,000 population			Average length of stay (in days) in a short-term hospital			Days of care in short-term hospitals per 1,000 population
	1965	1970	1972	1965	1970	1972	1972
All Ages	153.4	146.2	154.9	7.8	8.0	7.7	1,199.9
Less than 15 years	77.0	68.0	73.7	5.3	4.9	4.5	329.5
15-44	176.5	156.1	156.0	5.9	5.8	5.7	886.8
45-64	174.0	161.7	177.2	9.8	9.6	9.3	1,642.7
65+	264.0	306.1	332.9	13.0	13.1	12.2	4,076.8

Source: U.S. Department of Health, Education, and Welfare (1967, pp. 9-10; 1973b, pp. 19-21; 1975a, p. 7).

tion, and Welfare, 1972b, p. 29). For all conditions requiring hospitalization, the average length of stay for older people is 12.6 days; for patients between fifteen and forty-four years of age, it is 5.7 days; and for those under fifteen it is only 4.7 days (U.S. Department of Health, Education, and Welfare, 1974a, p. 27).

—Following hospitalization, older people are more likely to require longer rehabilitation periods and more continuing medical care than younger people. Thus, even those older people who are eventually able to return home are more likely to need a stay in some sort of nursing home or extended care facility or to require home care.

—Many older people eventually become unable to care for themselves. Since they are less likely to be able to live with younger relatives than they were in earlier times, they must often end their days in some sort of nursing home. About fifty-five of every 1,000 persons over sixty-five are residents of nursing care and related homes, and 89 percent of the residents of such facilities are in this older age group (U.S. Department of Health, Education, and Welfare, 1973c). The growing number of elderly people, changes in disease patterns, and changes in family living arrangements will continue to increase the demand for the level of care provided by nursing homes.

—Older people suffer from different kinds of maladies and therefore require different kinds of medical care than do younger people. For example, older people are more likely to suffer from "chronic conditions," that is, medical problems which persist over a prolonged period, while younger people suffer more from "acute conditions," that is, infections, injuries, and the like, which usually can be cured in a relatively short time.

URBANIZATION

American society is becoming increasingly urbanized. More and more of its citizens are moving from the farms and small towns into metropolitan areas. In 1950 the percentage of the population living in urban areas was 64 percent; by 1970 this had increased to 73.5 percent (U.S. Department of Commerce, 1974).

The urbanization of American society is having its impact on the health care system, too (see table 5.2).

—Urban inhabitants are more susceptible to acute illness, particularly respiratory diseases. Presumably this is at least in part a reflection of the air pollution in our cities.

—On the other hand, fewer inhabitants of metropolitan areas have their activities limited by chronic conditions. This may possibly reflect the fact that people living in cities are more likely to be in sedentary occupations where physical problems can be less of a handicap than in manual jobs.

—People living on farms pay a visit to the doctor far less often than people living in metropolitan areas. This may in part be due to the lower incidence of

TABLE 5.2

DIFFERENTIAL IN THE DEMANDS PLACED ON THE HEALTH
CARE SYSTEM BY POPULATIONS IN METROPOLITAN
VERSUS NONMETROPOLITAN AREAS

Residence of population	Incidence of acute conditions per 100 persons per year (1972-73)	Age-adjusted percent of population with limitation of activity due to chronic conditions (1972)	Physician visits per person per year (1973)	Persons hospitalized per 1,000 persons per year (1968)
Metropolitan areas (SMSAs)	200.8*	12.2%	5.2	93
Nonmetropolitan areas				
Nonfarm	197.0	13.5	4.6	103
Farm	161.1	13.2	3.7	88

*The high incidence of acute conditions in metropolitan areas is due primarily to respiratory diseases.

Source: U.S. Department of Health, Education, and Welfare (1971, p. 4; 1975b, p. 5; 1973d, p. 3; 1974b, p. 6).

acute illnesses in rural areas, but an important factor is undoubtedly the shortage of doctors in many areas outside the big cities.

—A study in New Mexico found that hospital admission rates increase as urbanization occurs in a county. Much of the increased hospital usage appears to be the result of the increased availability of hospital services to urban dwellers. However, while hospitalization is low among people living on farms, the highest rate of hospitalization nationally occurs among people living in small towns (see table 5.2). The fact that hospital admission rates are even higher in small towns than in metropolitan areas may be due in part to the shortage of doctors in many small towns, for the New Mexico study indicated that, in areas where the physician-to-population ratio is low, inpatient hospital care is substituted for ambulatory care normally provided by physicians (Anderson, 1973, pp. 104-20).

—The fact that population continues to be drained from nonmetropolitan areas makes it difficult to attract doctors and to maintain occupancy levels in hospitals in such areas. The high rate of hospitalization in small towns may be due in part to the fact that hospitals there may not be too crowded, and doctors may admit patients more readily than in crowded urban hospitals. As the New Mexico study found, the supply of hospital beds (in relation to the size of the population) is a major determinant of utilization in an area.

OCCUPATIONAL PROFILE

The occupational profile of the American people has undergone consider-able change in recent years. The proportion of white-collar workers—professional, managerial, sales, and clerical—has risen from 37.5 percent of employed persons in 1950 to 48.8 percent in 1974. On the other hand, farm workers have declined from 12.4 percent of employed persons in 1950 to 3.6 percent in 1974. The percentage of people employed as blue-collar workers (craft workers, operators, and nonfarm laborers) dropped almost five percentage points between 1950 and 1974, while service workers increased somewhat (U.S. Department of Commerce, 1974).

These changes in the occupational profile of the population will affect health care institutions in two ways.

—Disease patterns will change somewhat. For example, there will be fewer industrial accidents as the proportion of the population employed in blue-collar jobs declines. On the other hand, there will be an increase in those maladies aggravated by the sedentary occupations pursued by a growing percentage of the population. For example, white-collar workers have a higher ratio of observed to expected cases of coronary heart disease than do blue-collar or agricultural workers. On the other hand, chronic conditions afflict only 3.7 percent of professional, technical, and kindred workers but 19.0 percent of farmers and farm managers (Wan, 1972).

—Attitudes toward health care will change. White-collar workers, particularly those employed in the professions and in managerial positions, tend to be better educated than blue-collar workers and are, therefore, more likely to be knowledgeable about, and demanding of, medical care. Thus, the growth in the size of the white-collar force will undoubtedly stimulate the need for sophisticated medical care.

EDUCATION

The population of the United States is becoming increasingly better educated. Only thirty-five years ago, the median number of school years completed was 8.6. Currently it is slightly over twelve years, for 60 percent of the population over age twenty-five has graduated from high school. The median number of school years completed is expected to continue rising as more and more people are going to college. Furthermore, those who do go to college are tending to get higher degrees. While the number of bachelor of arts degrees conferred annually rose 373 percent between 1940 and 1971, the number of doctorates rose 970 percent (U.S. Department of Commerce, 1974).

As the American public becomes better educated, it becomes more knowledgeable about medical care, more demanding of good care, less in awe of the medical profession, more inclined to view the hospital care system with a critical eye, and more articulate in expressing criticism and in pressing for reform. Levels of aspiration are rising in health care as elsewhere. This pattern of change will have several consequences for the health care system.

1. Better educated people generally make greater use of health services, for there is increased awareness of the value and importance of seeking prompt medical treatment.

—Physicians are visited more often by people with a high educational level. In 1966-67, there were 3.7 physician visits per person per year in families headed by someone with less than five years of education; but there were 5.0 physician visits per person per year in families headed by someone with thirteen years or more of education (Bice, Eichorn, and Fox, 1972).

—Not only general physician use but also use of preventive services are significantly higher for those with some education beyond high school than for others (Schweitzer, 1974, p. 39).

—Better educated women are more likely to visit a doctor during the first trimester of pregnancy (U.S. House of Representatives, 1974, p. 268).

—Education (and race) have over the years remained consistently related to the use of physician services, but studies show that relationships between income and use have diminished considerably over the past four decades (Bice, Eichorn, and Fox, 1972).

2. People with a higher educational level are more likely to carry hospital insurance. Among families under age sixty-five headed by someone with less than eight years of education, only 56.7 percent of the families carried hospital insurance in 1968; but when the head of the family had thirteen or more years of education, 89.5 percent of the families had hospital insurance (U.S. Department of Health, Education, and Welfare, 1972c, p. 5).

3. Education about health care (good nutrition, preventive care, etc.) is usually more successful among people with high educational attainments.

4. The increasing educational level of the population has stimulated the demand for technologically advanced methods of care and for higher apparent quality of care.

5. Health care institutions can expect increasing public examination and criticism of their operations and growing insistence that the public be given some voice in determining their policies. Steven Strickland's (1971) survey of a representative cross-section of the U.S. population, for example, indicated a public demand for a greater role for consumers in the administration of the health care system, especially at the local level.

6. Doctors will be subject to more criticism, especially about the efficacy and efficiency with which they provide medical care to the public. This is one reason for the rise in the malpractice suits in recent years.

AFFLUENCE

The population of the United States is enjoying rising affluence. Since World War II, the economy has generally flourished, enjoying a growth in the Gross National Product (GNP) of 353 percent between 1950 and 1973. To be sure, much of this increase was attributable to rising prices; but, even in constant 1958 dollars, the GNP increased 92 percent between 1950 and 1973. Because the GNP has grown more rapidly than the population, per capita disposable income has increased from $1,364 in 1950 to $4,195 in 1973, an increase of 208 percent. In constant 1958 dollars, the increase in per capita disposable personal income was 76 percent (U.S. Department of Commerce, 1974).

The rise in per capita income does not, of course, mean that poverty has been eliminated in the United States. However, the percentage of persons considered to be living below the poverty level was cut in half between 1959 and 1972. While 22.4 percent of the United States population was classified as below the "low income level" in 1959, this percentage had dropped to 11.9 percent in 1972 (U.S. Department of Commerce, 1974).*

The growing affluence of much of the population is changing the character of the demands on the U.S. health care system.

1. As incomes rise and as the percentage of the population living in poverty declines, some of the diseases associated with poverty, malnutrition, and unsanitary living conditions should diminish. The impact of poverty on health problems is dramatic (see table 5.3 and figure 5.4).†

—A poor child has half the chance of a more affluent child to live to his first birthday. The poor child's chances of contracting communicable diseases are far greater; for example, only half of all poor children are now immunized against polio. Poor children have five times more mental illness, seven times more visual impairment, six times more hearing defects, and three times more heart disease than their more affluent contemporaries (Congressional Record, 1974).

—Tuberculosis, venereal disease, heart disease, hypertension, arthritis, mental disease, visual impairment, and orthopedic disability are far more common among the poor (Greene, 1970; Herman, 1972).

—The poor are far more likely to have their activity impaired because of chronic health problems. Of those with a family income of less than

*The "low income level" is defined by the "poverty index" adopted by the Federal Interagency Committee in 1969 and updated each year to reflect changes in the Consumer Price Index.

†Of course, health problems can *create* poverty if they drain away a family's savings or make it difficult for wage earners in a family to work. So poverty and the associated health problems can be a vicious circle, with each feeding on the other.

TABLE 5.3
IMPACT OF INCOME ON NEED FOR HEALTH CARE: 1973

Family income level	Percent of population with limitation in major activity due to chronic conditions*	Number of short-stay hospital discharges per 100 persons per year	Average length of stay (in days) for discharges from short-stay hospitals
All family income levels	10.2%	13.9	8.1
Under $5,000	22.9	19.3	9.8
$5,000-$9,999	10.7	15.1	8.3
$10,000 and over	5.6	11.7	6.9

*Among these chronic conditions are such things as heart conditions, high blood pressure, arthritis and rheumatism, orthopedic impairments, visual impairments, and mental and nervous conditions. See figure 5.4.

Source: *Public Health Reports* (1974).

$5,000 a year, 22.9 percent have some limitation in major activity due to a chronic condition, while only 5.6 percent of those with an income of $10,000 or more are so handicapped.

—The poor are hospitalized far more often than more prosperous citizens. Among those with a family income of less than $5,000 a year, there were 19.3 discharges from a short-stay hospital per 100 persons in 1973, while the discharge rate was only 11.7 for those with incomes of $10,000 or more. The high rate of hospitalization among the poor is in part a reflection of their greater affliction with medical problems, but it is also a reflection of difficulty the poor encounter in getting preventive and ambulatory health services. One study showed, for example, that over a three-year period rheumatic fever in an urban area with comprehensive medical care was about a third lower than in comparable parts of the same city without such care (Gordis, 1973).

—When the poor are hospitalized, they generally require a longer stay in the hospital than those with a higher income. In 1973, the average length of stay for those with an income of less than $5,000 was 9.8 days, while the corresponding figure for those with an income of $10,000 or more was 6.9 days.

2. While rising incomes may alleviate some health problems associated with poverty, affluence is creating new health hazards. As we grow more prosperous, we tend to eat too much, drink too much, and exercise too little and, in consequence, to suffer from health problems that might be classified as "affluencia consumeritis syndrome" (Somers, 1971, p. 22). As Michael Halberstam (1969) wrote in the *New York Times*, "Our mortality figures reflect convincingly the fact that most Americans die of excess rather than neglect or poverty." One study found that while more education is associated with relatively low death rates, high income is associated with high mortality when education and medical care are held constant (Auster, Leveson, and Sarachek, 1969).

FIGURE 5.4
RELATIONSHIP BETWEEN FAMILY INCOME AND HEALTH PROBLEMS CAUSING ACTIVITY LIMITATION: JULY 1962-JUNE 1963

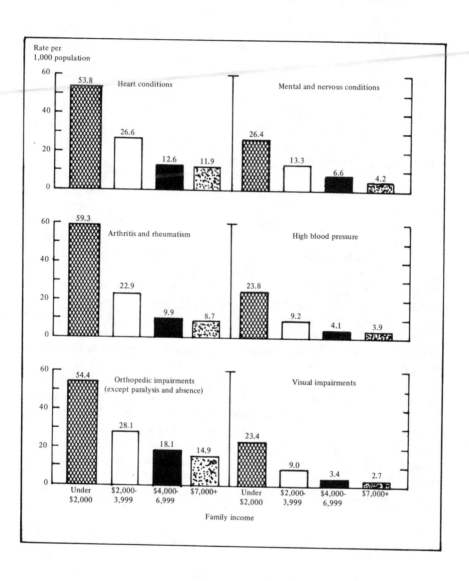

Source: U.S. Department of Health, Education, and Welfare (1964, p. 60).

3. Even though reducing the incidence of some medical problems, rising incomes stimulate demands on the health care system. The prosperous demand more and better health care than the poor. For sociological and psychological as well as financial reasons, the poor tend to seek less preventive care and less medical attention in the early stages of a disease.* In families with incomes of $10,000 or more, 76.5 percent of the children paid a visit to the doctor sometime in 1973; for families with incomes under $5,000 the percentage was only 65.6 percent (*Public Health Reports,* 1974). Of those with family incomes of $10,000 or more, 59 percent went to the dentist sometime in 1973, whereas only 32.8 percent did so from families with incomes under $5,000 (*Public Health Reports,* 1974). The poor are less likely to go to a doctor or dentist despite the fact that the poor tend to have greater health problems. And higher income people not only seek more medical attention, but they also tend to demand "better" and "more personal" care and thus are less likely to use a hospital emergency room or outpatient clinic.

4. Although rising incomes seem to stimulate the demand for health care, they may reduce the demand for hospital beds, for high income people generally require less hospitalization than those with low incomes (see table 5.3). There appear to be two reasons for this. In the first place, the poor tend to have more health problems. Secondly, poverty seems to be more of a barrier to ambulatory care than to hospital care, so the poor find it easier to get expensive hospital care than the simple care that might have made hospitalization unnecessary. If all financial barriers to health care were removed (by national health insurance, for example), the demand for ambulatory care is likely to rise more than the demand for hospital care (Newhouse, Phelps, and Schwartz, 1974).

5. From all the above, it is clear that the character of health problems and the nature of the demand for health care are affected by the socioeconomic status of the population served and thus can vary considerably from one area to another. And changes in the health status of the population can be affected as much by changes in its socioeconomic status as by changes in the medical care it receives. For example, deaths from tuberculosis dropped tenfold in Britain in the century before the first effective medical measures became available, and it is assumed that this dramatic drop was due largely to improved nutrition (Hiatt, 1975).

REDUCING INEQUITIES IN ACCESS TO HEALTH CARE

Heavier demands are being placed on the U.S. health care system not only because of the changing character of the population, but also because of accom-

---

*As indicated earlier, a study has shown that race and educational level remain consistently related to use of physician services, while the relationship between income and use have diminished over the past four decades (Bice, Eichorn, and Fox, 1972).

panying changes in our political and social values. With the growth of affluence has come a growing concern about the sizeable portion of the population still trapped in poverty.* "Equality of opportunity" is becoming a serious imperative, not just empty political rhetoric. A multitude of government programs have been instituted to translate this slogan into a reality, in voting rights, in education, in employment opportunities, and in access to health care.

Health care is increasingly regarded not as a privilege of the more prosperous, but as a right of all. And the government has assumed some responsibility for ensuring that right. Government monies have been poured into establishing neighborhood health centers, improving maternal and child health services, instituting programs to get doctors into underserved areas, and, above all, creating Medicaid and Medicare as a sort of government-supported health insurance for the medically indigent (Medicaid) and for the aged (Medicare). Let us look at how effective they have been in making it easier for the poor to obtain health care.

Hospital care is clearly more readily available to the poor today than it was a decade or so ago. As can be seen in table 5.4, hospitalization rates for low and high income people did not differ greatly in 1962-63 despite the fact that the poor are more likely to have health problems. By 1973, however, the poor were receiving substantially more hospital care than the more prosperous. During the intervening decade the hospitalization rate had increased only marginally for those with high incomes, while it had grown dramatically for those with low incomes, rising from about 13 to 19.3 hospital discharges per 100 persons per year, an increase of nearly 50 percent. Among low income people, hospitalization rates increased substantially for those in every age group; among high income people, hospitalization rates increased only slightly or even declined except for those over age sixty-five. Medicare would seem to have increased hospitalization among the elderly in all income groups, though much the biggest increase occurred among those with low incomes. The poor are receiving far more hospital care today than they did earlier, but it is not certain whether the increase has been large enough to meet the greater needs of the poor.

The poor would also appear to be getting more medical attention than they received earlier. In 1963, only 56 percent of those with low incomes had seen a physician during the year; by 1973 this figure had risen to nearly 74 percent. The percentage of those with high incomes who had seen a doctor during the year increased comparatively little during those years, and high income people actually had fewer physician visits per person per year in 1973 than they had

---

*It is interesting to note that during the 1974-75 recession, concern for the poor has tended to be deemphasized. The talk now is of providing health insurance for the unemployed, whose ranks include many from the middle classes. Proposals for national health insurance, which would extend insurance coverage to the poor and near poor, have dropped into the background for the time being, and Medicaid benefits for the poor are being reduced in many states.

TABLE 5.4

CHANGING DIFFERENTIALS IN MEDICAL CARE RECEIVED BY DIFFERENT INCOME GROUPS: SELECTED YEARS 1957-1973

Age and family income*	Number of physician visits per year per person		Percent seeing a physician during year			Discharges from short-stay hospitals per 100 persons per year		Percent seeing a dentist during year	
	July 1957-June 1959	1973	1963	1970	1973	July 1962-June 1963	1973	July 1957-June 1958	1973
All Ages									
All family incomes	5.0	5.0	65%	68%	74.5%	12.4	13.9	40%	48.9%
Low income	4.6	5.7	56	65	73.8	12.5	19.3	22	32.8
	4.6					13.2		31	
Middle income	5.1	4.8	64	67	72.9	13.0	15.1	44	40.8
High income	5.7	5.0	71	71	76.4	11.5	11.7	58	59.0
Under 17 years†									
All family incomes	4.6	4.2	NA	NA	73.0	6.5	7.0	NA	49.2
Low income	3.0	3.8	NA	51	65.6	4.8	9.5	13	31.3
	3.7					6.9		22	
Middle income	5.0	3.8	NA	62	70.0	6.8	7.1	36	37.6
High income	5.7	4.5	NA	73	76.5	6.6	6.2	54	59.7
17-44 years†									
All family incomes	4.8	5.0	NA	NA	76.2	15.5	15.6	NA	55.2
Low income	4.0	5.9	NA	NA	78.9	16.2	19.8	30	48.3
	4.5					17.5		38	
Middle income	4.9	4.8	NA	NA	75.3	16.8	18.2	48	47.4
High income	5.5	5.1	NA	NA	76.9	13.0	13.6	59	61.1

44-64 years									
All family incomes	5.4	5.5	NA	NA	72.6	13.9	16.6	NA	46.9
Low income	5.1	6.5	NA	NA	71.3	12.5	22.5	18	28.4
	5.4					13.3		25	
Middle income	5.4	5.6	NA	NA	70.5	15.6	17.9	33	38.1
High income	5.6	5.3	NA	NA	74.7	13.7	14.5	50	56.4
65+ years									
All family incomes	6.8	6.5	NA	NA	76.5	17.0	23.8	NA	27.3
Low income	6.5	6.6	NA	73	75.7	15.2	25.0	12	19.7
	6.6					16.5		17	
Middle income	6.9	6.5	NA	85	77.0	18.6	22.8	20	30.4
High income	8.7	7.1	NA	82	80.4	20.9	24.4	25	42.8

Note: NA = Not Available.

*Low income = Under $2,000 and $2,000-3,999 in 1957-59, 1957-58, and 1962-63; under $5,000 in 1973. Middle income = $4,000-6,999 in 1957-59, 1957-58, and 1962-63; $5,000 in 1973. High income = $5,000-9,999 in 1973. Income groups are not defined in 1963 and 1970.

†In 1957-59 and in 1962-63 two of the age groupings differed slightly from those given here; they were "under 15 years" (not "under 17 years") and "15-44 years" (not "17-44 years").

Sources: U.S. House of Representatives (1974, p. 263); U.S. Department of Health, Education, and Welfare (1964); *Public Health Reports* (1974).

in 1957-59. In every age group the number of physician visits per person declined for those with high incomes and rose for those with low incomes, with the biggest growth, surprisingly enough, occurring not among children or the elderly but among adults under the age of sixty-five. Low income adults under the age of sixty-five actually had more physician visits per year in 1973 than did their contemporaries with high incomes. *However, low income children and the aged poor even in 1973 were going to a doctor less often than those with high incomes and thus appear not to be getting as much medical attention as their greater health needs would warrant.* And the fact that only 65 percent of low income children saw a doctor during 1973 makes one wonder if these children are getting all the inoculations and other preventive care that modern medical practice recommends.

Inadequacies in the medical care received by the poor are not due solely to the financial barriers to care encountered by the poor. In some groups there are strong ethnic or cultural biases against professional medical services. The inner city ghetto resident may face a psychological barrier when he contemplates visiting an affluent white section of the city for a medical examination. Ignorance of where care can be obtained can be a problem in our scatter-site, atomistic, fee-for-service health care system (Schweitzer, 1974, pp. 34-51). And inner city ghettos and remote rural areas are generally inadequately supplied with doctors.

The improvement in the amount of dental care available to the poor has not been nearly so great as is the case with medical care or hospital care. Between 1957-58 and 1973 the percentage of the population that had seen a dentist some time during the year rose for all age groups—except for those in the middle income group. The increase in the percentage paying a visit to the dentist was greater for those with low incomes than for those with high incomes, but the gap between the two income groups remained substantial. Even in 1973 only 33 percent of those with a low income had paid a visit to the dentist during the year, while the figure for high income people was 59 percent. Poverty—or even a middle level income—would still appear to be a serious barrier to dental care. This is really not surprising since Medicare and Medicaid generally do not cover the ministrations of dentists, and even neighborhood health centers often do not make provision for dental care.

The current recession is creating pressures to economize on the various government programs to reduce inequities in access to health care. Presumably when the economy revives, these programs will again expand, and perhaps national health insurance will be instituted. *Whatever government programs are initiated or expanded will certainly increase the demands on the health care system, but the nature and the size of the increase will depend on the character and the thrust of the particular programs.* . . .

IMPACT OF SOCIAL CHANGES AND CHANGES IN LIFE STYLE

Social problems and changing mores have stimulated the growth of certain maladies:

—Drug addiction is clearly on the rise. The number of new narcotics addicts reported to the Drug Enforcement Administration by police authorities rose from 6,012 in 1965 to 24,692 in 1972. The total number of active addicts so reported on December 31, 1972 was 95,392, of which 90,494 were on heroin and 2,941 were on methadone (U.S. Department of Commerce, 1974). These numbers, of course, are simply the tip of the iceberg.

—Alcoholism is increasingly recognized as a serious problem, and along with the increase in alcoholism has come a rise in the death rate from cirrhosis of the liver from 9.2 per 100,000 population in 1950 to 15.7 per 100,000 in 1972. The death rate from cirrhosis of the liver varies greatly from state to state, ranging from 25.0 in Nevada and 24.3 in New York to 6.9 and 6.3 in Alabama and Mississippi (U.S. Department of Commerce, 1974). The consumption of alcohol also plays a role in automobile accidents, and heavy indulgence in alcohol, even among people not considered alcoholics, is increasingly thought to contribute to heart and circulatory problems and to do damage to the brain.

—Mental illness is growing. In 1955 there were 1,675,000 persons under treatment for such illnesses either in hospitals or through outpatient psychiatric services. By 1971 this figure had more than doubled to 4,038,000 (U.S. Department of Commerce, 1974). Some of this rise is simply attributable to the growing social acceptability of seeking psychiatric help: In the past people with problems tended to go to their friends or their ministers; today they are more likely to go to a mental health clinic or a psychiatrist. But obviously life in the United States today is creating a great deal of mental stress. Divorce rates have risen dramatically. Because of great mobility, people can no longer rely on extended families for psychological support. Women's new enthusiasm for careers may be creating some psychological problems for their children (and their husbands). The changing occupational profile of the country may also be playing a role in the increase in mental illness. A study of the statistics on disability insurance benefits awarded by the Social Security Administration in 1959-62 to men less than age sixty-five reveals that a much higher percentage of the awards made to accountants, auditors, and professional people were for mental illness as compared to the percentages of awards for such illnesses to people in various blue-collar occupations (*Public Health Service Bulletin* no. 1531).

—Deaths from suicide and homicide are rising. The suicide rate per 100,000 population declined from 11.4 in 1950 to 10.2 in 1955, but it has been rising steadily since then, reaching 11.7 in 1962. The suicide rate for white males between the ages of fifteen to twenty-four shot up from 6.6 per 100,000 population in 1950 to 13.9 in 1970; the figures for "Negro and other" males in this age group were 5.3 in 1950 and 11.3 in 1970. The suicide rate for white males rises steadily with age, but, for white males over forty-five, the suicide rate is lower today than it was in 1950. The suicide rate for females has risen somewhat since 1950 but has remained far below that of men. For both sexes and in every age group, the suicide rate is lower for "Negroes and others" than it is for "Whites" (U.S. Department of Commerce, 1974). The homicide trend in recent years is alarming: There was a decrease in the age-adjusted rate during the 1950s and then an increase of 84 percent between 1964 and 1973 (Klebba, 1975).

—The incidence of venereal diseases has reached epidemic proportions, at least in part because our changing sexual mores. Civilian cases of gonorrhea declined from 1945 to 1955, but since then they have more than tripled. The gonorrhea rate per 100,000 population jumped from 139.6 in 1960 to 420.1 in 1974. Syphilis cases among civilians declined steadily from 1945 to 1970 and have held fairly steady since then. However, the National Center for Disease Control indicates that the rate of primary and secondary syphilis per 100,000 population rose from 7.1 in 1960 to 11.9 in 1974, and these rates reflect only cases reported to the Center.*

—Heavy cigarette smoking is increasingly being indicated as a contributor to such health problems as lung cancer, heart diseases, peptic ulcers, and chronic sinusitis. It is at least partially responsible for the fact that the death rate for chronic respiratory diseases has grown faster than any other. The combined death rate from emphysema and chronic bronchitis among males rose from 12.6 per 100,000 population in 1960 to 21.4 per 100,000 in 1965 (*Health, Education, and Welfare Trends*). In 1970 the death rate from emphysema alone was 19.1 for males of all ages and 160.0 for men sixty-five and older (U.S. Department of Commerce, 1974).

—Cancer, second only to heart disease as the leading cause of death in this country, has continued to rise steadily. Between 1950 and 1969, the total increase in the age-adjusted death rate for cancer was 3.4 percent, reflecting rises in cancer-caused deaths among men but a decline in the death rate for women (Schmeck, 1974). The cancer rate without the age adjustment showed a more striking increase, growing from 149.2 per 100,000 population in 1960 to 166.6 in 1972 (U.S. Department of Commerce, 1974). Some of the rising incidence of cancer is due to the medical profession's success in preventing deaths from other diseases, which in an earlier era killed people off before they reached the cancer-prone years. Some of the increase in cancer, however, is due to our changing mode of life. Cigarette smoking, for example, certainly has increased the incidence of lung cancer and is one reason for the higher cancer death rate among men than among women. Some research indicates that our soft diet may play a role in the development of bowel cancer. Certain pollutants in the air and water, certain additives put in food, and even certain medications prescribed by doctors are thought to stimulate cancer. Some experts estimate that as much as 90 per-

*Figures supplied by the National Center for Disease Control in Atlanta, Ga.

cent of all cancer in this country is the result of environmental factors (Hiatt, 1975).

—The prevalence of major cardiovascular diseases in this country has grown significantly (heart diseases, high blood pressure, strokes, arteriosclerosis, etc.). In 1969, about 27 million Americans had major cardiovascular diseases (American Heart Association, 1971, p. 9), whereas just three years later the estimated prevalence of these diseases was 28.4 million (American Heart Association, 1974, p. 2). The growing prevalence of such problems is in part attributable to the fact that people are living longer. But it also appears to be related to our changing occupational profile, for white collar workers have a higher ratio of observed to expected cases of coronary heart disease than do blue-collar or agricultural workers (Wan, 1972). Our high speed, high pressure life style and our rich diet may also be playing a role in the rising incidence of cardiovascular diseases.

Despite the rising incidence of these diseases, the death rate from them is declining. The death rate from heart diseases did rise from 356.8 per 100,000 population in 1950 to 366.1 in 1969. However, if adjustments are made for the changing age distribution of the population, the age-adjusted death rate from heart disease fell 14 percent during those years, dropping from 307.6 in 1950 to 262.3 in 1969. "It is generally considered unlikely that changes in medical practice during the last few decades could account [for this drop] . . . . Even the current enthusiasm for exercise and dieting seems an inadequate explanation. Those have come too recently to affect the basic process responsible for most heart disease deaths. It is generally assumed that heart disease is a slow process, so that the death trends of the 1950s and 1960s would have to have their roots in factors that began to work at least five or ten years earlier" (Schmeck, 1974). Some crucial changes in our life style seem inexplicably to be lowering our heart disease death rate.

Even without age adjustment there has been a drop in the death rate for other major cardiovascular diseases, high blood pressure, strokes, and arteriosclerosis. The death rate for these diseases fell between 1950 and 1972 despite the growing size of our retirement-age population (U.S. Department of Commerce, 1974). Apparently the incidence of these diseases is growing—or at least, awareness of the maladies is increasing—while the death rate is declining for reasons the experts find mysterious.

—The death rate from accidents is lower today than it was in 1950, but the rate of injuries from accidents has climbed considerably since 1966 (see table 5.5). On the surface this would seem to indicate that the medical profession is doing a better job of treating those who are injured. However, many of the changes in accident rates are due to changes in our laws and mode of living, not to changes in health care. For example, the rate of injuries occurring on the job has fallen partly because of the diminishing proportion of our population in blue-collar jobs and partly because of higher safety standards being enforced in

TABLE 5.5
RATE OF INJURIES AND DEATH RATE FROM ACCIDENTS:
SELECTED YEARS 1950-1972

A. Injuries from accidents per 100 persons per year

Type of accident	1959-61	1962	1964	1966	1968	1970	1972
Total*	25.5	27.9	28.6	23.7	24.7	28.0	31.5
Moving motor vehicle	1.6	1.2	2.1	2.1	1.4	1.8	2.3
While at work		4.7	5.4	4.9	4.7	3.9	3.9
Home	23.9	12.7	13.5	9.5	11.9	10.8	11.8
Other		10.5	9.3	8.4	9.6	12.3	14.5

B. Deaths from Accidents per 100,000 Population per Year

Type of accident	1950	1955	1960	1965	1970	1972
Total	60.6	56.9	52.3	55.8	56.4	54.6
Motor vehicle accidents	23.1	23.4	21.3	25.4	26.9	27.2
All other accidents	37.5	33.5	31.0	30.4	29.5	27.4

*The sum of the rates for the four classes of accidents may be greater than the total because the classes are not exclusive.

Sources: U.S. House of Representatives (1974, p. 245); U.S. Department of Commerce (1974); *Health, Education, and Welfare Trends, 1966-67 Edition. Part 1: National Trends* (p. 22).

our factories and mines. Home injury rates have risen since 1966, presumably because of the growing array and increasing complexity of apparatus found in modern homes and perhaps also because of home owners' greater enthusiasm for doing home improvement projects themselves.

The death rate from automobile accidents—deaths per 100,000 population —has risen steadily since 1960, but the fatality rate—deaths per 100 million vehicle miles—dropped from 5.7 in 1966 to 4.2 in 1973, a decrease of 26 percent (Stevens, 1974). The incidence of disabling injuries from auto accidents has shown a similar decline. Many of these decreases, however, are due, not to improved medical care, but to better road signs, better law enforcement, driver training, and the like, which have steadily driven the fatality rate down since 1934. Lap and shoulder belts, combined, are shown in tests to reduce serious and fatal injuries by 50-60 percent, but study after study has shown that most people fail to use seat belts. Forcing people to use seat belts would presumably reduce the death rate from automobile accidents; but, when the interlock system was required in cars to compel the use of seat belts, at least 40 percent of drivers found ways of disconnecting or evading the system (Stevens, 1974). The gasoline shortage and the resultant lowering of speed limits reduced the automobile accident death rate, but prospects of a renewal of the gas shortage and/or a further escalation in gas prices are causing consumers to switch to smaller cars, which, most experts believe, are less safe than large ones because there is less safety room inside a compact. When Massachusetts lowered its drinking age to 18, the accident rate for teenage drivers shot up. The automobile accident rate is a dramatic example of the impact on the health status of factors that have nothing to do with the health care system—of factors as remote as the Arab oil embargo.

The above statistics on medical problems give some indication of how much the population's health is affected by elements outside the traditional province of the health professions. The physical environment, sanitation, diet, differences in occupations and in life styles, social customs, work regulations, the education provided by schools, abortion laws, FHA mortgages, television, speed limits, laws about alcohol consumption, the design of automobiles, the availability of public transportation, the condition of the economy, the Vietnam war—a multitude of factors have an impact on the health status of either the general population or certain segments of the population.

This is illustrated dramatically in figure 5.5, which shows the uneven distribution around the country of certain types of cancer. Bladder cancer mortality rates, for example, are particularly high in New Jersey, where a substantial number of people are employed in the chemical and allied industries. High rates of stomach cancer are found in North Dakota, Minnesota, Wisconsin, and Upper Michigan, where there is a concentration of people with ancestors from Austria, the Soviet Union, and Scandinavia, countries with higher stomach cancer rates than the United States. Interestingly enough, excessive deaths from lung cancer are not limited to densely populated urban areas where cigarette smoking and air pollution are creating health problems. Some of the highest death rates from lung cancer occur along the Gulf of Mexico, particularly in Louisiana. Not only cancer death rates but death rates from many ills vary greatly from state to state. The variations in the mortality and morbidity rates bear no clear relationship to differences in the delivery of health care in various parts of the country. Not even John Lindsay ever dubbed New York "health city" despite the unusually heavy concentration of physicians in that metropolis.*

Improving the health care system is not necessarily the most effective way of improving health. Sometimes a change in laws might have a more dramatic impact, though a change in the law that reduces one health problem may inadvertently create another. Regulations designed to reduce one form of pollution may cause increased emissions of other pollutants. Providing food stamps to the poor should in theory improve their diet and thus their health, but, if not

---

*The Canadian Government has concluded that "There is no evidence to suggest that the standard of health care is improved when the ratio of 1 [physician] to 600-650 [population] is exceeded," a ratio greatly exceeded in places like New York City. See Lalonde (1974, p. 29).

FIGURE 5.5
CANCER GEOGRAPHIC PATTERN
(1950-1969 by county for white men and women)

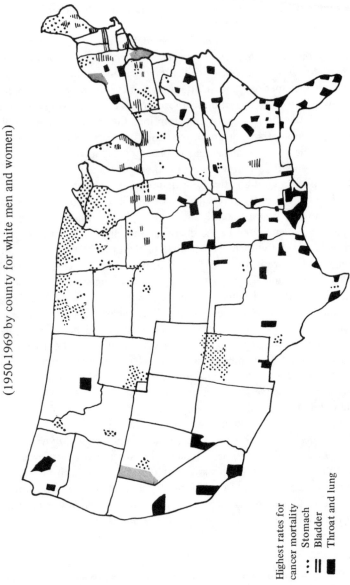

Highest rates for
cancer mortality
∴ Stomach
≣ Bladder
■ Throat and lung

Source: U.S. Department of Health, Education, and Welfare, National Institutes of Health, *Atlas of Cancer Mortality for U.S. Counties: 1950-1969* (Publication no. NIH 75-780).

coupled with education about nutrition, may simply increase the consumption of nutritionally undesirable foods such as potato chips and soft drinks.

There are also limits on what the government can legislate. A democracy cannot readily regulate people's life styles, to prevent them from indulging in practices deleterious to their own health. Our experience with Prohibition should make us cautious about enacting laws that run counter to the values and mores of a sizeable number of the population. Our regulations requiring the installation of seat belts have not been successful in getting people actually to use these safety devices. Behavioral scientists feel that "self-control procedures in which people change their own behavior to achieve long-range benefits are more likely to succeed [than governmental attempts] to modify behavior by simply trying to remove misused substances from the environment, as is demonstrated by the lack of success in legislating self-control by raising the price of cigarettes through taxation or by prohibiting the sale of alcoholic beverages" (Pomerleau, Bass, and Crown, 1975).

Another approach to controlling the nonmedical factors that affect health is the work of the Public Health Action Center to lower the nicotine content of cigarettes and to reduce other elements in the environment that appear to be harmful. The Public Health Action Center is part of the American Health Foundation, which is doing research to determine exactly which factors put people at risk of certain maladies and undertakes educational programs to warn people about these risk factors. However, educating people about health hazards is generally not too effective, as indicated by the seemingly limited impact of drug education programs in the schools. Television advertising on the dangers of cigarettes does not appear to have had any major effect on the nation's smoking habits: Domestic cigarette consumption in 1972 rose nearly 3 percent from the 1971 level (Bauer, 1974). One possible approach might be to increase health insurance premiums for those who smoke, drink heavily, etc., although this would create the problem of accurately determining people's habits. In sum, there are no easy answers to the problem of inducing people to change their life styles in the interest of improving their health. And life styles can have a greater impact on health than the health care system.*

IMPACT OF THE CHANGING AGE DISTRIBUTION OF THE POPULATION

Disease patterns in this country are also being affected by the trend toward an older population. As can be seen in figure 5.6, the incidence of heart conditions, hypertension, arthritis and rheumatism, and visual impairment rises steeply with age. The incidence of diabetes and malignant neoplasms (cancer) also rises with age but not so sharply. On the other hand, older people are less

*The Canadian government has become greatly concerned about the impact of life styles on health. See Lalonde (1974).

FIGURE 5.6
INCIDENCE OF SELECTED CHRONIC CONDITIONS CAUSING ACTIVITY LIMITATION BY AGE: 1972

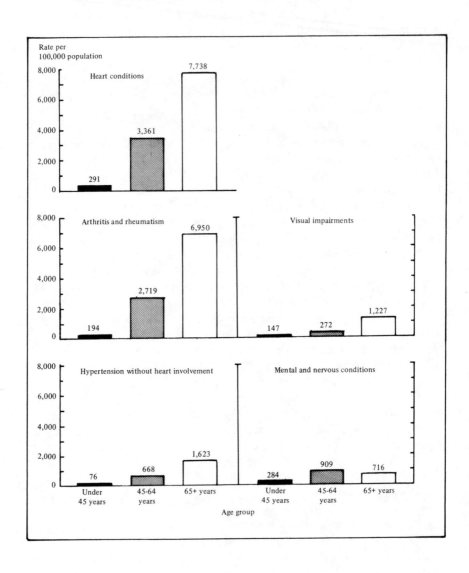

Source: U.S. Department of Commerce (1974).

susceptible to respiratory diseases, infective and parasitic maladies, problems with the digestive system, and injuries (see figure 5.7). Overall, older people are more likely to suffer from "chronic conditions," that is, medical problems which persist over a prolonged period, while younger people more often fall prey to "acute conditions," that is, infections and injuries, which usually can be cured in a relatively short time.

The different disease patterns of the different age groups has a marked effect on the character and the size of their demand for hospital care. Older people tend to be hospitalized for quite different maladies than young people. When the Commission on Professional and Hospital Activities studied the fifty most common diagnoses of patients discharged from hospitals, striking differences were found between patients sixty-five and over as compared with younger patients. The rates of discharges per 10,000 patients were far higher for patients over sixty-five for the following diagnoses: heart diseases, cerebrovascular diseases, hypertensive diseases, cataracts, arthritis and rheumatism, prostate diseases, and diseases of the intestine and peritoneum (except appendix and hernia). On the other hand, patients under sixty-five had far higher discharge rates for the following diagnoses: hypertrophy of tonsils and adenoids, acute appendicitis, upper respiratory infections, diseases of the teeth and jaws, injuries, neuroses, and personality and other nonpsychotic mental disorders. Younger patients, of course, also had far higher discharge rates for such things as abortions, diseases of the female genitalia, etc.

The maladies for which the elderly are hospitalized tend to be ones requiring a lengthier hospital stay than is necessary with such problems of the young as appendicitis or upper respiratory conditions. Even when the diagnosis is the same, the elderly generally spend more days in the hospital. When a person over sixty-five is hospitalized for an infective or parasitic disease, his average length of stay is 17.2 days, while the average length of stay for all patients with this diagnosis is 8.9 days. When an older person is hospitalized for a fracture or dislocation, his average length of stay is 27.5 days; the average length of stay for all patients with this problem is 15.7 days.

All of this means, of course, that the demand for medical care and particularly for hospital care is very much affected by the age distribution of the population in the area. An area with a large number of young families may need a sizeable obstetric unit and good facilities for treating accident victims. An area with a goodly proportion of elderly people will need more hospital beds, particularly in its coronary care unit and in its units treating cancer, strokes, and diabetes. *A sophisticated analysis of the hospital beds needed in a given area requires a projection not only of the overall population size but also of the age distribution of the population and even of its socioeconomic status.* Some weight, too, should be given factors in the environment likely to affect the demand for hospital care, such as air pollution and the traffic accident rate.

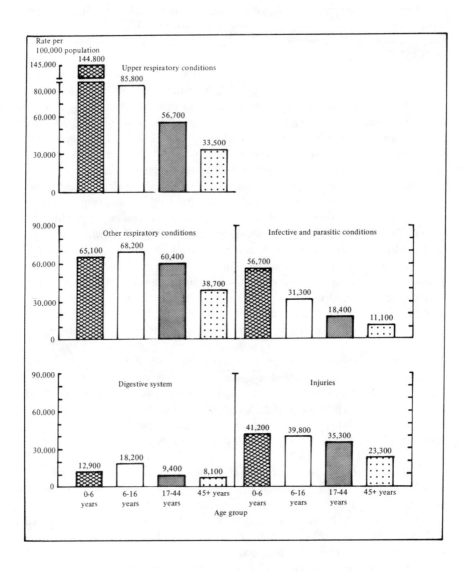

FIGURE 5.7
INCIDENCE OF SELECTED ACUTE CONDITIONS BY AGE: 1972

Source: U.S. Department of Health, Education, and Welfare (1973a, p. 9).

REFERENCES

American Heart Association. *Heart Facts 1972.* New York: American Heart Association, 1971.

American Heart Association. *Heart Facts 1975.* New York: American Heart Association, 1974.

Anderson, J. G. "Demographic Factors Affecting Health Service Utilization: A Causal Model." *Medical Care* (March/April 1973): 107.

Auster, R.; Leveson, I.; and Sarachek, D. "The Production of Health, an Exploratory Study." *Journal of Human Resources* (Fall 1969): 430.

Barnett, M. "Legalized Abortion Credited with Some Health Advances." *Hospital Tribune* (February 11, 1974).

Bauer, K. "Averting the Self-Inflicted Nemeses (Sins) from Dangerous Driving, Smoking, and Drinking." *Consumer Incentives for Health Care,* edited by S. Mushkin. New York: Milbank Memorial Fund, 1974.

Bice, T.; Eichorn, R.; and Fox, P. "Socioeconomic Status and Use of Physician Services: A Reconsideration." *Medical Care* (May/June 1972): 262-66.

Chase, H. (ed.). "A Study of Risks, Medical Care, and Infant Mortality." *American Journal of Public Health* (September 1973 Supplement).

Congressional Record (July 16, 1974). "HEW's Child Health Failure." Quoted in *Medical Care Review* (September 1974): 825.

Gold, E. "Public Health Aspects of Future OB-GYN Services." *Obstetrics and Gynecology* (March 1973): 462.

Gordis, L. "Effectiveness of Comprehensive-Care Programs in Preventing Rheumatic Fever." *New England Journal of Medicine* 289 (1973): 331-35.

Greene, C. "Medical Care for Underprivileged Populations." *New England Journal of Medicine* (May 21, 1970): 1187.

Halberstam, M. "The MD Should Not Try to Cure Society." *New York Times Magazine* (November 9, 1969): 62.

Herman, M. "The Poor: Their Medical Needs and the Health Services Supplied Them." *Annals of the American Academy of Political and Social Science* (January 1972): 12-21.

Hiatt, H. H. "Protecting the Medical Commons: Who Is Responsible?" *New England Journal of Medicine* (July 31, 1975): 238.

Jaffe, F. S. "Low Income Families: Fertility Changes in the 1960's." *Family Planning Perspectives* (January 1972).

Klebba, J. "Homicide Trends in the United States, 1900-1974." *Public Health Reports* (May/June 1975): 197.

Lalonde, M. *A New Perspective on the Health of Canadians.* Ottawa: Government of Canada, 1974.

New York Times. "Birth, Fertility Rates at a New Low in U.S." (April 16, 1974, p. 1).

New York Times. "In 1974, the Birth Rate Moved Up" (March 16, 1975, section 4, p. 5).

Newhouse, J.; Phelps, C.; and Schwartz, W. *Policy Options and the Impact of National Health Insurance.* Santa Monica, Calif.: Rand, 1974.

Pomerleau, O.; Bass, F.; and Crown, V. "Role of Behavior Modification in Preventive Medicine." *New England Journal of Medicine* (June 12, 1975): 1278.

Public Health Reports. "Profile of American Health, 1973: Based on Data Collected in the Health Interview Survey" (November/December 1974, pp. 504-24).

Schmeck, H. "Declines in Deaths from Nine Leading Diseases Show a Surprising Trend." *New York Times* (May 6, 1974): 16.

Schweitzer, S. "Incentives and the Consumption of Preventive Health Care Services." *Consumer Incentives for Health Care,* edited by S. Mushkin. New York: Milbank Memorial Fund, 1974.

Somers, A. *Health Care in Transition: Directions for the Future.* Chicago: Hospital Research and Educational Trust, 1971.

Stevens, W. "S.N. (Since Nader), Cars Are Safer, But . . . ." *New York Times* (March 24, 1974, p. E-9).

Strickland, S. "U.S. Health Care: What's Wrong and What's Right." National poll commissioned by Potomac Associates (October 1971).

U.S. Department of Commerce. Bureau of the Census. *Statistical Abstract of the United States, 1974.* Washington, D.C.: Government Printing Office, 1974.

U.S. Department of Health, Education, and Welfare. *Medical Care, Health Status, and Family Income: United States* (Public Health Service Publication no. 1000, Series 10). Washington, D.C.: HEW, 1964).

U.S. Department of Health, Education, and Welfare. National Center for Health Statistics. *Utilization of Short-Stay Hospitals: Summary of Nonmedical Statistics, United States, 1965* (Public Health Service Publication no. 1000, Series 13). Washington, D.C.: HEW, 1967.

U.S. Department of Health, Education, and Welfare. Public Health Service. *Persons Hospitalized by Number of Hospital Episodes and Days in a Year, United States, 1968* (Publication no. HSM 72-1029). Rockville, Md.: HEW, 1971.

U.S. Department of Health, Education, and Welfare. National Center for Health Statistics. *Infant Mortality Rates: Socioeconomic Factors, United States* (Publication no. HSM 72-1045). Rockville, Md.: HEW, 1972a.

U.S. Department of Health, Education, and Welfare. National Center for Health Statistics. *Age Patterns in Medical Care, Illness and Disability, United States, 1968-1969* (Publication no. HSM 72-1026). Washington, D.C.: HEW, 1972b.

U.S. Department of Health, Education, and Welfare. National Center for Health Statistics. *Hospital and Surgical Insurance Coverage, United States, 1968* (Publication no. HSM 72-1033). Rockville, Md.: HEW, 1972c.

U.S. Department of Health, Education, and Welfare. National Center for Health Statistics. *Current Estimates from the Health Interview Survey, United States, 1972* (Publication no. HRA 74-1512). Rockville, Md.: HEW, 1973a.

U.S. Department of Health, Education, and Welfare. *Utilization of Short-Stay Hospitals: Summary of Nonmedical Statistics, United States, 1970* (Publication no. HRA 74-1765). Rockville, Md.: HEW, 1973b.

U.S. Department of Health, Education, and Welfare. National Center for Health Statistics. *Characteristics of Residents in Nursing and Personal Care Homes, United States, June-August 1969* (Publication no. HSM 73-1704). Rockville, Md.: HEW, 1973c.

U.S. Department of Health, Education, and Welfare. *Acute Conditions: Incidence and Associated Disability, United States, July 1972-June 1973* (Publication no. HRA 75-1525). Rockville, Md.: HEW, 1973d.

U.S. Department of Health, Education, and Welfare. National Center for Health Statistics. *Utilization of Short-Stay Hospitals: Summary of Nonmedical Statistics, United States, 1972* (Publication no. HRA 75-1768). Washington, D.C.: HEW, 1974a.

U.S. Department of Health, Education, and Welfare. *Limitation of Activity and Mobility Due to Chronic Conditions, United States, 1972* (Publication no. HRA 75-1523). Rockville, Md.: HEW, 1974b.

U.S. Department of Health, Education, and Welfare. *Utilization of Short-Stay Hospitals: Summary of Nonmedical Statistics, United States, 1972* (Publication no. HRA 75-1770). Rockville, Md.: HEW, 1975a.

U.S. Department of Health, Education, and Welfare. *Physician Visits: Volume and Interval Since Last Visit, United States, 1971* (Publication no. HRA 75-1524). Rockville, Md.: HEW, 1975b.

U.S. House of Representatives. Committee on Ways and Means. *National Health Insurance Resource Book.* Washington, D.C.: Government Printing Office, 1974.

Wan, T. "Social Differentials in Selected Work-Limiting Chronic Conditions." *Journal of Chronic Diseases* (1972): 365-74.

6

Rising Public Expenditures

Selection by the Executive Office of the President

INTRODUCTION

During 1975, price increases for health services outpaced increases in the overall economy by a substantial margin. Prices for medical care services jumped by 10.3 percent during the year, substantially higher than the 7.7 percent increase in the prices of other services. While hospital charges showed the largest increases, physician fees also rose at rapid rates. In addition, drug prices climbed in 1975 at rates unprecedented for that industry.

The Council on Wage and Price Stability has the statutory responsibility to monitor and analyze inflationary developments in individual sectors of the economy. The substantial rates of inflation the nation has experienced in the health care sector have had serious repercussions throughout the economy. In the twelve months ending June 1975, the United States spent $118.5 billion for health care, up 13.9 percent from the previous year. Health expenditures accounted for 8.3 percent of the nation's Gross National Product, the highest level in history, compared to 5.9 percent ten years ago—an increase of 41 percent in one decade. Federal outlays for health now comprise 11.3 percent of the federal budget; only national defense, interest on the national debt, and income security programs have a larger share. Steadily increasing portions of employer labor expenses are absorbed by increasing health insurance premiums for employees rather than actual wage payments as both premium rates and benefit levels con-

Reprinted from "The Problem of Rising Health Care Costs" (Washington, D.C.: Executive Office of the President, Council on Wage and Price Stability, 1976).

tinue to rise. Despite the growth of public health programs and private health insurance, direct payments for health care by individuals continue to rise.

This report will attempt to document the extent of inflation in this sector and assess its impact upon the individual household, labor, industry, and government. It will also review possible explanations for the unusual behavior of prices in this sector, including the unique structural characteristics of the industry and how they may have contributed to these rapid increases. These include the prevalence of third party payments; the peculiarities of public and private health insurance financing; the high levels of government support; the key decision-making role of the physician; the incentive structure in the industry; and rapid but costly technological change. The impact of the controls period of 1971 through 1974, of the high rates of inflation in other sectors in 1974 upon the medical care sector, and of changes in the nature and overall quality of medical care are also considered.

Double-digit inflation is but one of several problems troubling the existing health care delivery and financing system. Many of the poor, aged, and those living in rural areas still do not receive, or cannot afford, adequate medical attention. Catastrophic medical expenses continue to strike numerous households every year, and are a constant concern for all. While this report focuses on the problem of inflation, these other problems are close related. Finally, in reviewing this report, the reader should note that some increases in prices for health care reflect improvements in the quality of service as well as "pure" price increases. As with any service, it is extremely difficult to assess whether changes in medical care techniques constitute improvements in quality of the service and thus to separate out these two factors.

I. WHAT IS THE PROBLEM?

How Rapidly Have Health Care Costs Been Rising?

Whether stated in terms of total expenditures or in terms of various price and cost measures, the increase in what the nation has paid for health care is remarkable.

Rising expenditures

At the $118.5 billion level recorded for fiscal year 1975, health care expenditures have increased almost tenfold since 1950 ($12 billion) and have tripled since 1965 ($39 billion), the year before Medicare and Medicaid were introduced. In the 1970s alone, expenditures have increased $49 billion, or an average of almost $10 billion per year. The increase from 1974 to 1975 of $14.5 billion was the largest the nation has ever experienced. These increases reflect a combination of increases in price, population growth, increases in utilization of medical services, and quality improvements.

Table 6.1 illustrates that while expenditures under federal health programs

TABLE 6.1
PER CAPITA EXPENDITURES FOR PERSONAL HEALTH CARE

	1965	1975	Percent increase 1965-1975
Direct payments	$89.37	$155.10	73.5%
Private insurance benefits	42.10	126.21	199.8
Federal	14.44	131.92	813.6
State and local	20.94	56.99	172.2

Source: U.S. Department of Health, Education, and Welfare, Social Security Administration.

have shown the most remarkable increase in the past decade, private health insurance benefits and direct payments by individuals, as well as state and local health expenditures, have also continued to grow.

Despite the enormous growth in public and private insurance benefits, direct payments by individuals have also increased from $89.37 to $155.10 annually over the decade. Direct payments, while declining from 52.5 percent to 32.6 percent of spending for personal health care during the decade, remain the largest single component of personal health care spending.

Rising prices

The prices charged for medical care increased much faster during 1975 than prices for other consumer goods and services, as table 6.2 illustrates.

The 9.9 percent increase registered in the medical care sector is substantially higher than the 6.8 percent increase for the rest of the economy. This increase was spread throughout the sector.

Hospitals: The increase in hospital service charges was both the largest (13.0 percent) and the most significant, since expenditures for hospital care comprise almost 40 percent of all health spending. Among hospital services, the most substantial increases were for semiprivate room charges (14.7 percent) and for operating room charges (13.8 percent). Revenue per adjusted patient day, an alternate measure compiled by the American Hospital Association, showed an even sharper increase in 1975, 18.4 percent.

Physician fees: The overall increase in physician fees (11.8 percent) was substantially higher than that for services in other sectors (7.7 percent). The largest price increases were registered for general office visits (12.0 percent) and for obstetrical cases (13.9 percent).

Drugs and prescriptions: The rate of price increases here (7.4 percent), though not excessive relative to the rest of the economy, is highly unusual since, even before price controls were imposed from 1971 through 1974, drug and prescription prices had rarely increased more than 1 percent annually. From 1966 to 1971, drug and prescription prices inched up 1.0 percent annually while the

TABLE 6.2
HEALTH CARE PRICE INCREASES: 1975*

	Percentage change 12/74-12/75	Percentage of total health care spending
CPI, all items	7.0%	
(less medical care)	6.8	
CPI, all services	8.1	
(less medical care)	7.7	
CPI, medical care services	10.3	
Hospital service charges	13.0	39.3%
Physician fees	11.8	18.6
Dentist fees	7.8	6.3
Drugs and prescriptions	7.4	8.9
CPI, medical care, total	9.9	

*The Consumer Price Index for Medical Care and its various components have frequently been criticized as not adequately accounting for changes in quality and product mix; to the extent they understate these changes, they may overstate true price increases. Similar problems are encountered in measuring price changes for other services. The Council staff recognizes these shortcomings, and plans to work in the future with appropriate government agencies and the medical care sector to improve the measures of medical care prices.

Source: U.S. Department of Labor, Bureau of Labor Statistics; U.S. Department of Health, Education and Welfare, Social Security Administration.

overall consumer price index rose at a 4.5 percent annual rate (see table 6.4 and figure 6.1).

Rising outlays for treatment

The impact of these trends upon the consumer is reflected in the substantial increases in expenses for the average hospital stay, as measured by the American Hospital Association. In 1965, the average expense per stay was $311; by 1974, this had almost tripled to $873. The average expense per stay in 1975 was $1017, an increase of 16 percent from the 1974 average. This increase is all the more remarkable since the average length of hospital stays declined steadily from 1969 through 1974; thus, the average expense per day in the hospital has actually risen more rapidly.

Similarly, the price of going to see one's physician has escalated rapidly. The average fee for an initial office visit, as measured by the American Medical Association, increased from $12.80 in 1969 to $19.55 in 1974, an increase of 53 percent, even though price controls were in effect for much of that period (Eisenberg, 1976).

Another measure of the impact of rising health care costs on the consumer is the average aggregate cost of treatment for particular illnesses—including hospital charges, physician fees, and other expenditures—taking into account changes in techniques for diagnosis and treatment over time. One recent study, based upon actual case records, shows substantial increases in the period from 1964 to 1971 (Scitovsky and McCall, 1975). The most remarkable increase was for treatment of heart attacks, from $1449 in 1964 to $3280 in 1971, an increase of 126 percent. Other sizeable increases were noted for breast cancer treatment, from $1559 to $2557 (64 percent); maternity care, from $527 to $807 (53 percent); and for simple appendicitis, from $592 to $1063 (80 percent). This study did not attempt to measure whether these increases in the cost of treatment resulted in better quality care.

Have Health Prices Been Increasing Faster Than Other Consumer Prices?

The importance of rising prices in this sector as an issue deserving public attention is all the more apparent when compared to other sectors where inflation has been perceived to be a significant problem. As noted above, the rate of increase in health prices in 1975 outpaced that for other consumer prices in general. But as table 6.3 illustrates, it has also exceeded the rate for other important consumer goods and services.

TABLE 6.3
COMPARATIVE RATES OF PRICE INCREASE: 1975

	Percentage change 12/74-12/75
Hospital service charges	13.0%
Physician fees	11.8
Food	6.5
Home ownership	7.9
Rent	5.2
Fuel and utilities	11.2
New cars	7.3
Used cars	8.1
Gasoline and motor oil	10.5
All services (other than medical)	7.7
Dry cleaning	7.6
Domestic services	5.4
Auto repairs	9.3
Recreational services	3.5
Personal care services	6.4

Source: U.S. Department of Labor, Bureau of Labor Statistics.

Only increases in energy-related prices have approached the rate of increase for hospital and physician services. The rates of price increase for food, home ownership and rental expenses, new and used cars, and for other consumer services have been lower. That the much more rapid increases in hospital and physician prices have until recently received less public attention than smaller increases in other sectors may reflect the hidden nature of health care spending. The individual often does not purchase health care with the same attitudes or through the same mechanisms as he buys other goods and services. These differences, to be reviewed later in this report, obscure the impact of rising health care prices on the household budget.

How Long Has This Been Going On?

An inflation rate significantly higher than that prevalent in the rest of the economy has been characteristic of the health sector for several years, as table 6.4 illustrates. As can be seen from table 6.4, price increases in this sector

TABLE 6.4
ANNUAL RATES OF PRICE INCREASE

	Pre-Medicare 7/59-6/66	Post-Medicare 6/66-6/71	Controls 8/71-4/74	1974 Post-controls 4/74-12/74	1975 12/74-12/75
CPI, all services					
(less medical care)	2.0%	5.8%	5.2%	9.5%	7.7%
CPI, medical care services	3.2	7.9	4.9	12.1	10.3
Hospital service					
charges	n.a.	n.a.	4.6	14.6	13.0
Semiprivate room					
charge	6.0	14.8	5.7	16.9	14.7
Physician fees	2.9	6.9	4.0	12.8	11.8
Dentist fees	2.3	5.9	4.2	9.6	7.8
Drugs and prescriptions	−0.7	1.0	0.7	7.8	7.4

Source: U.S. Department of Labor, Bureau of Labor Statistics.

jumped significantly with the introduction of Medicare and Medicaid in 1966. Medical care services prices rose at a 7.9 percent annual rate from 1966 to 1971, compared to a 3.2 annual rate for the prior six-year period. However, even before 1966, health care prices were increasing substantially faster than other consumer prices suggesting that forces were already operating to cause a relatively rapid rate of price increase in this sector. This trend was particularly noticeable for hospital charges: semiprivate room charges, for example, rose 6.0 percent annually from 1959 to 1966 while service prices outside the medical sector were increasing 2.0 percent annually.

From August 1971 to April 1974, when various forms of mandatory economic controls were in effect for the health sector, health care prices rose more slowly than other prices. Since controls ended in April 1974, health care prices have again risen more rapidly than other prices—and at faster rates than ever before, hovering in the double digit range throughout the period. In addition, substantial price increases are now spread throughout the sector: while previously most concern was focused on hospital charges, physician fees and drug prices have also been escalating at unprecedented rates since the end of controls (see figure 6.1).

FIGURE 6.1
ANNUAL RATES OF PRICE CHANGE, 1965-1975

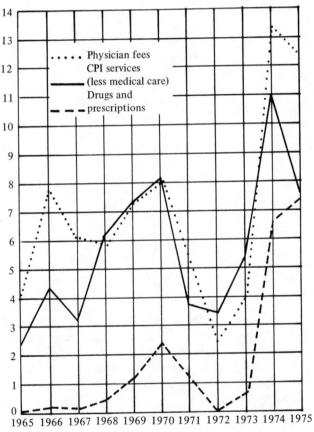

Source: U.S. Department of Labor, Bureau of Labor Statistics.

Summary

Health care prices have been increasing much faster than other prices in our economy. As figure 6.2 illustrates, price increases for medical care services

FIGURE 6.2
RELATIVE PRICE CHANGES, 1965-1975

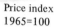

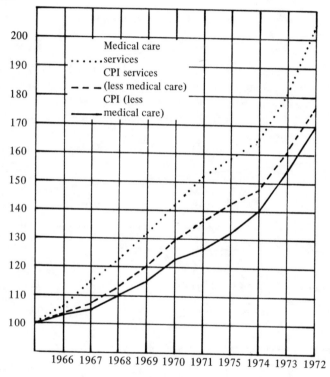

Source: U.S. Department of Labor, Bureau of Labor Statistics.

over the past decade have significantly outpaced increases in other consumer prices. This disparity has been accelerating rapidly in the past year. The 8.3 percent of our Gross National Product now devoted to health care is unprecedented. Continued growth in health care spending is expected: the Department of Health, Education, and Welfare estimates that by 1990, 10 to 12 percent of our Gross National Product will be spent for health care.

In part this growth in health care prices and spending reflects changes in the mix and level of services provided. To the extent these changes constitute improvements in the quality or delivery of care, price increases would not be "inflationary" in a technical sense. However, whether such a change is a quality improvement is particularly difficult to evaluate. As a result, there is considerable debate whether the overall quality and delivery of the medical care received by the American people has improved in step with the rapid rises in expenditures and prices. This question is integral to an understanding of the behavior of prices in this sector.

II. IS THERE A SIMPLE EXPLANATION?

The Bulge: Are We Still in It?

As table 6.5 indicates, the rate of increase in health care service prices escalated rapidly after mandatory controls expired in April 1974: starting from an average annual rate of 4.9 percent during the controls period, medical care price increases rose at an annual rate of 16.6 percent in the third quarter (July through September) of 1974. During that period hospital service charges rose at a 20.0 percent annual rate and physician fees at a 15.8 percent annual rate.

TABLE 6.5
ANNUALIZED RATES OF PRICE INCREASE: POST-CONTROLS

	1974:3	1974:4	1975:1	1975:2	1975:3	1975:4
CPI, all services (less medical care services)	13.1%	11.3%	6.7%	5.8%	8.1%	10.5%
Medical care services*	16.6	11.4	14.5	9.2	10.5	7.2
Hospital service charges	20.0	14.2	19.1	8.7	13.8	10.7
Physician fees	15.8	9.6	14.5	9.5	10.1	13.1

*Seasonally adjusted.
Source: U.S. Department of Labor, Bureau of Labor Statistics.

Then during the last quarter in 1974, the so-called catch-up period seemed to be over, with medical service prices rising at approximately the same rate as other services. However, the first quarter in 1975 saw another dramatic increase to 14.5 percent annually, while inflationary pressures in the rest of the economy seemed to be abating. Medical care price increases slowed somewhat in the balance of 1975; however, rates of increase for hospital service charges and for physicians fees remained in the double-digit range, exceeding rates for other services.

While a "bulge" would account for the rapid escalation of prices in the third quarter of 1974, it is not particularly helpful in explaining subsequent developments. Furthermore, we have noted previously that price increases higher than those in the rest of the economy were characteristic of the health sector long before the controls period, suggesting that other factors peculiar to this industry are at play.

Are Provider's Expenses Growing Rapidly?

Another possible explanation for the relatively high price increases in the health sector would be unusually high rates of increase in wages and prices of nonlabor inputs peculiar to this industry. Through 1973, this does not appear to have been the case. A review of increases in hospital costs by the Social Security Administration indicates that, through 1973, while wages and prices paid by hospitals have been increasing, such increases only account for approximately half of the increase in total costs. The balance can be attributed to expenditures for changes in type and level of service provided, which have increased the amount of labor and nonlabor inputs used per day of care and per patient.

TABLE 6.6
RELATIVE CONTRIBUTION OF WAGE AND PRICE INCREASES
AND RELATED FACTOR USE TO RISING HOSPITAL COSTS,
1951-1973

	1951-60	1960-65	1965-67	1967-69	1969-71	1971-73
Average annual increase in average expense per patient day	7.5%	6.7%	10.3%	13.8%	14.8%	11.5%
Portion of increase due to:						
Increases in wages and prices of nonlabor inputs	50.0%	51.5%	39.7%	58.2%	55.3%	51.3%
Increased use of labor and non-labor inputs	50.0%	48.5%	60.3%	41.8%	44.7%	48.7%

Source: U.S. Department of Health, Education, and Welfare, Social Security Administration, *Medical Care Expenditures, Prices and Costs: Background Book* (September 1975, p. 39).

The same review showed that the most rapidly growing component of costs has been expenditures for additional equipment and supplies, which grew at approximately 10 percent annually from 1965 through 1973. Economists at the Brookings Institution and Harvard University who have studied hospital cost increases have reached similar conclusions, i.e., that increased wages and prices are only a partial explanation of increases in hospital costs and that increased expenditures for new equipment and supplies are a crucial factor (Davis, 1974; Feldstein, 1971).

However, preliminary data for 1974 and 1975 on hospital costs provided by the American Hospital Association indicate that, while real inputs continue to rise rapidly, the relative contribution of increased input prices to rising costs has grown dramatically. Increases in input prices accounted for 73.1 percent of rising hospital costs in 1974 and 73.3 percent in the first six months of 1975, far exceeding the historical pattern. A breakdown of the 1975 data by the American Hospital Association indicates that price increases for nonlabor inputs are the key driving factor, accounting for 44.8 percent of hospital cost increases in the first six months of 1975. This reflects primarily the impact of the high general rate of inflation in 1974 upon input prices, particularly in the energy area and increases in malpractice premiums. The potential impact of this latter development (malpractice premium increases) upon hospital charges is of serious concern; however, adequate data to assess this impact are not yet available.

Research on physician charges, while not as extensive and based upon less comprehensive data, indicates a similar conclusion to that reached for hospitals, i.e., that increased use of real inputs, including laboratory tests, X-rays, support personnel, and the like is a prime determinant of increased expenditures (Worthington, 1975). Substantial increases in malpractice premiums in 1975 and 1976 are likely to have an impact upon fees, but it is still too early to quantify this impact.

There is a need for further research and analysis of the components of increases in medical costs and their relative contribution to inflation in the sector. The long-term trend towards additions to equipment and supplies and the impact of recent developments such as higher labor costs resulting from expanded minimum wage laws and collective bargaining, increased malpractice insurance premiums, and higher energy costs all deserve special attention. However, a full understanding of the long-standing inflation in this sector also requires analysis of the inflationary pressures generated by the unusual structural characteristics of the mechanisms through which consumers demand and suppliers provide health care.

Summary

Can rapidly rising health care costs be explained as a "bulge" effect following the controls period of the early 1970s, or as a result of sharp increases in factor costs unique to this industry? While these explanations account for some of the rise in health care costs, they cannot fully account for the long-standing inflation in this sector or its recent acceleration.

III. WHAT IS UNIQUE ABOUT THE STRUCTURE OF THIS SECTOR TO HAVE CAUSED COSTS TO GO UP SO RAPIDLY?

Third-Party Payment

The purchase of health care services typically differs from the usual consumer transaction where the consumer pays directly to the provider the price for the goods or services received. Instead, the health care sector is characterized by a system of third-party payments to providers on behalf of consumers through health insurance, public insurance, or public health programs.

In fiscal year 1975, such third-party payments constituted 67.4 percent of total expenditures for personal health care. 92.0 percent of expenditures for hospital care and 65.5 percent of payments to physicians were from third-party sources. Much smaller, but growing, percentages of expenditures for dentists and drugs were paid by third parties.

Private health insurance pays for 26.5 percent of total personal health care expenditures. In 1974, 85.2 percent of the population under age 65 had some coverage for hospital care and 81.4 percent for surgical fees. The rapid growth of private health insurance began in the late 1940s, with the portion of expenditures met by private health insurance expanding from 8.5 percent in 1950 to 24.7 percent in 1965. Since 1965, expenditures under private health insurance plans have increased 229 percent—from $8.3 billion in 1965 to $27.3 billion in 1975. However, the portion of total personal health care expenditures met by private health insurance has been relatively stable, reaching 26.5 percent of expenditures in 1975.

The rapid growth in private third-party payments in the last decade is dwarfed by the growth in public expenditures resulting from Medicare and Medicaid. Government expenditures for personal health care jumped 484 percent, from $7.0 billion to $40.9 billion, between 1965 and 1975. Government sources thus accounted for 39.7 percent of personal health care expenditures in 1975, compared to 20.8 percent in 1965. The government's impact is particularly noticeable in the hospital sector, where it met 55.0 percent of expenditures in 1975.

This absence of direct payments by consumers, particularly in the hospital sector, is an important feature of the health care industry. There has been considerable analysis of the impact of widespread insurance coverage upon demand and prices in the health sector; the consensus is that the prevalence of third-party payments is a significant factor affecting decision making by consumers and providers.

A key link in this conclusion is the typical "first dollar" form of coverage for hospital care and related surgical fees, i.e., full coverage of all expenses up to a predetermined ceiling. When a consumer pays out-of-pocket either none or a small fraction of the total cost of providing health services, economic theory and common sense suggest that he will tend to demand more services than if his out-of-pocket cost reflected the full cost of providing that care. Several studies have confirmed this effect, i.e., that the insured patient is willing to buy more care or more expensive care than he would if not insured (see, for example, Ginsburg and Manheim, 1973; Newhouse and Phelps, 1974; Phelps, 1975). One possible advantage of the "first dollar" form of coverage, however, is that it may enable lower income individuals who would otherwise shun "necessary" medical care to get that care and thus avoid possibly greater medical expenditures in the long run.*

Hidden Premium Costs

Increasing insurance expenditures are, of course, reflected in increasing health insurance premiums, and were the consumer aware of premium costs and increases, he or she might choose a different form of paying for medical care. However, under the current system of financing health insurance premiums, the individual is often unaware of premium costs.

Approximately 80 percent of health insurance premiums are paid through employment-related group insurance plans. Another 3.0 percent is paid through other group insurance policies; only 17.5 percent of premiums are for individual policies. Under such group insurance plans, the employer pays, on the average, 67 percent of the total premium, and in 41 percent of such policies, the employer pays the total premium (Mitchell and Phelps, 1975).

This prevalence of employment-related group insurance plans derives, in large part, from collective bargaining agreements negotiated over the past thirty years that include employer-provided health insurance as a jointly negotiated fringe benefit. The federal tax structure also plays a key role. Health insurance premium payments are subsidized in two ways. First, employer payments for group insurance premiums are not counted in the employee's income. This creates a tax incentive for employees to bargain for generous employer-provided health benefits: the employer dollar spent for health insurance buys more coverage than were the same dollar paid as a wage, taxed, and the balance spent by the employee for health insurance. Second, one-half (and in some cases, all) of individual payments for health insurance are deductible. While not as attractive a tax break as the first, this does further reduce the financial impact of health insurance premiums. With premium costs obscured in this fashion, the individual is likely to demand more comprehensive coverage through employer group insurance coverage than if he bore premium costs directly.

---

*For example, a study of the impact of consumer cost sharing under public health insurance in the Province of Saskatchewan, Canada, shows utilization falling 18 percent among lower-income beneficiaries in contrast to an overall 7 percent decrease. See Beck (1974).

Heavy Government Involvement

The combination of direct and tax-related federal, state, and local payments to the health industry make this one of the most heavily supported industries in the country.

In fiscal year 1975, 42.2 percent of health expenditures came from public funds. Federal payments for Medicare and Medicaid totalled $21.8 billion; total federal payments, including VA and DOD hospitals and various construction and research programs, were $33.8 billion. State and local outlays for health were $16.1 billion for the same period, including $6.0 billion in state Medicaid payments and $4.4 billion for public hospitals.

Another significant source of support flows from the federal income tax subsidies for health insurance premiums discussed in the previous section. The Office of Management and Budget estimates that the income tax revenues foregone as a result of these and of the medical expenses deduction in fiscal year 1975 were $5.6 billion. When foregone Social Security tax revenues are added in, the total tax support may be as high as $8 billion (see U.S. Office of Management and Budget, 1977; Mitchell, 1976).

Finally, additional government support flows from a variety of federal, state, and local tax exemptions provided to nonprofit hospitals and to Blue Cross-Blue Shield plans. It would be difficult to calculate these with any accuracy. Even if these are not counted, however, table 6.7 indicates that the total annual level of government support to this industry is approximately $58 billion, almost half of total health expenditures.

TABLE 6.7
GOVERNMENT SUPPORT TO THE HEALTH INDUSTRY:
FISCAL 1975

Source	Amount ($ billion)
Federal expenditures	$33.8
State and local expenditures	16.1
Federal tax preferences	8.0
Total	$57.9

In addition, government regulation of the industry is varied and widespread: licensing requirements for health care professionals; restrictions on development and marketing of drugs and medical devices; minimum health and safety standards for hospitals and other health care facilities; prohibitions against advertising by health care providers; certificate-of-need laws; and so on. This government role is expanding: the National Health Planning and Resources Development Act of 1974, signed in 1975 and now being implemented in stages, calls for an extensive federal, state, and local role in planning for health services delivery.

Provider's Choice

One unique aspect of medical care is the extent to which the provider of the service determines the nature and extent of services provided. To some extent this may reflect the third-party payment system in the sector which minimizes consumer awareness of what he or she is spending for the services received. On the other hand, it also derives in part from the patient's typical attitude towards medical care, one which is characterized by confidence in (or dependence upon) a particular physician and that physician's recommendations.

The physician's diagnosis determines the extent to which his or her own services are required as well as the utilization of diagnostic tests, therapeutic drugs, and hospitals. The patient usually lacks sufficient information or expertise, even if so inclined, to question a physician's recommendation or to seek possible alternatives.

Some economists contend that the peculiar consumer psychology prevalent in this sector has created a situation where physician "supply creates its own demand," i.e., where individual physicians are able to command certain amounts of resources and income regardless of the total number of physicians (see, for example, Feldstein, 1970; Fuchs and Kramer, 1972). This runs directly contrary to usual expectations of the impact of increased supply.

While there is some controversy over this conclusion, it is nevertheless clear that whatever the impact, the physician, rather than the consumer, is in most cases the key decision maker. The professional training of physicians has traditionally not emphasized this role of the physician as a manager of health care resources confronted with complex issues of cost and efficiency.

Providers' Incentives

In traditional markets, incentives to providers to be efficient would exist and would presumably restrain inflation. In the health sector, by contrast, the incentive structure of the industry appears to encourage greater quantity of service rather than efficiency.

Physician fees are, for the most part, paid on a fee-for-service basis, even though health maintenance organizations and various forms of prepaid group practice have expanded in recent years. The physician thus has little financial incentive to seek the most cost-effective utilization of hospital facilities in an individual case. This lack of incentives appears to encourage overutilization. Recent studies sponsored by the Department of Health, Education, and Welfare comparing federal employees covered under fee-for-service plans with those enrolled in a prepaid group health plan showed surgery rates 44 to 54 percent higher among the former groups. A recent Social Security Administration study of Medicaid recipients reached similar results. Such findings as well as studies of various programs requiring a second opinion for surgery,* have fueled a controversy over whether some of the surgery performed in this country may be unnecessary.

Hospital costs, as noted above, are commonly paid by public or private third parties, and these typically adopt a cost-reimbursement approach. Within certain limits, all the costs incurred by a hospital in treating a patient will be reimbursed. Under such a payment mechanism, there is little incentive for the hospital to be efficient. In addition, almost half of all hospitals (49 percent) are private, nonprofit institutions. Another 38 percent are public, and only 12 percent are proprietary. Nonprofit and public institutions have little incentive to seek or maximize profit; rather, it is commonly theorized and observed that such institutions tend to compete by increasing in size, in technological sophistication, or in prestige.

The medical care sector is also characterized by limited price competition. Advertising by physicians (on price or other matters) has been curtailed by medical societies and by some state laws. State law has also prohibited the advertising of prescription drug prices and of prices for eyeglasses and other optical equipment. While there is no empirical evidence on physician fees, recent studies looking at prices for drugs and eyeglasses have found that, where advertising is permitted, retail prices are generally lower (Cady, 1976; Benham and Brozen, 1975). Hospitals also rarely advertise—there is little reason to do so when consumers do not pay directly for hospital services. The Federal Trade Commission and Justice Department have recently taken action to remove some of these restraints on advertising and competition.

An additional factor affecting the incentive structure of the sector in recent years is the increasing size and number of malpractice judgments or settlements against hospitals and physicians. One impact of this trend may be a tendency towards so-called "defensive medicine," i.e., providing more thorough and expensive care than otherwise, in anticipation of possible malpractice claims.

Medical Innovation and Technological Change

Medical innovations in recent years have been characterized by an emphasis upon complex diagnostic and therapeutic techniques usually requiring hospi-

---

*See, for example, McCarthy and Widmer (1974). While this study showed significant declines in surgery rates, the author's qualifications should be noted:

> The findings of this report should be considered preliminary. Several questions need to be explored before the full value of the screening program can be determined. It is important to know how many of the members whose operations were not confirmed later had an operation for the condition screened, and how many required continued medical treatment; for confirmed cases, one should determine if presurgical screening affects the length of the hospital stay. Selected demographic characteristics and attitudes about presurgical screening of members using the program should also be surveyed.

talization and complicated, expensive equipment. Examples of this trend include chemotherapy, cancer radiation therapy, renal dialysis, open-heart surgery, organ transplants, intensive care units for heart attacks, burns, and trauma, and electronic brain and whole-body scanners. This trend has been associated with considerable advances in medical technology as well as the spread of existing technology.

As noted previously, new and sophisticated equipment has been a crucial factor in rising medical care outlays. New technology in medicine, unlike that in other industries, has unfortunately tended, on the whole, to be cost-raising rather than cost-saving. The initial expense for the new equipment and its installation is often high. There is evidence of widespread duplication in the purchase of expensive equipment by several institutional providers within the same geographic area. Once the equipment is in place, operating costs, including the cost of the highly trained personnel usually required, can be substantial. Finally, new technology often creates new demands on the part of both the patient and physician.

The use of intensive care units for treating heart attack victims provides one example of this expansion of medical technology and its impact on medical costs. In 1960, only 11 percent of private nonprofit hospitals had intensive care units; by 1973 such units were in place in approximately 71 percent. These units increase the costs of treating heart attacks dramatically: a recent study found the average cost escalating from $1449 per case in 1964 to $3280 per case in 1971, an increase of 126 percent, or 12 percent per year. Although this sharp increase in cost may reflect improved care, some clinical studies reported in several medical journals have questioned the effectiveness of such units compared to less expensive forms of treatment.*

That this rapid and widespread technological change can take place in the medical care sector despite its high cost is a telling indicator of the peculiar economics of this sector. Most advanced medical technological change is centered in the hospitals—where 92 percent of expenses are paid by third parties, who usually pay on a cost-reimbursement basis. Decisions as to the purchase and utilization of advanced technology thus need not turn on considerations of cost and efficiency.

Summary

Because of its institutional peculiarities, the economics of the health care sector differ markedly from American industry in general. Overall demand is increased by a payments structure that obscures the impact of health care spending upon the household budget. The nature and extent of services provided is

---

*See discussion and studies cited in Scitovsky and McCall (1975, p. 35). None of these studies is generally regarded as conclusive by the medical profession, and no opinion is expressed here on the merits of the issue of the effectiveness of coronary care units.

usually determined by the physician in a transaction in which the patient is often a passive participant. The economic rewards for efficiency and cost-reducing innovation that are characteristic of our economic system seem to be lacking. Heavy levels of government support have altered the economics of this sector even further. Any attempts to mitigate the rapid rise of inflation in health care must take account of these institutional peculiarities.

IV. WHAT IS THE IMPACT OF RISING HEALTH CARE EXPENDITURES?

Who Is Paying for What and How Much?

Rising health care expenditures are having a significant impact upon the individual household. In the twelve months ending in June 1975, the nation's expenditures for health were $547 per capita, an increase of 13 percent in just one year. For an average household of four, this translates into $2188 annually. Per capita personal income for the same period was $5633; thus, on the average, Americans spent almost 10 percent of their income for health care (see figure 6.3).

Given the complex way in which health care is financed, however, aggregate data of this nature may understate the actual economic impact of the health care system upon the individual household. Due to the complexity of this financing system, it is extremely difficult to calculate the total amount people pay for health care.

Figure 6.4 outlines the major components of our health care financing system, indicating the major sources of funds, intermediaries, and recipients. The major sources of funds, and their flows are as follows:

1. *Direct payments* from consumers to health care providers totalled $33.6 billion in fiscal year 1975, accounting for 32.6 percent of personal health care expenditures in that period. This is the primary means of paying for drugs (85.0 percent) and dental services (84.6 percent). However, only 34.5 percent of physicians services and 8.0 percent of hospital care are paid directly by the consumer.

2. *Premium payments (direct)*. 35.8 percent of hospital care and 39.0 percent of physicians services are paid for through various private health insurance plans; the total amount paid through these plans in fiscal year 1975 was $27.3 billion. These insurance plans are financed through premium payments by individuals or by employers on their behalf. Approximately 17.5 percent of premiums are paid for individual health insurance policies; in 59 percent of the plans, individuals also share in expenses for group policy premiums. Similarly, elderly persons enrolled in the Supplementary Medical Insurance (SMI) part of the Medicare program, which pays for various physician charges, also pay an insurance premium to the federal government. In addition, some portion of individual payments for automobile liability insurance premiums should be added in to the extent that such insurance pays for medical expenses resulting from automobile accidents.

FIGURE 6.3
NATIONAL HEALTH CARE EXPENDITURES
AS A PERCENT OF PERSONAL INCOME

Percent

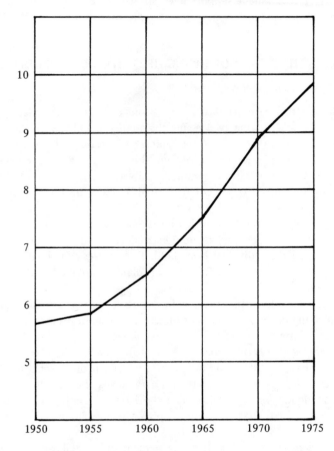

Source: U.S. Department of Commerce; U.S. Department of Health, Education, and Welfare, Social Security Administration, Office of Research and Statistics.

3. Premium payments (indirect). The balance of health insurance premiums derive from employer payments on behalf of employees. These payments also affect the household budget eventually, but their impact is difficult to predict or to measure. Health insurance premium expenses increase employer labor costs. Employers may strive to adjust by limiting wage rate increases, limiting further hiring, by pursuing other cost-reduction strategies, or by raising prices if market conditions allow. They may choose to, or have to, earn lower profits. In

FIGURE 6.4
THE FLOW OF HEALTH CARE DOLLARS

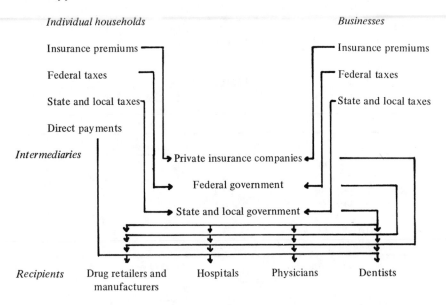

Sources of funds

Individual households   *Businesses*

Insurance premiums   Insurance premiums

Federal taxes   Federal taxes

State and local taxes   State and local taxes

Direct payments

Intermediaries   Private insurance companies

                                    Federal government

                                    State and local government

Recipients   Drug retailers and   Hospitals   Physicians   Dentists
                  manufacturers

most cases, however, an indirect cost is imposed on the individual household through lower wages or higher prices.

4. *Federal taxes (personal).* According to the Social Security Administration, the federal government spent $33.8 billion in fiscal year 1975 for health; this included expenditures for Medicare, portions of Medicaid, operation of VA and DOD hospitals and Public Health Service programs, research, and health facilities construction. Federal health spending is financed both from general revenues and from the 1.8 percent payroll tax for Medicare shared equally by employers and employees. Thus individuals also pay for health care through personal income and payroll taxes.

5. *Federal taxes (corporate).* Businesses also pay federal income taxes and share in the payroll tax for Medicare. These taxes are also frequently passed on to the individual either through lower wages or higher prices.

6. *State and local taxes.* State and local governments spent $16.1 billion for health care in fiscal year 1975, primarily for Medicaid payments and for public hospitals. This is financed through a variety of income, sales, and property taxes on both individuals and businesses.

Given the complexity of this system for financing health care, it would be difficult to calculate with any precision the actual impact of health care costs upon the average household at various income levels, and the Council is not aware of any definitive studies measuring this impact. Some indication of the impact of out-of-pocket expenditures can be derived from a survey conducted by researchers at the University of Chicago in 1971. Based upon 1970 data, this survey found that out-of-pocket expenditures (i.e., direct payments to providers, employee share of health insurance premiums) constituted a decreasing percentage of family income as income increased.

TABLE 6.8
OUT-OF-POCKET EXPENSES AS PERCENTAGE
OF FAMILY INCOME: 1970

		Average amount
Under $2,000	14.5%	
$2,000-3,499	9.3	$256.00
$3,500-4,999	7.7	327.00
$5,000-7,499	6.1	381.00
$7,500-9,999	4.6	402.00
$10,000-14,999	3.8	475.00
$15,000 and over	3.3	

Source: Ronald Anderson et al., *Expenditure for Personal Health Services: National Trends and Variations 1953-1970* (October 1973).

These data, of course, fail to reflect the substantial increases in medical care costs since 1970: data based upon 1975 would still surely show much higher expenditures. Even these updated data would understate the impact of medical care costs, however, particularly for middle income groups. Employer contributions to group insurance premiums and employer tax payments are ultimately passed on to the public through higher prices for the public as a whole, through lower wages for employees or through lower profits and dividends. When the burden of tax payments to finance federal, state, and local government health expenditures is considered, it is clear that all income groups, particularly the middle class and lower middle class, pay much higher portions of their income for health care than out-of-pocket expenditure data would indicate.

What Is the Cost? What Is the Return?

In the twelve months ending June 1975, 8.3 percent of our Gross National Product was spent for health care—the highest level in history. As figure 6.5 illustrates, the portion of our Gross National Product devoted to health has increased 41 percent in the past decade. While health care spending as a portion of Gross National Product had been rising steadily before 1965, never has the increase been so rapid. Two crucial questions flow from this growing allocation of re-

FIGURE 6.5
NATIONAL HEALTH EXPENDITURES AS A PERCENT OF
GROSS NATIONAL PRODUCT

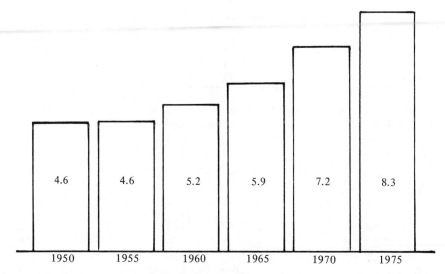

4.6	4.6	5.2	5.9	7.2	8.3
1950	1955	1960	1965	1970	1975

Source: U.S. Department of Health, Education, and Welfare, Social Security Administration, Office of Research and Statistics.

sources to health care. First, what are the opportunity costs—what are we giving up in order to spend this increased amount for health care? Second, what return is the nation receiving from this drastically increased spending—has our overall health improved; has the overall quality and delivery of health care improved?

The realization that continued growth in health care spending will limit the opportunity to use available resources for other purposes is rapidly spreading among various groups in our society. The rising cost of health care promises to be a major issue at the bargaining table this year. 1976 brings a heavy schedule of collective bargaining negotiations in major industries, and the impact of escalating health insurance premiums upon the employer's ability to pay increased wages is a matter of common concern. Data submitted to the Council concerning the automobile, rubber, and steel industries indicate that between 1965 and 1974, the cost of negotiated employee benefits (including health insurance) increased much more rapidly than wages.

A broader survey of American industry, conducted by the Bureau of Labor Statistics, shows that between 1966 and 1972, total employer payments for insurance and health benefits jumped 100 percent while wages increased only 47.7 percent. These data, of course, include the cost of life and other types of insurance as well as health benefits (Council on Wage and Price Stability, 1976).

TABLE 6.9
RELATIVE GROWTH OF WAGES AND COSTS OF
NEGOTIATED BENEFITS IN SELECTED INDUSTRIES:
PERCENTAGE GROWTH 1965-1974

	Autos	Rubber	Steel
Gross average hourly earnings	83%	59%	85%
Negotiated employee benefits	240	150	160
Total compensation costs	116	83	103

Source: Data provided by companies. These data reflect changes in the cost of providing benefits, not in the level of benefits received by workers. See Council on Wage and Price Stability, *1976 Collective Bargaining Negotiations: A Background Paper.*

A recent study conducted by the Social Security Administration indicates that health benefit costs have risen even more rapidly: between 1965 and 1973, annual contributions to employee health benefit plans (including both employer and employee shares) jumped 164 percent from $7.5 billion to $19.8 billion (Koludrubetz, 1975). Health benefits are thus becoming an ever larger portion of total compensation costs. Both union and management leaders have expressed concern over further cost increases in the health benefit component of labor compensation and their potential impact upon prices, wages, and profits.

In the public sector, increasing expenditures have led to proposals to limit undue expansion of public health programs. The portion of the federal budget expended for health has increased from 8.9 percent in 1969 to 11.3 percent in 1975 and is projected to be 11.7 percent in 1977. Only national defense, interest on the national debt, and income security programs now consume a larger share. The fiscal year 1977 federal budget includes proposals for limiting further growth in Medicare costs by imposing limits on increases in hospital charges to 7 percent and physician fees to 4 percent in 1977 and 1978 and by increasing certain deductible and coinsurance requirements. Several states are considering proposals to limit Medicaid costs.

In light of the ever-increasing allocation of resources to health care, is society reaping sufficient benefits compared to alternative uses of those resources? The evidence is mixed and difficult to evaluate and it would be impossible to resolve that question here. Studies of the factors affecting individual health status in industrialized nations seem to indicate that increases in national expenditures for health care and in utilization of hospital and physician services have, in the aggregate, only a minor impact. Some studies have found that in the United States, differences in heredity, education, life style, and the environment have a more significant impact upon health status than differences in utilization of medical care.* This research suggests that large additional expenditures on medical care, even though they may enhance the apparent quality of the care received, may be a very costly way of achieving improved national health. However, any attempt to compare these costs to the benefits of marginally improved health is hampered by complex medical and ethical issues. Potentially more cost-effective means than increased expenditures for medical care for improving the general health of the populace are available, such as programs to further reduce smoking, reckless or drunken driving, contamination in foods, and the like. Many of these, however, may not be socially or politically acceptable.

CONCLUSION

This report has reviewed inflationary trends in the medical care sector and has explored some possible explanations. It is to be hoped that it will contribute to public understanding of the serious economic problem presented by inflation in this sector, and provide the basis for cooperation with the medical care sector, as well as industry and labor in other sectors, and other government agencies in addressing this problem.

REFERENCES

Beck, R. G. "The Effects of Co-Payment on the Poor." *Journal of Human Resources* IX, no. 1 (Winter 1974).

Benham, L., and Benham, A. "The Impact of Incremental Medical Services on Health Status 1963-1970." *Equity in Health Services,* edited by R. Anderson et al. Cambridge, Mass.: Ballinger, 1975.

Benham, L., and Brozen, Y. *Advertising, Competition and the Price of Eyeglasses* (Reprint no. 36). Washington, D.C.: American Enterprise Institute for Public Policy Research, 1975.

Cady, J. F. *Restricted Advertising and Competition: The Case of Retail Drugs.* Washington, D.C.: American Enterprise Institute for Public Policy Research, 1976.

Council on Wage and Price Stability. *1976 Collective Bargaining Negotiations: A Background Paper.* Washington, D.C.: The Council, 1976.

Davis, K. "The Role of Technology, Demand and Labor Markets in the Determination of

---

*See U.S. Council of Economic Advisers, *Annual Report 1976,* chapter 3; Benham and Benham (1975); Fuchs (1974).

The measurement of health status and the study of factors that influence it are both exceedingly difficult. First, health status cannot be measured directly, but only through such surrogate measures as mortality and morbidity trends. Second, it is difficult, if not impossible, to conduct rigorous studies that isolate the impact over time of medical care as a variable, excluding the influence of other factors.

Much of the basic data on indicators of health status have recently been compiled by the Department of Health, Education, and Welfare in a three-volume publication, *Health— USA: 1975.*

Hospital Costs." *The Economics of Health and Medical Costs,* edited by R. Perlman. Washington, D.C.: Brookings Institution, 1974.

Eisenberg, B. S. *Trends in Physician Incomes, Expenses, and Fees, 1969-1974.* Chicago: Center for Health Services Research and Development, American Medical Association, 1976.

Feldstein, M. S. "The Rising Price of Physicians' Services." *Review of Economics and Statistics* 52 (May 1970).

Feldstein, M. S. *The Rising Costs of Hospital Care.* Washington, D.C.: Information Resources Press, 1971.

Fuchs, V. R. *Who Shall Live?* New York: Basic Books, 1974.

Fuchs, V. R., and Kramer, M. J. *Determinants of Expenditures for Physicians' Services in the United States, 1948-68* (Publication no. HSM 73-3013). Washington, D.C.: HEW, 1972.

Ginsberg, P. B., and Manheim, L. M. "Insurance Copayment and Health Services Utilization: A Critical Review." *Journal of Economics and Business* 25 (Winter 1973).

Koludrubetz, W. "Employee Benefit Plans, 1973." *Social Security Bulletin* (May 1975).

McCarthy, E. G., and Widmer, G. W. "Effects of Screening by Consultants on Recommended Elective Surgical Procedures." *New England Journal of Medicine* 291, no. 25 (December 1974).

Mitchell, B. N. *Basic Elements of Financing National Health Insurance.* Santa Monica, Calif.: Rand, 1976.

Mitchell, B. N., and Phelps, C. E. *Employer-Paid Group Health Insurance and the Costs of Mandated National Coverage.* Santa Monica, Calif.: Rand, 1975.

Newhouse, J. P., and Phelps, C. E. *On Having Your Cake and Eating It Too: Economic Problems in Estimating the Demand for Health Services.* Santa Monica, Calif.: Rand, 1974.

Phelps, C. E. "Effects of Insurance on Demand for Medical Care." *Equity in Health Services,* edited by R. Anderson et al. Cambridge, Mass.: Ballinger, 1975.

Scitovsky, A. A., and McCall, N. *Changes in the Cost of Treatment of Selected Illnesses 1951-1964-1971.* Discussion paper, University of California at San Francisco Health Policy Program (September 1975).

U.S. Office of Management and Budget. "Special Analysis F." *Special Analyses Budget of the United States Government, Fiscal Year 1977.* Washington, D.C.: Government Printing Office, 1977.

Worthington, N. "Expenditures for Hospital Care and Physicians' Services: Factors Affecting Annual Changes." *Social Security Bulletin* (November 1975).

Selection by John K. Iglehart

The explosive rise in medical care costs—the most pressing health issue facing the federal government—is emerging again at a time President Ford says the
federal government should curb its intervention in the private sector.

This combination of factors—sharply increasing prices and a government
policy of nonintervention—is leading to sizable federal and state budget overruns
and sharply higher private health insurance premiums.

During the twenty-three months since health cost controls under the federal economic stabilization program expired, the medical care component of the
consumer price index has increased at an annual rate of 12 percent—almost three
times the rate of increase during the period of economic controls and almost
twice the rate during the pre-freeze period.

The annual spending increase in the federal government's two major health
financing programs—Medicare and Medicaid—alone could exceed the size of the
remainder of the health budget request of the Department of Health, Education,
and Welfare in fiscal 1977.

HEW now estimates that Medicare and Medicaid expenditures will jump
from $25 billion in fiscal 1976 to $30.4 billion in fiscal 1977, an increase of
$5.4 billion.

Medicare expenditures alone will rise to $21 billion in fiscal 1977 from
$11.3 billion in fiscal 1974—just three years.

Reprinted by permission from "Health Care Cost Explosion Squeezes Government
Programs, Insurers," *Health Conference Issues* (Washington, D.C.: National Journal, 1976).

Ford requested $4.5 billion for all HEW health programs except Medicare and Medicaid in fiscal 1976, though Congress appropriated $6 billion. The administration requested $5.4 billion for these programs in fiscal 1977.

HEW now spends considerably more to purchase health services for the nation's poor through Medicaid than it does for cash assistance to this same population, although the cash payments represent the bulk of most welfare families' budgets.

The increase in health costs will be a major factor in shaping the Ford Administration's entire domestic policy agenda in election year 1976.

"The health cost increases will put a squeeze on every other program budget in town," a ranking HEW official predicted.

Concern. The cost issue has become a prevailing concern of HEW policy makers. They are raising fundamental questions over what the government's ever-growing investment in personal health services is buying.

Dr. Theodore Cooper, assistant HEW secretary for health, said June 14, 1975, in a speech to interns and residents at the American Medical Association's annual meeting: "Let us be frank with the American people, with their lawmakers, and with ourselves. . . . It is one of the great and sobering truths of our profession that modern health care probably has less impact on the health of the population than economic status, education, housing, nutrition, and sanitation. . . . Yet knowing that, I think we have fostered the idea that abundant, readily available, high quality health care would be some kind of panacea for the ills of society and the individual. That is a fiction, a hoax."

In a series of "health transition papers" prepared for HEW Secretary David Mathews when he took office, the department's office of planning and evaluation said: "As the percentage spent on health care rises, it is necessary to question where these funds come from and what the benefits really are from the additional spending. . . . Throughout this and most other discussions of our health care system there is an implicit, if not explicit, equation between better or more medical care and better health. This proposition must be challenged."

Issue. The rapid rise in health care costs poses a dilemma for the Ford Administration. Though the federal government is by far the nation's largest purchaser of personal health services, it has not been able to translate this economic leverage into controlling costs.

"In essence," HEW's office of planning and evaluation reported to Mathews, "the capacity of the federal government at the present time to control the rate of increase in medical costs is extremely limited."

Ford's oft-stated antipathy toward government regulation presumably will preclude the administration from reimposing broad economic controls on the health industry, the only constraints Washington has ever applied on medical services that seem to have had the desired effect of keeping prices down.

Yet, unless the administration takes some action to curb the uncharted and uncontrollable growth of the medical sector, HEW's two health-financing programs will gobble up even more of the department's health budget—Medicare and Medicaid already absorb 80 percent of it. In any event, private insurance premiums will increase significantly.

For example, the Blue Cross and Blue Shield plans, more than half of which lost money in the first six months of 1975, and commercial health insurers are seeking premium increases ranging from 10 percent to 60 percent to cover their costs.

At this point, the administration is not seriously considering any major new proposals to curb medical spending generally. HEW officials who are seeking action are pessimistic about winning White House support for a broad controls program.

An HEW policy maker said: "Surrounding the President is a group led by Alan Greenspan (chairman of the Council of Economic Advisers) who are so fundamentally opposed to controls of any kind that they find it hard, perhaps impossible, to separate out health from any other sector. Greenspan is trying to deregulate the economy."

Congress. In the decade since the federal government moved heavily into the financing of health care through Medicaid and Medicare, Congress has expressed its concern over rising costs in a sporadic fashion.

Its major expression of concern came in enactment of the Social Security Amendments of 1972 (86 Stat 1329), which contained a number of controversial provisions intended to control federal health expenditures.

Cost control pressures also were a driving force behind the enactment of the Health Maintenance Organization Act of 1973 (87 Stat 2994) and the National Health Planning and Resources Development Act of 1974 (88 Stat 2994).

But Congress also has been sensitive to pressures from the health industry. For example, it refused to accept the Nixon Administration's plan to continue health cost controls after expiration of the Economic Stabilization Act. And it has responded sympathetically to the hospital lobby's strong objection to Medicare cost controls.

Legislators rarely hear from any other force except the administration on the subject of controlling costs. Virtually all congressional witnesses testify in favor of expanding federal subsidies, not controlling them. In this milieu, legislators find few incentives to support controls.

"When we proposed controls we stepped on the toes of every interest in the industry; the ensuing pressures were relentless," said former Rep. James F. Hastings (R-N.Y.), a member of the House Interstate and Foreign Commerce Subcommittee on Health and the Environment.

Hastings sought to convince his fellow committee members that they should take a closer look at costs and how the health system operates.

TREND

Rising health care costs have been watched and debated extensively for almost a decade. But, day in and day out, it is an issue that holds little appeal for politicians who operate in a system that rewards advocates of new and expanded programs and benefits, rather than those who try to control costs.

The latest chapter in the medical care cost saga—a further documentation of the view that without controls the health system's appetite is unquenchable—indicates strongly that legislators will have to address the fundamental question of resource allocation as they consider national health insurance legislation.

The simple issue is how much money federal policy makers are prepared to invest in medical care at the expense of other needs and in a climate that increasingly questions the value of personal health services as a determinant of health status.

Pattern. Just since 1970, when the Nixon Administration and powerful congressional Democrats rekindled the government's flirtation with national health insurance, public and private national health expenditures have increased from $69.2 billion to $118.4 billion without the enactment of any major new program.

The focus of federal concern is on the twenty-three months since expiration of the medical price controls that were imposed as part of the Nixon Administration's economic stabilization program.

While the depressed business climate eased inflationary pressures in the general economy during this period, no similar let-up stemmed health care cost inflation. The health sector was left largely unharmed by the recession.

The gross national product (GNP), the total value of goods and services produced, dropped by more than $65 billion during the recession, but that portion of it absorbed by health expenditures increased from 7.7 percent in fiscal 1974 ($104.2 billion) to an estimated 8.3 percent ($118.4 billion) in fiscal 1974.

Since expiration of the economic stabilization program April 30, 1974, health care costs have risen at an annual rate of 12 percent, according to the Social Security Administration's office of research and statistics. Prices for all goods and services during this period rose at an annual rate of 10.1 percent.

HEW attributes the bulk of this cost increase to attempts by the health industry to recoup for the period when doctors and hospitals were under economic controls.

During the last quarter of 1974, this so-called catch-up period seemed to end; medical prices rose only slightly faster than the overall consumer price index (CPI). But during the first half of 1975, medical care prices shot forward again, helping to fuel a return to double-digit inflation for the economy as a whole (see table 6.10).

Hospitals. The most troublesome element in the CPI's medical care component was hospital service charges, which have increased at an annual rate of 15.3 percent since controls ended.

During the post-controls period, according to figures compiled by the Social Security Administration, semiprivate room charges increased at an annual rate of 18 percent; X-ray and diagnostic services were up 11.3 percent and oper-

TABLE 6.10
RATES OF COST INCREASE

Item	Prefreeze 1969-71	Economic controls	First half of 1975
CPI, all items	4.6%	6.4%	6.7%
Medical care	6.7	4.3	11.8
Medical care services	7.6	4.9	12.1
Hospital service charges	N.A.	4.6	13.8
Semiprivate room	13.0	5.7	15.0
Physician fees	7.4	4.0	12.0
Dentist fees	6.4	4.2	9.8
Drugs and prescriptions	2.0	0.7	9.2

Note: The 32½ months (Aug. 15, 1971-April 30, 1974) during which the health industry lived under government controls is the only period cost increases have slowed markedly since the enactment of Medicare and Medicaid in 1965. This table from the Bureau of Labor Statistics compares the annual rate of cost increases for items in the medical care component of the consumer price index (CPI) before controls were imposed, during controls, and after controls were lifted. "Medical care" includes all other categories plus health insurance: "medical care services" includes professional fees and hospital costs.

ating room charges rose 20.1 percent. For all three of these service charges, the increase was substantially higher than any previous comparable period.

The rate of increase in daily hospital costs was 18.8 percent in May 1975, the latest monthly figure available, equaling the previous high recorded in March 1975.

Hospital cost increases have been stoked by inflation, higher payroll costs, and malpractice premiums. Patient use, as measured by the number of days a person is hospitalized, has declined, requiring institutions to spread their rising costs over a shrinking patient population.

Inpatient hospital use declined 1.6 percent in May, compared with a year earlier. Hospital admissions were down 2.1 percent and the occupancy rate dropped 3.3 percent in May—the third consecutive month in which both these latter measures declined.

The annual increase in both outpatient visits and surgical operations also slowed somewhat in 1974.

Physicians. During the post-controls period, physicians' fees have risen at an annual rate of 13 percent—higher than any previous recorded period. All of the components of the physicians' fee index have risen sharply.

Fees for dentists' services have increased at an annual rate of 9.4 percent during the last twenty-one months. This is double the rate during the pre-freeze period, according to the Social Security Administration.

Fees for eye examinations and the prescription and dispensing of eyeglasses have increased at an annual rate of 8.8 percent during the post-controls period, almost double the rate during any previous period.

Similarly, the annual post-controls increase for routine laboratory tests was 15.2 percent, far surpassing the rate of the increase during the pre-freeze and controlled periods.

The combined consumer price index of drugs and prescriptions increased at an annual rate between May 1974 and January 1976 of 8 percent, four times the pre-freeze increases.

STRUCTURE

In striving to control medical care costs, the federal government must deal with an area of the economy that has unique characteristics which make it exceedingly difficult to limit growth short of imposing pervasive controls.

When the government has sought to modify characteristics of the medical system, elements of the industry have strongly resisted such changes.

A classic example of such resistance was the American Medical Association's fight to kill the Health Maintenance Organization Act of 1973. This law authorizes HEW to subsidize the development of health care facilities that reverse the traditional economic incentive of doctors—that is, the more services they provide the more their incomes rise.

Cost Analysis. Walter J. McClure, a health economist at InterStudy, a Minneapolis health policy research organization, said in an analysis of the cost issue: "The powerful cost raising incentives are intrinsic in the way the present medical care system is organized . . . the problem is structural, not conspiratorial. The great bulk of medical professionals are honorable, committed people. Even a group of saints placed in the present medical care system would produce the same malperformance. The system is doing exactly what society rewards it to do."

No other sector produces goods and services in American society under an economic system comparable to that of the health industry.

"Health services are for many reasons unique," HEW's office of planning and evaluation told Mathews in its transition papers. It continued: "At the lifesaving extreme there are no services which a society values more. We have granted to the practitioner of medical care a special place in the occupational hierarchy—the physician stands next to the clergy as our most respected occupation and his earnings are on average double those of his nearest competitor. Health care, at least in principle, is recognized as the service most deserving of the term 'a right.' Thus utilization could be unlimited."

Unlike other economic sectors, the key decision maker in health care is the producer of the product—the doctor—rather than the consumer—the patient.

Physicians make the decision to send a consumer to the hospital for services, to the drug store for a prescription, and to a laboratory for tests. In essence, it is the physician who decides what and how much care shall be consumed and paid for by the patient.

Insurance. Health policy makers generally agree that the rapid growth of insurance has generated increased spending because it makes physicians and consumers alike less sensitive to the true cost of treatment.

Testifying July 24 before the House Ways and Means Subcommittee on Health, Martin S. Feldstein, professor of economics at Harvard University, said: "There is now substantial evidence that . . . patients, guided by their doctors, demand more services and more expensive services when a large part of their costs are offset by insurance."

The growth of private health insurance dates to World War II when labor unions, forced to live under wage controls, received expanded health plans as a fringe benefit in the absence of higher wages.

Feldstein offered this explanation for the growth in costs:

In 1950, when the average cost per patient day was $16, private insurance paid 37 percent of hospital bills. That meant on the average the net cost to a private patient was $10.

In 1974, the average cost per patient day jumped to about $125, but private insurance was paying 77 percent of the private hospital bill, leaving a net cost to the patient of $28.50.

Thus, cost per day was up from $10 to $28.50. But $28.50 in 1974 really only bought $13 worth of goods and services based on 1950 prices. So in real terms, the net cost to the patient has hardly changed during that twenty-five year period.

Before 1965, the major part of the increase in insurance coverage occurred in the private sector. Since 1965, however, increases in coverage stem primarily from the enactment of Medicare and Medicaid.

By 1972, HEW estimates, about 90 percent of hospital bills were paid by third parties. Thus, most consumers pay only a small proportion of the total costs of medical care at the time they use the service.

The late Ray E. Brown, who was executive vice president of Northwestern University's McGaw Medical Center, said at the 1972 National Forum on Hospital and Health Affairs: "The economic consequences to the user are impersonalized by the fact that the tab is picked up by a third party. He can literally have his cake and eat it too. He does not need to forego his other options in order to have his health care. . . . At the same time, the provider is isolated from the punishment of a market that is monitored by individual choices."

Nonprofit system. The nation's 7,000 hospitals represent the heart of the health system. They are primarily a voluntary, nonprofit network of independent, autonomous units that under the existing cost-plus reimbursement system have few incentives to control expenditures.

The nonprofit status of these institutions has freed them from the usual economic profit constraint of private enterprise and left each hospital relatively free to expand, sometimes without serious consideration of true community needs.

In the last five years, for example, the nation's hospital bed supply has increased from 833,264 to 897,990, according to the American Hospital Association's bureau of research services. At the same time, the occupancy rate for all hospitals has dropped from 75.9 percent to 73.6 percent, thus exerting increased pressure on these institutions to raise their prices.

Brown said in his 1972 talk: "To a great extent hospitals have done what hospitals wanted to do. They have looked to their own institutional aspirations. Being a hybrid between a private and a public enterprise they have escaped the controls of both the marketplace and the government."

The cost-plus reimbursement system that private insurors traditionally have used to pay hospitals was adopted by Congress in 1965 for Medicare and Medicaid.

Former HEW Secretary (1973-1975) Caspar W. Weinberger told the House Ways and Means Subcommittee on Health on June 12: "I have said many times, and firmly believe, that the faulty design of Medicare and Medicaid is the principal culprit responsible for this super inflation in health care costs. The guaranteed government payment of health care costs in virtually any amount submitted by the provider, and with normal market factors absent in the health care area, inflation was bound to happen, and it did."

Other characteristics. HEW, in the June 1975 quarterly report of the Council on Wage and Price Stability, identified these other underlying structural characteristics of the health field, which it described as "inflationary pressures."

—The industry is labor intensive—about 60 percent of hospital expenses are made for labor and the salaries of these workers, traditionally low, have been rising faster than the average.

—Restrictive laws and practices have often limited the use of new categories of health manpower, e.g., physician extenders, and inhibited the growth of alternative organizational frameworks for delivering health services, e.g., prepaid group practices.

—There are tremendous pressures to spend money—technological advances are often introduced into hospital operations as soon as they are available, in some cases before there has been sufficient evidence of their efficiency or effectiveness.

—Hospitals receive over 50 percent of their revenues on the basis of actual costs incurred; since higher costs generate higher revenues, incentives for efficiency are lacking.

—Although consumers make the initial contact, subsequent determinations of the nature and amount of services are made by practitioners who are usually reimbursed on a fee-for-service basis.

Consumers frequently lack information on which to judge the prices and quality of health services making it difficult to evaluate the "product" or to compare prices.

PUBLIC PROGRAMS

Growing at a $5 billion a year clip, Medicare and Medicaid are "tearing the hell out of our budget," a ranking HEW official said in an interview.

HEW's budget office said that expenditures for Medicare and Medicaid totaled $10 billion in fiscal 1970; it estimates that spending for the programs will total $25 billion in fiscal 1976 and $52 billion in fiscal 1981.

HEW lacks a broad statutory mandate to curb spending in Medicare or, to a lesser extent, Medicaid. Most times when the administration has proposed steps to constrain their growth, Congress has rejected the measures.

The increase in Medicare expenditures stems largely from higher prices charged by hospitals and doctors and the utilization of more services. The size of the Medicare population has increased only 18 percent since 1967, while the number served by Medicaid has risen more than 100 percent.

Medicare and Medicaid were enacted in 1965 to provide public insurance to protect the elderly and the poor against the economic consequences of illness.

Although enacted together, Medicare and Medicaid reflect different historical perspectives. Proponents of Medicare view it as a social insurance program—similar to the social security cash payment program—to which a worker becomes entitled through personal payroll tax contributions while he is working.

The Social Security Administration strongly embraces this view of Medicare. Its resistance to efforts by the HEW Secretary's office to constrain Medicare spending stems in part from this attitude.

Medicaid, in contrast, is an extension of the federally supported state welfare programs.

Medicare. About 98 percent of all persons over sixty-five, or 23.3 million persons, are eligible for social security cash benefits. These individuals are enrolled automatically in Medicare's Part A hospital insurance program. The remaining 2 percent of the aged may enroll and pay the full premium, which is $40 a month, for the same coverage.

The Social Security Amendments of 1972 extended Medicare coverage to those people under sixty-five who have received disability insurance cash benefits for twenty-four months and to anyone afflicted with end-stage renal disease (kidney failure).

Medicare's Part B program of physician services is available on a voluntary enrollment basis to any person who is either over sixty-five or who qualifies as a disabled individual.

Part A is financed through a 1.8 percent payroll tax paid equally by employers and employees. Part B is financed 40 percent from premium contributions ($6.70 a month per enrollee in fiscal 1976) and the remainder of the coverage from general revenue.

The health system's inflationary environment and a substantial—and unexpected—increase in the utilization of hospital services by the elderly are contributing to a massive Medicare budget overrun in fiscal 1976. These factors also are forcing HEW to plan for a far larger fiscal 1977 Medicare budget than originally projected.

President Ford's fiscal 1976 budget estimated that Medicare expenditures would total $15.5 billion, not including cost saving legislative proposals that would have reduced that total by $1.4 billion. Congress never seriously considered these proposals.

HEW currently estimates that Medicare expenditures will be $1.1 billion higher in fiscal 1976. And its estimate for fiscal 1977 is that Medicare expenditures will run $4 billion, or 23.7 percent higher than that, for a total of about $21 billion.

Medicare's actuaries include an inflationary factor in their calculations. But a cost factor that caught everybody by surprise was a substantial increase in the use of hospital services by the elderly.

Preliminary indications are that hospital services per Medicare beneficiary were 5 percent higher in fiscal 1975 than a year earlier, following declines ranging between 0.5 percent and 3 percent during each of the previous five years.

Thomas M. Tierney, director of the Medicare program, said that the use of hospital services is higher for all age categories. "I don't know what the hell is happening but it is happening and not just in Medicare."

The budget overrun will have several consequences, including placing great pressure on HEW to cut spending in its controllable health programs.

It also will eliminate any prospect of legislators being able to turn to the Medicare trust fund, as recommended by the Social Security Advisory Council, to bail out the underfunded social security case benefit program.

Conflict. The offices of the assistant secretaries for budget and for planning evaluation engaged in a bureaucratic debate with the Social Security Administration over whether HEW again should propose Medicare cost controls in the President's fiscal 1977 budget.

The stewards of Medicare traditionally have resisted the imposition of cost controls on their program, arguing that it generates conflict with participating hospitals and doctors. Moreover, Medicare officials maintain that its statutory mandate is to finance health benefits for the elderly, not strive to control medical costs.

Tierney said: "We can and do control expenditures from Medicare funds (fraud), but we have no authority to control medical costs."

Reflecting this attitude, the Social Security Administration submitted no new cost control proposals along with its fiscal 1977 budget estimates. Tierney said that HEW should focus its cost control efforts on a massive jawboning campaign—"organized from the highest level of government down to the local medical societies."

The jawboning proposal first was advanced by James B. Cardwell, social security commissioner, in a meeting with Weinberger shortly before he resigned August 10.

John D. Young, assistant secretary-comptroller, and William A. Morrill, assistant secretary for planning and evaluation, opposed as inadequate the proposed jawboning campaign as the only federal initiative to control costs.

They pressed Mathews to embrace a broader set of controls. Young, in particular, advocated a revision of the way Medicare reimburses hospitals for the services they provide elderly beneficiaries.

Young pressed for development of a proposal through which hospitals would be reimbursed on a prospective basis.

Under such a scheme, hospitals would be told prior to the beginning of their fiscal year the level of reimbursement Medicare and Medicaid would pay for services. Such an approach, presumably, would grant the government increased leverage to control costs.

But the words "prospective reimbursement" have come to mean different things to different interests. Stuart H. Altman, deputy assistant HEW secretary for health planning and analysis, said June 2 at the International Conference on Health Care Costs and Expenditures: "We talk about prospective reimbursement in this country. Well, one thing that I have learned is that when everybody likes something, you are obviously talking about a different thing. In this country the hospitals like prospective reimbursement, the doctors like prospective reimbursement, the states like prospective reimbursement, the federal government likes prospective reimbursement, and even patients walking down the street talk about prospective reimbursement. When this happens you know that people view prospective reimbursement quite differently."

The major pressure on Young was the expectation that Medicare hospital reimbursements, if left alone, would increase 24.3 percent in fiscal 1977 over the administration's fiscal 1975 budget.

Young favored the development of legislation permitting HEW to reshape the mechanism through which it pays hospitals, thus giving it some control over costs.

In a draft memorandum prepared to sell the prospective reimbursement idea to the Office of Management and Budget (OMB), HEW's budget office said: "The major new (cost control) proposal we would recommend is prospective reimbursements to hospitals. The level of reimbursement would be set by a composite index allowing an overall increase that takes into account both payroll and nonpayroll hospital costs. . . . This kind of prospective system would allow the hospital to choose its own area of spending, but would prevent the kind of increases we are currently experiencing because we reimburse retrospectively. If the limit was set conservatively—disallowing 2 percent of the expected 24.2 percent increase in hospital costs between fiscal 1976 and fiscal 1977—we could expect to save $300 million in fiscal 1977. The effect of this index would be compounded each year so that savings in 1981 would exceed $2.1 billion."

The draft memorandum concluded: "If this proposal is not enacted we recommend that the proposal introduced last year—to limit the rate of increase of 80 percent of similar hospitals—be resubmitted. This proposal would disallow costs retrospectively and therefore be less effective as a control than prospective reimbursement. This would save $175 million in fiscal 1977 and, through the compounding effect on program outlays, $500 million by 1981."

The Social Security Administration preferred that the administration not advance a prospective reimbursement proposal at this time. The agency is financing a number of prospective reimbursement experiments and would rather wait for the results of these projects before plunging ahead with a broader proposal.

Ultimately, OMB rejected HEW's cost containment ideas and opted instead for a more arbitrary approach to the problem. The President's budget contained proposals that would limit increases in Medicare fees to 7 percent a year for hospitals and 4 percent for doctors.

HEW Secretary Mathews said the medical marketplace is "not a true market" and, as a result, "these control proposals make sense."

Mathews said it was his hope that doctors, instead of increasing their fees to elderly patients to offset the 4 percent limitation, would be "motivated . . . to absorb some of these costs themselves."

The Washington lobbies for hospitals and doctors strongly opposed the Administration's control proposals.

Medicaid. The federal-state Medicaid program finances the principal health care needs of 24 million poor people. The program will cost an estimated $14.2 billion in fiscal 1976, of which $7.8 billion is federal and $6.4 billion is state and local expenditures.

Medicaid expenditures have grown far more rapidly than Congress originally anticipated because of three factors: increases in enrollment, rising medical costs, and changes in services.

Medicaid, in contrast to Medicare, attributes the bulk of its expenditure growth to increasing enrollment, particularly between 1967 and 1972. The use of Medicaid services per beneficiary actually has declined somewhat over time, HEW says.

Under the law, states must extend Medicaid benefits to individuals eligible for aid to families with dependent children and, with certain exceptions, beneficiaries of supplementary security income, the new federalized program for the aged, blind, and disabled.

States may, at their option, extend Medicaid coverage to the so-called medically needy—individuals who make too much money to make them eligible for cash assistance but still are unable to pay their medical bills.

The Social and Rehabilitation Service (SRS), the bureaucratic umbrella under which Medicaid operates, estimates in its revised fiscal 1976 budget calculations that federal Medicaid expenditures will run $121 million higher than the President's initial budget, or a total of $7.9 billion.

In fiscal 1977, SRS estimates, federal Medicaid expenditures will increase $1.5 billion more than its revised fiscal 1976 spending level, for a total of $9.4 billion.

Rising Medicaid costs have generated substantial pressures at both the federal and state levels to control expenditures. Some states have attempted to constrain expenditures by reducing the scope of benefits offered and clamping down on physicians' reimbursement.

Congress, in its 1967, 1969, and 1972 amendments to the Social Security Act, approved proposals designed to control costs such as mandating utilization review in hospitals, allowing states to cut back optional services, and imposing cost sharing requirements on beneficiaries.

The President's fiscal 1976 budget requested legislation to eliminate federal matching fund requirements for adult dental services and to reduce the minimum federal Medicaid matching rate from 50 percent to 40 percent. Neither proposal received a hearing on Capitol Hill.

The effort to cut costs has in some instances actually added expenses, according to M. Keith Weikel, director of the federal Medicaid program.

The Medicaid law requires that states reimburse hospitals on the same cost-plus basis as does the federal government. But states have the option of reducing the payments doctors receive.

In New York, for example, only 38 percent of the doctors will see Medicaid patients. Many other doctors regard the compensation paid by Medicaid as inadequate and thus refuse to serve the program's eligible population.

As a result, Medicaid patients "are pushed into emergency rooms to receive ambulatory care that could more economically be rendered in a doctor's office," Weikel said. "We really get clipped in the emergency room setting."

PRIVATE PROGRAMS

Commercial and private, nonprofit health insurance carriers are experiencing medical price increases that are larger, for the most part, than those of 1971 before President Nixon imposed a wage-price freeze on the economy.

The health care cost increases are being translated into premium hikes that range from 10 percent to 60 percent for employers who offer their employees group health insurance.

The rise in medical costs that has occurred thus far in 1975 caught both commercial insurers and the Blue Cross Association and the National Association of Blue Shield Plans by surprise. Their explanations for the increases vary.

The rise in malpractice insurance premiums, an oft-cited reason, seems to be having a two-edged impact. Insurance company officials attribute to it an increase in doctors' fees and a rise in the utilization of services as practitioners turn to so-called "defensive medicine."

Blue Cross. The Blue Cross and Blue Shield plans, private, nonprofit organizations that insure 80 million people, lost more than $400 million in the first half of 1975.

Ninety-four of its 132 local plans suffered losses, according to a survey taken by the association's headquarters office in Chicago.

Like HEW, the Blues anticipated a bulge in prices following the end of the economic stabilization program. The health industry was controlled more tightly than virtually all other sectors of the economy. Following this bulge in the spring and summer of 1974, the rate of cost increases diminished.

But, the association's survey said, "without warning, hospital service charges began a rapid increase in the fourth quarter of 1974. Physician charges and rates of professional service utilization also increased dramatically during the quarter. this sudden increase in Blue Cross and Blue Shield plan cost trends, in conjunction with relatively low trend factors then employed in rating procedures, produced losses for many plans."

The association's report shows that in the second quarter of 1975, ninety-four plans had net financial losses totaling $210.4 million; thirty plans reported net gains of $22.6 million. The net loss for the organization was $188 million. This loss, added to a little larger first quarter deficit, produced a total loss of an estimated $402 million in the first half.

Almost all of the increase in Blue Cross plan expenditures was attributable to higher hospital costs. The plans reported that per diem costs were up from about 15 percent to 25 percent, with a median increase of 18.3 percent.

The survey revealed an entirely different picture for Blue Shield plans. The increasing cost of care "seems to be due to changes in both utilization and unit costs, in approximately equal amounts."

Blue Cross and Blue Shield plan presidents were asked by their national office for their explanations of the dramatic increases in cost.

Two explanations were mentioned most frequently. One, products and services upon which hospitals depend still are subject to inflation. Included in the list of items were salaries, supplies—especially petrochemicals and derivatives -energy, and fringe benefits.

Two, malpractice insurance, "both in the rising cost of premiums and the threat it poses against the physician and hospital to force more defensive practices such as more diagnostic tests."

Asked about their predictions for the next year, the plan presidents were almost evenly divided between those who foresaw some leveling off of costs and those who saw no signs of leveling off. "Professional liability (malpractice) is anticipated to be a continued problem during the year both for Blue Cross and Blue Shield plans," the survey said.

Federal employees. Blue Cross and Blue Shield insure approximately 63 percent of the workers enrolled in the federal health benefits program.

The medical cost increases have forced the Blues to seek a premium increase of about 35 percent from the Civil Service Commission, which oversees the administration of the federal program.

Aetna Life and Casualty, which insures 15 percent of the workers enrolled in the federal program, is seeking a premium increase of a similar size.

Robert J. Laur, vice president and director of Blue Cross's federal employee program, said in an interview that the program never before has experienced the kind of cost increases it experienced in the last nine months.

On the physician side, Laur attributed the Blues' request for a substantial premium increase to higher utilization of services and inflation.

"I suspect a defensive medicine trend, but I couldn't prove it," Laur said. "Providers may also be anticipating another round of price controls and are building their financial bases up."

Laur said the Blues "are doing as good a job of claims cost control as it's possible to do," thus suggesting that the increases could not be held in closer check by improved management of the program.

Commercial insurers. Commercial health insurance carriers are being forced to seek premium increases from their group customers that range to 60 percent.

Burton E. Burton, a senior vice president of Aetna Life and Casualty, expressed "considerable alarm" at the sharp rise in medical costs.

Burton said that Aetna is seeking from its group health insurance customers premium increases that average 25 percent but range to 60 percent. One year ago, he said, Aetna's premium increases ranged from 7 percent to 9 percent.

Asked whether insurers are able to cope with the health cost increases because they are passed along to customers, Burton replied: "Yes, in our group business it is largely a pass-through business where our group policy holders have to pay the costs."

Nevertheless, he said, Aetna's profits have been "impacted severely" by the increases in health care costs.

OUTLOOK

The sharp rise in health costs and the government's recognition that controlling them is an extremely difficult assignment may be having its greatest policy impact in significantly slowing the drive toward national health insurance.

Sen. John V. Tunney (D-Calif.) symbolized the concern among many of his colleagues when he announced August 5 that he now opposes the national health insurance bill (S 3) advocated by his law school roommate, Sen. Edward M. Kennedy (D-Mass.).

Tunney said the measure carries "a price tag of somewhere between $25 and $35 billion. That's just too much at this point in time. I mean, we just can't afford it now," he said in a California speech.

Ford put to rest in his State of the Union message any speculation that in an election year he would feel compelled to urge action on national health insurance. "We cannot realistically afford federally dictated national health insurance providing full coverage for all 215 million Americans. The experience of other countries raises questions about the quality as well as the cost of such plans," he said.

Nevertheless, the President did not totally reject the idea of an expanded federal role in providing medical services. Appealing to a key voting bloc in an election year, Ford proposed a "catastrophic" health insurance scheme for the elderly.

Ford's plan would limit the liability of 25 million aged and disabled Medicare eligibles to an annual maximum of $500 per year for covered hospital and nursing home care and $250 a year for doctor's fees. The proposal was sharply criticized by most members of Congress because it would cost the vast bulk of Medicare beneficiaries more money, but afford only a few added protection.

The House Ways and Means Subcommittee on Health resumed public hearings September 19, 1975, on possible changes in Medicare, but there was no indication then or in subsequent sessions that its activities would lead to cost savings in Medicare. If anything, the panel is likely to embrace amendments that could cost more money.

The Senate Finance Subcommittee on Health may take up the issue of Medicare costs this spring. The discussions would center on a measure that Sen. Herman E. Talmadge (D-Ga.), the subcommittee chairman, introduced on March 25.

Talmadge's proposal, he said last June 20, 1975, in a Senate speech, will be designed to correct "administrative deficiencies . . . assure effective investigation of fraud and abuse (in Medicaid) and . . . resolve some of the reimbursement and related problems in Medicare and Medicaid, and some of the more arbitrary and inequitable regulations which have been promulgated by HEW."

The likelihood of final action on Talmadge's bill this year, though, looks remote. Moreover, the problem of costs that rise uncontrollably is broader than Medicare and Medicaid. The government must either impose a broader set of controls or be prepared to accept the budgetary consequences.

7

The Diminishing Marginal Benefit of High-Technology Services

Selection by Renée C. Fox

The statement that American society has become "medicalized" is increasingly heard these days. During the past decade or so, the allegation has been made by social scientists, jurists, politicians, social critics, medical scientists, and physicians. In many instances, it has been accompanied by the claim that the society is now "overmedicalized," and that some degree of "demedicalization" would be desirable. There are those who not only espouse "demedicalizing the society," but who also predict that, in fact, it will progressively come to pass.

One of the most extreme statements of this kind is Ivan Illich's monograph, *Medical Nemesis*, which opens with the assertion that "the medical establishment has become a threat to health," and goes on to develop the many damaging ways in which the author considers modern medicine to be responsible for "social" as well as "clinical" and "structural" iatrogenesis:

The technical and nontechnical consequences of institutional medicine coalesce and generate a new kind of suffering: anesthetized, impotent, and solitary survival in a world turned into a hospital ward. . . . The need for specialized, professional health care beyond a certain point can be taken as an indication of the unhealthy goals pursued by society. . . . The level of public health corresponds to the degree to which the means and responsibility for coping with illness are distributed amongst the total population. This ability to cope can be enhanced but never replaced by medical intervention in the lives of people or by the hygienic characteristics of the environment. The society which can reduce professional intervention to the minimum will provide the best conditions for

Reprinted by permission from "The Medicalization and Demedicalization of American Society," *Daedalus* (Winter 1977), pp. 9-22.

health. . . . Healthy people are those who live in healthy homes on a healthy diet; in an environment equally fit for birth, growth, work, healing, and dying: sustained by a culture which enhances the conscious acceptance of limits to population, of aging, of incomplete recovery and ever imminent death. . . . Man's consciously lived fragility, individuality, and relatedness make the experience of pain, of sickness, and of death an integral part of his life. The ability to cope with this trio autonomously is fundamental to his health. As he becomes dependent on the management· of his intimacy, he renounces his autonomy and his health *must* decline. The true miracle of modern medicine is diabolical. It consists not only of making individuals but whole populations survive on inhumanly low levels of personal health. That health should decline with increasing health service delivery is unforeseen only by the health managers, precisely because their strategies are the result of their blindness to the inalienability of life (Illich, 1975, pp. 165-69).

There are numerous grounds on which Illich's thesis can be criticized. He minimizes the advances in the prevention, diagnosis, and treatment of disease that have been made since the advent of the bacteriological era in medicine, and he attributes totally to nonmedical agencies all progress in health that has ensued. He implies that modern Western, urban, industrialized, capitalist societies, of which the United States is the prototype, are more preoccupied with pain, sickness, and death, and less able to come to terms with these integral parts of a human life, than other types of society. Although his volume appears to be well documented, a disturbing discrepancy exists between the data presented in many of the works that Illich cites in his copious footnotes and the interpretive liberties that he takes with them. Perhaps most insidious of all is the sophistry that Illich uses in presenting a traditional, orthodox, Christian-Catholic point of view in the guise of a vulgar Marxist argument. For he repeatedly claims that "when dependence on the professional management of pain, sickness, and death grows beyond a certain point, the healing power in sickness, patience in suffering, and fortitude in the face of death must decline." In Illich's view, this state is not only morally dubious, but also spiritually dangerous. Because it entails the "hubris" of what he deems arrogant and excessive medical intervention, it invites "nemesis": the retribution of the gods.

But whatever its shortcomings, Illich's essay is a kind of lightning rod, picking up and conducting the twin themes of medicalization and demedicalization which have become prominent in the United States and a number of other modern Western societies. These themes will concern us here. We shall begin by identifying the constellation of factors involved in what has been termed "medicalization," offer an interpretation of these phenomena, and consider and evaluate certain signs of demedicalization. Finally, some speculative predictions about the probable evolution of the medicalization-demedicalization process in American society will be offered.

One indication of the scope that the "health-illness-medicine complex" has acquired in American society is the diffuse definition of health that has increasingly come to be advocated: "a state of complete physical, mental, and social well-being," to borrow the World Health Organization's phrase. This conception of health extends beyond biological and psychological phenomena relevant to the functioning, equilibrium, and fulfillment of individuals, to include social and cultural conditions of communal as well as personal import. Such an inclusive perspective on health is reflected in the range of difficulties that persons now bring to physicians for their consideration and help. As Leon Kass (1975) picturesquely phrased it: "All kinds of problems now roll to the doctor's door, from sagging anatomies to suicides, from unwanted childlessness to unwanted pregnancy, from marital difficulties to learning difficulties, from genetic counseling to drug addiction, from laziness to crime. . . ." A new term has even been coined by medical practitioners to refer to those clients who seem to have some legitimate need of their therapeutic services, but who technically cannot be considered to be ill. With discernible ambivalence, such persons are often called "the worried well."

Accompanying the increasingly comprehensive idea of what constitutes health and what is appropriate for medical professionals to deal with is the growing conviction that health and health care are rights rather than privileges, signs of grace, or lucky, chance happenings. In turn, these developments are connected with higher expectations on the part of the public about what medicine ideally ought to be able to accomplish and to prevent. To some extent, for example, the rise in the number of malpractice suits in the United States seems not only to be a reaction to the errors and abuses that physicians can commit, but also a reflection of the degree to which the profession is being held personally responsible for the scientific and technical uncertainties and limitations of their discipline. The vision of an iatrogenesis-free furthering of health, which social critics such as Illich hold forth, is also an indicator of such rising expectations.

One significant form that the process of medicalization has taken is the increase in the numbers and kinds of attitudes and behaviors that have come to be defined as illnesses and treatment of which is regarded as belonging within the jurisdiction of medicine and its practitioners. In an earlier, more religiously oriented era of a modern Western society like our own, some of these same kinds of attitudes and behaviors were considered sinful rather than sick, and they fell under the aegis of religious authorities for a different kind of diagnosis, treatment, and control. In a more secular, but less scientifically and medically oriented, stage of the society than the current one, certain of these ways of thinking, feeling, and behaving were viewed and dealt with as criminal. Although sin, crime, and sickness are not related in a simple, invariant way, there has been a general tendency in the society to move from sin to crime to sickness in categorizing a number of aberrant or deviant states to the degree that the concept of the "medicalization of deviance" has taken root in social-science writings. The sin-to-crime-to-sickness evolution has been most apparent with respect to the conditions that are now considered to be mental illnesses, or associated with serious psychological and/or social disturbances.* These include, for example, states of hallucination and delusion that once would have been interpreted as signs of possession by the Devil, certain forms of physical violence, such as the type of child abuse that results in what is termed the "battered child syndrome," the set of behaviors in children which are alternatively called hyperactivity, hyperkinesis, or minimal brain dysfunction, and so-called addictive disorders, such as alcoholism, drug addiction, compulsive overeating, and compulsive gambling.

This "continuing process of divestment" (Kittrie, 1971, pp. 1-49) away from sin and crime as categories for abnormality, dysfunction, and deviance and toward illness as the explanatory concept has entailed what Peter Sedgwick (1973) calls "the progressive annexation of not-illness into illness." "The future belongs to illness," he proclaims, predicting that "we . . . are going to get more and more diseases, since our expectations of health are going to become more expansive and sophisticated." If we include into what is considered to be sickness or, at least, nonhealth in the United States, disorders manifested by subjective symptoms which are not brought to the medical profession for diagnosis and treatment, but which do not differ significantly from those that are, then almost everyone in the society can be regarded as in some way "sick."

At least two . . . studies have noted that as much as 90 percent of their apparently healthy sample had some physical aberration or clinical disorder. . . . It seems that the more intensive the investigation, the higher the prevalence of clinically serious but previously undiagnosed and untreated disorders. Such data as these give an unexpected statistical picture of illness. Instead of it being a relatively infrequent or abnormal phenomenon, the empirical reality may be that illness, defined as the presence of clinically serious symptoms, is the statistical *norm*. (Zola, 1966)

Such a global conception of illness acutely raises the question of the extent to which illness is an objective reality, a subjective state, or a societal construct that exists chiefly in the minds of its social "beholders," a question that will be considered in greater detail below.

The great "power" that the American medical profession, particularly the physician, is assumed to possess and jealously and effectively to guard is another component of the society's medicalization. In the many allusions to this medical "power" that are currently made, the organized "autonomy" and "dominance"

---

*In his novel *Erewhon*, written in 1872, Samuel Butler satirized this evolution, and the degree to which what is defined as illness is contingent on social factors. In Erewhon (the fictitious country that Butler created by imagining late nineteenth- and early twentieth-century England stood on its head), persons afflicted with what physicians would call tuberculosis are found guilty in a court of law and sentenced to life imprisonment, whereas persons who forge checks, set houses on fire, steal, and commit acts of violence are diagnosed as suffering from a "severe fit of immorality" and are cared for at public expense in hospitals.

of the profession are frequently cited, and, in some of the more critical statements about the physician, these attributes are described as constituting a virtual "monopoly" or "expropriation" of health and illness. The "mystique" that surrounds the medical profession is part of what is felt to be its power: a mystique that is not only spontaneously conferred on its practitioners by the public but, as some observers contend, is also cultivated by physicians themselves through their claim that they command knowledge and skills that are too esoteric to be freely and fully shared with lay persons.

However, it is to the biotechnological capacities of modern medicine that its greatest power is usually attributed: both its huge battery of established drugs and procedures and its new and continually increasing medical and surgical techniques. Among the actual or incipient developments that are most frequently mentioned are the implantation of cadaveric, live, or mechanical organs, genetic and other microcellular forms of "engineering," and *in vitro* fertilization, as well as various chemical, surgical, and psychophysiological methods of thought and behavior control. The potentials of medicine not only to prevent and to heal, but also to subjugate, modify, and harm are implicated in such references.

The high and rapidly growing cost of medical and health care is still another measure of increased medicalization. In 1975, Americans spent $547 per person for health care and related activities such as medical education and research. This represented 8.3 percent of the GNP. In 1950, 4.6 percent and in 1970, 7.2 percent of the GNP was spent. From 1963 to the present, health expenditures have risen at a rate exceeding 10 percent annually while the rest of the economy as reflected in the GNP has been growing at a rate between 6 and 7 percent.

In addition to allocating an ever increasing proportion of society's economic resources for health care, greater amounts of political and legal energy are also being invested in health, illness, and medical concerns. The pros and cons of national health insurance, which continue to be vigorously debated in various arenas, are as much political, ideological, and legal issues, as they are economic ones. The volume of legislation relevant to health care has grown impressively. In 1974, for example, more than 1,300 health care bills were introduced in the Congress, and more than 900 such bills in the state legislature in New York alone. The health subcommittees of the Senate and the House of Representatives are particularly active, and they have become prestigious as well. Furthermore, partly as a consequence of various congressional investigations and hearings, the federal government is now significantly involved in bioethical questions (especially those bearing on human experimentation) in addition to their more traditional interests in medical economic and health care delivery problems.

During the past few years, a number of medico-legal decisions have been made that are of far-reaching cultural importance, affecting the society's fundamental conceptions of life, death, the body, individuality, and humanity. These include: the Supreme Court's decisions in favor of the legal right of women to decide upon and undergo abortion; the Court's ruling against the involuntary, purely custodial confinement of untreated, mentally ill persons; the Uniform Anatomical Gift Act, adopted in fifty-one jurisdictions, which permits persons to donate all or parts of their bodies to be used for medical purposes after their death; death statutes passed in various states which add the new, "irreversible coma" criterion of "brain death" to the traditional criteria for pronouncing death, based on the cessation of respiratory and cardiac function; and, in the case of Karen Ann Quinlin, the New Jersey Supreme Court's extension of "the individual's right of privacy" to encompass a patient's decision to decline or terminate life-saving treatment, under certain circumstances.

One other, quite different, way in which medical phenomena have acquired central importance in the legal system is through the dramatic escalation of malpractice suits against physicians. An estimated 20,000 or more malpractice claims are brought against doctors each year, and the number seems to be rising steadily. In New York, for example, the number of suits filed against physicians rose from 564 in 1970 to 1,200 in 1974; in the past decade, the average award for a malpractice claim grew from $6,000 to $23,400, with far more very large awards being made than in the past (*Newsweek,* June 9, 1976, p. 59).

Increasing preoccupation with bioethical issues seems also to be a concomitant of the medicalization process. Basic societal questions concerning values, beliefs, and meaning are being debated principally in terms of the dilemmas and dangers associated with biomedical advances. Consideration of particular medical developments such as genetic engineering, life-support systems, birth technology, organ implants, and population and behavior control have opened up far-reaching ethical and existential concerns. Problems of life, death, chance, "necessity," scarcity, equity, individuality, community, the "gift relationship," and the "heroic" world-view are being widely discussed in medical, scientific, political, legal, journalistic, philosophical, and religious circles. A bioethics "subculture" with certain characteristics of a social movement has crystallized around such issues.

The unprecedented number of young people who are attempting to embark on medical careers is also contributing to the medicalization process. In this country, on the average, more than three persons apply for each medical-school place available to entering first-year students, and there is as yet no sign of a leveling off. Paradoxically, this is happening during a period when medicine and the medical profession are being subjected to increased scrutiny and criticism.

Complex, and by no means consistent, the process of medicalization is not an easy one to analyze. Several preliminary *caveats* seem in order. In part, they are prompted by two sorts of assumptions made by critics of medicalization in America: one is that the central and pervasive position of health, illness, and medicine in present-day American society is historically and culturally unique, and the other, that it is primarily a result of the self-interested maneuvers of the medical profession. Neither of these assumptions is true without qualification.

To begin with, in all societies, health, illness, and medicine constitute a nexus of great symbolic as well as structural importance, involving and interconnecting biological, social, psychological, and cultural systems of action. In every society, health, illness, and medicine are related to the physical and psychic integrity of individuals, their ability to establish and maintain solidary relations with others, their capacities to perform social roles, their birth, survival, and death, and to the ultimate kinds of "human condition" questions that are associated with these concerns. As such, health, illness, and medicine also involve and affect every major institution of a society, and its basic cultural grounding. The family, for example, is profoundly involved in the health and illness of its members, and, especially in nonmodern societies, the kinship system is as responsible for health and illness as are specialized medical practitioners. The institutions of science, magic, and religion are the major media through which the "hows" and "whys" of health and illness, life and death are addressed in a society, and through which culturally appropriate action for dealing with them is taken. The economy is also involved in several ways: the allocation of resources that health, illness, and medicine entail; the occupational division of labor relevant to diagnosis and therapy; and the bearing of health and illness on the individual's capacity and motivation for work. The deviance and social-control aspects of illness have important implications for the polity which, in turn, is responsible for the organized enforcement of health measures that pertain to the community or public welfare. And in all societies, the influence, power, and prestige that accrue to medical practitioners implicate the magico-religious and stratification systems as well as the polity.

As the foregoing implies, there are certain respects in which health, illness, and medicine are imbued with a more diffuse and sacred kind of significance in nonmodern than in modern societies. For example, in traditional and neotraditional Central African societies, the meaning of health and illness, the diagnosis and treatment of sickness, and the wisdom, efficacy, and power of medical practitioners are not only more closely linked with the institutions of kinship, religion, and magic than in American society; they are also more closely connected with the overarching cosmic view through which the whole society defines and orients itself. One indication of the larger matrix into which health, illness, and medicine fit in such a society is that in numerous Central African languages the same words can mean medicine, magico-religious charms, and metaphysically important qualities such as strength, fecundity, and invulnerability, which are believed to be supernaturally conferred.

In the light of the multi-institutional and the cultural significance of health, illness, and medicine in all societies it is both illogical and unlikely to believe that the current process of medicalization in American society has been engineered and maintained primarily by one group, namely, the physicians. What the manifestations of medicalization that we have identified do suggest, however, is that the health-illness-medical sector has progressively acquired a more general cultural meaning in American society than it had in the past (Knowles, 1977).

Within this framework, the medicalization process entails the assertion of various individual and collective rights to which members of the society feel entitled and which they express as "health," "quality of life," and "quality of death." The process also involves heightened awareness of a whole range of imperfections, injustices, dangers, and afflictions that are perceived to exist in the society, a protest against them, and a resolve to take action that is more therapeutic than punitive. Medicalization represents an exploration and affirmation of values and beliefs that not only pertain to the ultimate grounding of the society, but also to the human condition, more encompassingly and existentially conceived.

Thus, in American society, health and illness have come to symbolize many positively and negatively valued biological, physical, social, cultural, and metaphysical phenomena. Increasingly, health has become a coded way of referring to an individually, socially, or cosmically ideal state of affairs. Conversely, the concept of illness has increasingly been applied to modes of thinking, feeling, and behaving that are considered undesirably variant or deviant, as well as to more forms of suffering and disability. In turn, this medicalization of deviance and suffering has had a network of consequences.

Talcott Parsons' well-known formulation of the "sick role"* provides important insights into what these effects have been. According to him, the sick role consists of two interrelated sets of exemptions and obligations. A person who is defined as ill is exonerated from certain kinds of responsibility for his illness. He is not held morally accountable for the fact that he is sick (it is not considered to be his "fault"), and he is not expected to make himself better by "good motivation" or high resolve without the help of others. In addition, he is viewed as someone whose capacity to function normally is impaired, and who is therefore relieved of some of his usual familial, occupational, and civic activities and responsibilities. In exchange for these exemptions which are conditionally granted, the sick individual is expected to define the state of being ill as aberrant and undesirable, and to do everything possible to facilitate his recovery from it. In the case of illness of any moment, the responsibility to try to get well also entails the obligation to seek professionally competent help. In a modern Western society, such as the United States, this obligation involves a willingness to confer with a medically trained person, usually a physician, and to undergo the modes of diagnosis and treatment that are recommended, including the ministrations of other medical professionals and hospitalization. Upon entering this relationship with institutionalized medicine and its professional practitioners, an

---

*Talcott Parsons' formulation of the sick role is the most important single concept in the field of the sociology of medicine. For his own elaboration of this concept, see, especially, Parsons (1964, pp. 428-79; 1975).

individual with a health problem becomes a patient. By cooperating and collaborating with the medical professionals caring for him, the patient is expected to work toward recovery, or, at least, toward the more effective management of his illness.

The fact that the exemptions and the obligations of sickness have been extended to people with a widening arc of attitudes, experiences, and behaviors in American society means primarily that what is regarded as "conditionally legitimate deviance" has increased. Although illness is defined as deviance from the desirable and the normal, it is not viewed as reprehensible in the way that either sin or crime is. The sick person is neither blamed nor punished as those considered sinful or criminal are. So long as he does not abandon himself to illness or eagerly embrace it, but works actively on his own and with medical professionals to improve his condition, he is considered to be responding appropriately, even admirably, to an unfortunate occurrence. Under these conditions, illness is accepted as legitimate deviance. But this also implies that medical professionals have acquired an increasingly important social-control function in the society. They are the principal agents responsible for certifying, diagnosing, treating, and preventing illness. Because a greater proportion of deviance in American society is now seen as illness, the medical profession plays a vastly more important role than it once did in defining and regulating deviance and in trying to forestall and remedy it.

The economic, political, and legal indicators of a progressive medicalization cited above also have complex origins and implications. For example, the fact that activities connected with health, illness, and medicine represent a rising percentage of the gross national product in the United States is a consequence of the fee-for-service system under which American health care delivery is organized; the central importance of the modern hospital in medical care; the mounting personnel, equipment, and maintenance costs that the operation of the hospital entails; and the development of new medical and surgical procedures and of new drugs, most of which are as expensive as they are efficacious. Some of this increase in costs results from the desire for profits that medical professionals, hospital administrators, and members of the pharmaceutical industry share to varying degrees. But how much is difficult is ascertain, though radical ideological criticisms and defensive conservative statements on the point are both rife at present.

In addition to such political and economic factors, the heightened commitment to health as a right and the medicalization of deviance have also contributed to the growth of health expenditures. Because health is both more coveted and more inclusively defined, and because a greater amount of medical therapeutic activity is applied to deviance-defined-as-illness, increasing economic resources are being invested in the health-illness-medicine sector of the society.

The political and legal prominence of questions of health care and medicine in American society at the present time reflects in part a widespread national discontent with the way medical care is organized, financed, and delivered, and with some of the attitudes and behaviors of physicians. The inequities that exist in access to care, and in its technical and interpersonal excellence, are among the primary foci of political and legal activities. Another major area of current political and legal action concerns the internal and external regulation of the medical profession better to insure that it uses its knowledge and skill in a socially as well as medically responsible way, and that it is adequately accountable both to patients and to the public at large. Various new measures, which represent a mixture of controls from within the medical profession and from outside it, have been set into motion. For example, in 1972, the Professional Standards Review Organization was established through the passage of amendments to the Social Security Act which were designed to provide quality assessment and assurance, utilization review, and cost control, primarily for Medicare and Medicaid patients. Over the course of the years 1966 through 1971, a series of government regulations were passed which mandate peer review for all biomedical research involving human subjects, supported by the Department of Health, Education, and Welfare (and its subunits, the National Institutes of Health and the Public Health Service), as well as by the Food and Drug Administration. In 1975, the American College of Surgeons and the American Surgical Association set forth a plan for systematically decreasing the number of newly graduated doctors entering surgical training. In part, this plan represented an organized, intraprofessional attempt to deal with what appears to be an oversupply of surgeons in the United States, and thereby to reduce the possibility that federal health manpower legislation would have to be passed to remedy this maldistribution.

The fact that an extraordinary number of young people are opting for careers in health, particularly as physicians, is the final concomitant of medicalization previously mentioned. Reliable and valid data are not available to explain the mounting wave of young persons who have been attracted to medicine since the 1960s. We do not know as much as we should about how they resemble their predecessors, or differ from them. We are aware that more women, blacks, and members of other minority groups are being admitted to medical school than in the past, partly because of "affirmative action" legislation. But we do not have overall information about the characteristics of those who are accepted as compared with those who are not. Only sketchy materials are available on the impact of those changes in medical school curricula during the past decade that were designed to make students more aware of the social and ethical dimensions of their commitment to medicine. We do not know whether their attitudes, their professional decisions, or their medical practice actually changed. More data are needed before we can interpret the short- and long-term implications of the rush of college youth toward medicine. As premedical and medical students themselves are first to testify, the prestige, authority, "power," autonomy, and financial rewards of medicine attract them and their peers to medicine, along with scientific interests, clinical impulses, and humanitarian concerns. But there is also evidence to suggest that even among those who readily contend that their reasons for choosing medicine are self-interested, a "new" medical-student orientation has been emerging. In fact, the very candor that medical students exhibit —and in some cases flaunt—when they insist that, regrettably, like their predecessors, their competitiveness, desire for achievement, and need for security have drawn them into medicine is part of this new orientation. Activist and meditative, as well as critical and self-critical, the "new medical student" not only wants to bring about change in the medical profession, but to do so in a way that affects other aspects of the society as well. The structural and symbolic meaning acquired by health, illness, and medicine has led such students to hope that their influence will be far-reaching as well as meliorative. How many students with this ostensibly "new" orientation will maintain it throughout their medical training and whether their entrance into the profession will significantly alter the future course of medicalization in American society remain to be seen (Fox, 1974, pp. 197-227).

Along with progressive medicalization, a process of demedicalization seems also to be taking place in the society. To some extent the signs of demedicalization are reactions to what is felt by various individuals and groups to be a state of "*over*medicalization." One of the most significant manifestations of this countertrend is the mounting concern over implications that have arisen from the continuously expanding conception of "sickness" in the society. Commentators on this process would not necessarily agree with Peter Sedgwick (1973) that it will continue to "the point where everybody has become so luxuriantly ill" that perhaps sickness will no longer be "in" and a "backlash" will be set in motion; they may not envision such an engulfing state of societally defined illness. But many observers from diverse professional backgrounds have published works in which they express concern about the "coercive" aspects of the "label" illness and the treatment of illness by medical professionals in medical institutions (in addition to Illich, 1975, and Kittrie, 1971, see, for example, Carlson, 1975; Foucault, 1967; Freidson, 1970; Goffman, 1961; Laing, 1967; Scheff, 1966; Szasz, 1961; and Waitzkin and Waterman, 1974). The admonitory perspectives on the enlarged domain of illness and medicine that these works of social science and social criticism represent appear to have gained the attention of young physicians- and nurses-in-training interested in change, and various consumer and civil rights groups interested in health care.

This emerging view emphasizes the degree to which what is defined as health and illness, normality and abnormality, sanity and insanity varies from one society, culture, and historical period to another. Thus, it is contended, medical diagnostic categories such as "sick," "abnormal," and "insane" are not universal, objective, or necessarily reliable. Rather, they are culture-, class-, and time-bound, often ethnocentric, and as much artifacts of the preconceptions of socially biased observers as they are valid summaries of the characteristics of the observed. In this view, illness (especially mental illness) is largely a mythical construct, created and enforced by the society. The hospitals to which seriously ill persons are confined are portrayed as "total institutions": segregated, encompassing, depersonalizing organizations, "dominated" by physicians who are disinclined to convey information to patients about their conditions, or to encourage paramedical personnel to do so. These "oppressive" and "countertherapeutic" attributes of the hospital environment are seen as emanating from the professional ideology of physicians and the kind of hierarchical relationships that they establish with patients and other medical professionals partly as a consequence of this ideology, as well as from the bureaucratic and technological features of the hospital itself. Whatever their source, the argument continues, the characteristics of the hospital and of the doctor-patient relationship increase the "powerlessness" of the sick person, "maintain his uncertainty," and systematically "mortify" and "curtail" the "self" with which he enters the sick role and arrives at the hospital door.

This critical perspective links the labeling of illness, the "imperialist" outlook and capitalist behavior of physicians, the "stigmatizing" and "dehumanizing" experiences of patients, and the problems of the health care system more generally to imperfections and injustices in the society as a whole. Thus, for example, the various forms of social inequality, prejudice, discrimination, and acquisitive self-interest that persist in capitalistic American society are held responsible for causing illness, as well as for contributing to the undesirable attitudes and actions of physicians and other medical professionals. Casting persons in the sick role is regarded as a powerful, latent way for the society to exact conformity and maintain the status quo. For it allows a semi-approved form of deviance to occur which siphons off potential for insurgent protest and which can be controlled through the supervision or, in some cases, the "enforced therapy" of the medical profession. Thus, however permissive and merciful it may be to expand the category of illness, these observers point out, there is always the danger that the society will become a "therapeutic state" that excessively restricts the "right to be different" and the right to dissent. They feel that this danger may already have reached serious proportions in this society through its progressive medicalization.

The criticism of medicalization and the advocacy of demedicalization have not been confined to rhetoric. Concrete steps have been taken to declassify certain conditions as illness. Most notable among these is the American Psychiatric Association's decision to remove homosexuality from its official catalogue ("nomenclature") of mental disorders. In addition, serious efforts have been made to heighten physicians' awareness of the fact that because they share certain prejudiced, often unconscious assumptions about women, they tend to overattribute psychological conditions to their female patients. Thus, for example, distinguished medical publications such as the *New England Journal of Medicine* have featured articles and editorials on the excessive readiness with which medical specialists and textbook authors accept the undocumented belief that dysmenorrhea, nausea of pregnancy, pain in labor, and infantile colic are all psychogenic disorders, caused or aggravated by women's emotional problems. Another related development is feminist protest against what is felt to be a too great tendency to define pregnancy as an illness, and childbirth as a "technologized" medical-surgical event, prevailed over by the obstetrician-gynecologist. These sentiments have contributed to the preference that many middle-class couples have shown for natural childbirth in recent years, and to the revival of midwifery. The last example also illustrates an allied movement, namely a growing tendency to shift some responsibility for medical care and authority over it from the physician, the medical team, and hospital to the patient, the family, and the home.

A number of attempts to "destratify" the doctor's relationships with patients and with other medical professionals and to make them more open and egalitarian have developed. "Patients' rights" are being asserted and codified, and, in some states, drafted into law. Greater emphasis is being placed, for example, on the patient's "right to treatment," right to information (relevant to diagnosis, therapy, prognosis, or to the giving of knowledgeable consent for any procedure), right to privacy and confidentiality, and right to be "allowed to die," rather than being "kept alive by artificial means or heroic measures . . . if the situation should arise in which there is no reasonable expectation of . . . recovery from physical or mental disability."*

In some medical milieux (for example, community health centers and health maintenance organizations), and in critical and self-consciously progressive writings about medicine, the term "client" or "consumer" is being substituted for "patient." This change in terminology is intended to underline the importance of preventing illness while stressing the desirability of a nonsupine, nonsubordinate relationship for those who seek care to those who provide it. The emergence of nurse-practitioners and physician's assistants on the American scene is perhaps the most significant sign that some blurring of the physician's supremacy vis-à-vis other medical professionals may also be taking place. For some of the responsibilities for diagnosis, treatment, and patient management that were formerly prerogatives of physicians have been incorporated into these new, essentially marginal roles (Rogers, 1977).

Enjoinders to patients to care for themselves rather than to rely so heavily on the services of medical professionals and institutions are more frequently heard. Much attention is being given to studies such as the one conducted by Lester Breslow and his colleagues at the University of California at Los Angeles which suggest that good health and longevity are as much related to a self-

*This particular way of requesting that one be allowed to die is excerpted from the "Living Will" (revised April, 1974, version), prepared and promoted by the Euthanasia Educational Council.

enforced regimen of sufficient sleep, regular, well-balanced meals, moderate exercise and weight, no smoking, and little or no drinking, as they are to professionally administered medical care. Groups such as those involved in the Women's Liberation Movement are advocating the social and psychic as well as the medical value of knowing, examining, and caring for one's own body. Self-therapy techniques and programs have been developed for conditions as complicated and grave as terminal renal disease and hemophilia A and B. Proponents of such regimens affirm that many aspects of managing even serious chronic illnesses can be handled safely at home by the patient and his family, who will, in turn, benefit both financially and emotionally. In addition, they claim that in many cases the biomedical results obtained seem superior to those of the traditional physician-administered, health care delivery system.

The underlying assumption in these instances is that, if self-care is collectivized and reinforced by mutual aid, not only will persons with a medical problem be freed from some of the exigencies of the sick role, but both personal and public health will thereby improve, all with considerable savings in cost. This point of view is based on the moral supposition that greater autonomy from the medical profession coupled with greater responsibility for self and others in the realm of health and illness is an ethically and societally superior state.

We have the medicine we deserve. We freely choose to live the way we do. We choose to live recklessly, to abuse our bodies with what we consume, to expose ourselves to environmental insults, to rush frantically from place to place, and to sit on our spreading bottoms and watch paid professionals exercise for us. . . . Today few patients have the confidence to care for themselves. The inexorable professionalization of medicine, together with reverence for the scientific method, have invested practitioners with sacrosanct powers, and correspondigly vitiated the responsibility of the rest of us for health. . . . What is tragic is not what has happened to the revered professions, but what has happened to us as a result of professional dominance. In times of inordinate complexity and stress we have been made a profoundly dependent people. Most of us have lost the ability to care for ourselves. . . . I have tried to demonstrate three propositions. First, medical care has less impact on health than is generally assumed. Second, medical care has less impact on health than have social and environmental factors. And third, given the way in which society is evolving and the evolutionary imperatives of the medical care system, medical care in the future will have even less impact on health than it has now. . . . We have not understood what health is. . . . But in the next few decades our understanding will deepen. The pursuit of health and of well-being will then be possible, but only if our environment is made safe for us to live in and our social order is transformed to foster health, rather than suppress joy. If not, we shall remain a sick and dependent people. . . . The end of medicine is not the end of health but the beginning. . . .

The foregoing passage (excerpted from Rick Carlson's book, *The End of Medicine,* pp. 41, 141, 203-31) touches upon many of the demedicalization themes that have been discussed. It proclaims the desirability of demedicalizing

American society, predicting that, if we do so, we can overcome the "harm" that excessive medicalization has brought in its wake and progress beyond the "limits" that it has set. Like most critics of medicalization on the American scene, Carlson inveighs against the way that medical care is currently organized and implemented, but he attaches exceptional importance to the health-illness-medical sector of the society. In common with other commentators, he views health, illness, and medicine as inextricably associated with values and beliefs of American tradition that are both critical and desirable. It is primarily for this reason that in spite of the numerous signs that certain *structural* changes in the delivery of care will have occurred by the time we reach the year 2000, American society is not likely to undergo a significant process of *cultural* demedicalization.

Dissatisfaction with the distribution of professional medical care in the United States, its costs, and its accessibility has become sufficiently acute and generalized to make the enactment of a national health insurance system in the foreseeable future likely. Exactly what form that system should take still evokes heated debate about free enterprise and socialism, public and private regulation, national and local government, tax rates, deductibles and co-insurance, the right to health care, the equality principle, and the principle of distributive justice. But the institutionalization of a national system that will provide more extensive and equitable health insurance protection now seems necessary as well as inevitable even to those who do not approve of it.

There is still another change in the health-illness-medicine area of the society that seems to be forthcoming and that, like national health insurance, would alter the structure within which care is delivered. This is the movement toward effecting greater equality, collegiality, and accountability in the relationship of physicians to patients and their families, to other medical professionals, and to the lay public. Attempts to reduce the hierarchical dimension in the physician's role, as well as the increased insistence on patient's rights, self-therapy, mutual medical aid, community medical services and care by nonphysician health professionals, and the growth of legislative and judicial participation in health and medicine by both federal and local government are all part of this movement. There is reason to believe that, as a consequence of pressure from both outside and inside the medical profession, the doctor will become less "dominant" and "autonomous," and will be subject to more controls.

This evolution in the direction of greater egalitarianism and regulation notwithstanding, it seems unlikely that all elements of hierarchy and autonomy will, or even can, be eliminated from the physician's role. For that to occur, the medical knowledge, skill, experience, and responsibility of patients and paramedical professionals would have to equal, if not replicate, the physician's. In addition, the social and psychic meaning of health and illness would have to become trivial in order to remove all vestiges of institutionalized charisma from the physician's role. Health, illness, and medicine have never been viewed casually in any society and, as indicated, they seem to be gaining rather than losing importance in American society.

It is significant that often the discussions and developments relevant to the destratification and control of the physician's role and to the enactment of national health insurance are accompanied by reaffirmations of traditional American values: equality, independence, self-reliance, universalism, distributive justice, solidarity, reciprocity, and individual and community responsibility. What seems to be involved here is not so much a change in values as the initiation of action intended to modify certain structural features of American medicine, so that it will more fully realize long-standing societal values.

In contrast, the new emphasis on health as a right, along with the emerging perspective on illness as medically and socially engendered, seems to entail major conceptual rather than structural shifts in the health-illness-medical matrix of the society. These shifts are indicative of a less fatalistic and individualistic attitude toward illness, increased personal and communal espousal of health, and a spreading conviction that health is as much a consequence of the good life and the good society as it is of professional medical care. The strongest impetus for demedicalization comes from this altered point of view. It will probably contribute to the decategorization of certain conditions as illness, greater appreciation and utilization of nonphysician medical professionals, the institutionalization of more preventive medicine and personal and public health measures, and, perhaps, to the undertaking of nonmedical reforms (such as full employment, improved transportation, or adequate recreation) in the name of the ultimate goal of health.

However, none of these trends implies that what we have called *cultural* demedicalization will take place. The shifts in emphasis from illness to health, from therapeutic to preventive medicine, and from the dominance and autonomy of the doctor to patient's rights and greater control of the medical profession do not alter the fact that health, illness, and medicine are central preoccupations in the society which have diffuse symbolic as well as practical meaning. All signs suggest that they will maintain the social, ethical, and existential significance they have acquired, even though by the year 2000 some structural aspects of the way that medicine and care are organized and delivered may have changed. In fact, if the issues now being considered under the rubric of bioethics are predictive of what lies ahead, we can expect that in the future, health, illness, and medicine will acquire even greater importance as one of the primary symbolic media through which American society will grapple with fundamental questions of value and belief. What social mechanisms we will develop to come to terms with these "collective conscience" issues, and exactly what role physicians, health professionals, biologists, jurists, politicians, philosophers, theologians, social scientists, and the public at large will play in their resolution remains to be seen. But it is a distinctive characteristic of an advanced modern society like our own that scientific, technical, clinical, social, ethical, and religious concerns should be joined in this way.

REFERENCES

Carlson, R. J. *The End of Medicine.* New York: John Wiley & Sons, 1975.

Foucault, M. *Madness and Civilization.* New York: Random House, 1967.

Fox, R. C. "The Process of Professional Socialization: Is There a 'New' Medical Student? A Comparative View of Medical Socialization in the 1950's and the 1970's." *Ethics in Health Care,* edited by L. R. Tancredi. Washington, D.C.: National Academy of Sciences, 1974.

Freidson, E. *Professional Dominance.* Chicago: Aldine, 1970.

Goffman, E. *Asylums.* New York: Doubleday, 1961.

Illich, I. *Medical Nemesis: The Expropriation of Health.* New York: Pantheon, 1975.

Kass, L. R. "Regarding the End of Medicine and the Pursuit of Health." *The Public Interest* 40 (Summer 1975): 11.

Kittrie, N. N. *The Right To Be Different: Deviance and Enforced Therapy.* Baltimore: Johns Hopkins, 1971.

Knowles, J. H. "The Responsibility of the Individual." *Daedalus* (Winter 1977).

Laing, R. D. *The Politics of Experience.* New York: Ballantine, 1967.

Parsons, T. *The Social System.* Glencoe, Ill.: Free Press, 1964.

Parsons, T. "The Sick Role and the Role of the Physician Reconsidered." *Milbank Memorial Fund Quarterly, Health and Society* (Summer 1975): 257-77.

Rogers, D. "The Challenge of Primary Care." *Daedalus* (Winter 1977).

Scheff, T. J. *Being Mentally Ill.* Chicago: Aldine, 1966.

Sedgwick, P. "Illness—Mental and Otherwise." *The Hastings Center Studies* 1, no. 3 (1973): 37.

Szasz, T. S. *The Myth of Mental Illness.* New York: Harper & Row, 1961.

Waitzkin, H. D., and Waterman, B. *The Exploitation of Illness in Capitalist Society.* Indianapolis: Bobbs-Merrill, 1974.

Zola, I. K. "Culture and Symptoms—An Analysis of Patients' Presenting Complaints." *American Sociological Review* 31, no. 5 (October 1966): 615-16.

Selection by Howard H. Hiatt

In 1968, in an article called "The Tragedy of the Commons," Garrett Hardin discussed a class of human problems that in his view had no technical solution. Focusing on the population problem, Hardin likened our present dilemma to that of a group of herdsmen whose cattle shared a common pasture. As long as the number of animals was small in relation to the capacity of the pasture, each herdsman could increase his holdings without detriment to the general welfare. As the number of cattle approached the capacity of the land, however, each additional animal contributed to overgrazing. Any single herdsman attempting to maximize his own gain could reasonably project that the addition of one or a few cattle to his holdings would have minimal effect on the general welfare. All herdsmen reasoning and acting individually in this fashion, however, would destroy the commons. "Ruin," concluded Hardin, "is the destination toward which all men rush, each pursuing his own best interest in a society that believes in the freedom of the commons. Freedom in a commons brings ruin to all."

The total resources available for medical care can be viewed as analogous to the grazing area on Hardin's commons, and the practices drawing on those resources to Hardin's grazing animals. Surely, nobody would quarrel with the proposition that there is a limit to the resources any society can devote to medical care, and few would question the suggestion that we are approaching such a limit. Yet there is almost universal recognition that among the additional demands that must be made on our resources are those designed to address the

Reprinted by permission from "Protecting the Medical Commons: Who Is Responsible?," *New England Journal of Medicine* 293, no. 5 (July 31, 1975), pp. 235-41.

current inadequacy of medical care for large sectors of the population. The dilemma confronting us is how we can place additional stress on the medical commons without bringing ourselves closer to ruin.

In our society, demands from both preventive and curative medicine are made upon the same commons and therefore must be regarded as in competition with each other and with needs for research and teaching. Priority setting is further complicated by the inadequacy of data that are critical to intelligent decision making. Failure to recognize these realities has in the past often led to unwise policy setting, without due consideration of long-term consequences. We need to consider problems arising from ways in which the medical commons has traditionally been used and the need for alternative approaches.

First of all, let us look at a principle on which medical practice has been based—that one should do everything possible for the individual patient. Let us then examine this principle in the context of our system, in which few constraints are placed upon the introduction of new medical practices. I believe this is a luxury we can no longer afford. As we develop more and more practices that may be beneficial to the individual but not to the interests of society, we risk reaching a point where marginal gains to individuals threaten the welfare of the whole.

Secondly, we must examine another consequence of freedom of access to the medical commons: the utilization of precious resources for practices that benefit neither the individual nor society, and that indeed are frequently harmful to both. Such practices are especially important in a campaign to reduce demands on the medical commons, for their elimination would benefit both individual and society.

Thirdly, there is a widely accepted but narrow interpretation of health as an exclusively medical concern, which, together with a failure to appreciate fully the limitations of curative medicine, contributes to continuing raids on the commons by expensive practices. At best, many of these deal imperfectly with conditions that could be prevented by less costly approaches.

Although no one should be optimistic that we can rapidly change existing practices and thereby redirect resources to other pressing needs, an examination of a few of our present problems may be useful, especially in preventing their replication, and possibly in contributing to their amelioration.

MEDICAL PRACTICES THAT POSE CONFLICTS BETWEEN THE INTERESTS OF THE INDIVIDUAL AND THOSE OF SOCIETY

An infant born with agammaglobulinemia has markedly reduced resistance to and may die from infection. The test for detecting the condition is simple and relatively inexpensive. Once the condition is diagnosed, one can immediately institute treatment that will prevent or ameliorate serious infections. However, the condition is so rare that in a society with limited resources it would be difficult to argue for a universal screening campaign, even though it might prevent serious illness and occasionally even death among a few infants.

Detection of agammaglobulinemia may be an extreme case, but a sensitive one nonetheless. Even more troubling are questions that arise concerning more prevalent conditions. A most poignant example today may be kidney dialysis and transplantation, access to which has been largely determined by economic and geographic considerations. Other procedures pose similar questions. If coronary-artery bypass graft operations were shown to be effective for all patients with coronary-artery disease, if an effective artificial heart were found, if the artificial pancreas now being investigated were shown to be potentially useful to the estimated four million Americans with diabetes, what fraction of our resources should be given to these measures, and at what cost to others dependent on the commons?

A decision that may shortly be before us provides another example. A recent report (Liberthson et al., 1974) suggested that trained prehospital rescue units may contribute to increased survival of patients with cardiac arrest. The report described 301 subjects with prehospital ventricular fibrillation for whom the rescue units were used. For the forty-two who survived to leave the hospital, the mean survival period was 12.7 months (and five of the survivors required long-term case for brain damage). For discussion purposes, let us grant that such an approach to patients with cardiac arrest did save these lives. Reasoned decision making would then require that society first ascertain the cost per life saved and determine whether a universal program of implementation were worthy of further consideration. Two critical questions would be: What can really be achieved? Are the benefits of wide application such as to warrant displacing something else? In raising such questions, it is essential to recognize the needs for continuing research in medical care, such as that represented by the study on the rescue units, on the one hand, and for decision making regarding the dissemination of new practices, once proved effective, on the other.

A deeply troubling (and perhaps insoluble) ethical dilemma comes sharply into focus when we attempt to set a monetary value on a human life. However, the dilemma is unnecessarily intensified by a widespread misconception that the principal objective of medical practice is the prevention of death. Bunker (1974) points out that only a small fraction of surgery and a much smaller fraction of nonsurgical encounters involve life-and-death decisions, most being directed at the provision of relief from physical or emotional discomfort or disability. In these circumstances we must think in such terms as which measures will provide greater relief, which conditions are more burdensome, and which patients are in greater need of help. Although these questions are obviously thorny ones, they provide a more common framework for discussion of tradeoffs than attempts to relate the value of a life to the resources of the commons. The latter question, too, must be dealt with, but much less often than the former.

The issues that arise with regionalization of medical resources seem so much easier to resolve that one wonders why they are so prevalent. Early in the 1960s, for example, it was found that of almost 800 hospitals in the United States equipped for closed heart surgery, over 90 percent did fewer than one case per week, and 30 percent had done none in the year studied (Maxwell, 1974). Although regionalization may sometimes lead to inconvenience and questions of "status" (some take pride in having "everything" locally available), the drawbacks seem trivial when compared, first, to the medical advantage of having such complicated procedures carried out by specialists whose skills are honed on a continuous basis and, second, to the obvious economic benefits.

MEDICAL PRACTICES OF NO VALUE OR OF UNDETERMINED VALUE

Nancy Mitford (1966) may have been indulging in literary license when she predicted that "in another two hundred and fifty years present day doctors may seem to our descendants as barbarous as Fagon and his colleagues seem to us. . . . In those days, terrifying in black robes and bonnets, they bled the patient; now, terrifying in white robes and masks, they pump blood into him." Wholesale bloodletting disappeared from our "therapeutic" kit long ago, but within my own professional lifetime, I recall seeing patients "treated" for multiple sclerosis by having blood pumped into them until they were polycythemic.

How do we determine which practices should be discarded and which continued? More than twenty years ago the British statistician Sir Austin Bradford Hill demonstrated the importance to medical investigation of the randomized controlled trial, which had been developed earlier in agriculture by R. A. Fisher. It was used for testing the Salk vaccine, and partly as a result, when the field trials of the vaccine were completed, the vaccine's usefulness had been unequivocally proved.

One could cite a substantial number of procedures that were at one time practiced rather widely in this country, many of them within relatively recent years, but that have now been virtually abandoned. Such a list might include gastric freezing for peptic ulcer, colectomy for epilepsy, bilateral hypogastric-artery ligation for pelvic hemorrhage, renal-capsule stripping for acute renal failure, sympathectomy for asthma, internal-mammary-artery ligation for coronary-artery disease, the "button" operation for ascites, adrenalectomy for essential hypertension, complete dental extraction for a variety of complaints thought to be the result of focal sepsis, lobotomy for many mental disorders, and wiring for aortic aneurysm. It is interesting that most of these practices disappeared not because better procedures came along (which would have been an appropriate reason) but because they were found ultimately to be without value. No careful pilot studies were undertaken to evaluate them at the time they were introduced. As a result, even though some merited introduction on an experimental basis, they remained on the medical commons much too long, at costs that went beyond those of the economic resources inappropriately used.

A number of other medical practices, shown or suggested to be without merit, remain with us. For example, treating critical phases of acute illnesses in intensive-care units has become an established practice in many general hospitals over the past decade. Griner (1972) compared adult patients suffering from pulmonary edema of nonsurgical causes who were admitted to the intensive-care unit of a university hospital with those admitted to a general medical floor immediately before the opening of the special unit. His studies revealed no difference in mortality and a slightly but not significantly increased duration of stay for patients in the unit. In Griner's words, "The most noticeable change in the overall experience of adult patients hospitalized with acute pulmonary edema . . . since the opening of an intensive care unit has been a marked increase in the cost of rendering care to these patients." (Note that charges for a day of care on the general medical services of one Boston teaching hospital at present average $250; charges for a day on the intensive-care unit exceed $400!) The Griner study requires confirmation, particularly since his "control" group may have differed from the experimental. But if it were proved valid, what steps might be taken to protect the commons?

Although tonsillectomy surely has a place in medical practice, some pediatricians suggest that over 90 percent of the one million children who underwent tonsillectomies last year in the United States did so unnecessarily. Consistent with this estimate, one study showed a greater than tenfold difference in the procedure from one area to another in the same state (Wennberg and Gittelsohn, 1973). If 90 percent is a reasonable approximation, the $400 million taken from the medical commons for this purpose might have been reduced to less than $40 million, the number of hospital days required for people undergoing this operation might have been reduced proportionately, and the number of deaths, using only a conservative estimate of deaths expected from general anesthesia alone, might have been cut from seventy to seven. The reduction in human suffering, of course, cannot be described in such quantitative terms.

Oral hypoglycemic agents were initially hailed as an alternative to insulin injections for many diabetic patients. Randomized clinical trials, however, gave evidence, first published over five years ago (University Group Diabetes Program, 1970; Knatterud et al., 1971), of increased cardiovascular disease, which in the view of most experts outweighs any possible short-term benefits of the drugs. Nonetheless, according to a rough estimate based on the number of prescriptions written and the prescription renewal rate, 1.4 million Americans were taking these compounds last year. This figure has gone up progressively over the years despite increasing adverse evidence concerning the usefulness of the drugs (Committee for the Assessment of Biometric Aspects of Controlled Trials of Hypoglycemic Agents, 1975).

It is important to recognize that randomized trials cannot always be done (Jaffe et al., 1974; Weinstein, 1974), but the problem is compounded in dealing with practices already adopted. Once disseminated, a practice is not quickly abandoned, even after it has been shown ineffective—another strong reason for careful evaluation before widespread adoption of new procedures. Let us consider the drain on resources resulting from a few practices whose true usefulness still remains to be established.

At present, there are few hospitals without coronary-care units. There is no disputing the cost they have added to our medical bills, but there is much debate about their effects on mortality from myocardial infarction (Astvad et al., 1974; Martin et al., 1974).

Cytologic examination of uterine cervical secretions is commonly assumed to be responsible for the acknowledged recent decline in deaths from carcinoma of the uterine cervix. However, this cause-and-effect connection has by no means been conclusively demonstrated. Since the death rate began falling some years before there was widespread use of the examination, and, further, since the rate of decline has been much the same in different areas, irrespective of the proportion of women screened (Mitchell, 1971; Kinlen and Doll, 1973), serious questions must be raised concerning the role of the procedure.

These data emphasize the need for further evidence and cast considerable doubt on the justifiability of the enormous drain of resources. However, both the coronary-care unit and cervical cytologic examination are so much a part of the medical culture that it now seems impossible to carry out proper evaluation. Indeed, one effect of premature adoption is to place ethical difficulties in the way of truly controlled trials.

A present case in point may be coronary-artery bypass graft operations. It is estimated that 38,000 such procedures were carried out in the United States in 1973, at a cost in excess of $400 million. Almost 400 hospitals are believed to have bypass teams, and one of the strongest proponents for this approach to management of coronary-artery disease was recently quoted as having said that the United States should prepare to do 80,000 coronary arteriograms a day (*Medical World News,* 1974). Rough calculations indicate that such a radiologic assessment alone would cost in excess of $10 billion a year and would average one catheterization for every American every ten years. If today's ratio of arteriograms to bypass surgery were to prevail, the cost of the resultant surgery would exceed $100 billion a year, a figure almost equivalent to the total resources now on the commons!

The current absence of regulatory mechanisms for dissemination of such procedures offers little hope for restraints, even long enough for proper evaluation. Ironically enough, in the absence of regulatory mechanisms, national health insurance, particularly if limited to catastrophic events, could accelerate premature application of this and similar costly procedures.

At an earlier stage of utilization is the computerized axial tomograph machine for radiologic examination. The capital cost of each machine is nearly $400,000. It permits extremely sophisticated diagnostic studies of the brain without the need for invasive procedures, and may prove an important addition to the diagnostic armamentarium. However, its role remains to be established. Furthermore, it requires more highly specialized personnel, and there already is evidence of its being used for purposes for which much simpler equipment is adequate. Will we be able to establish guidelines for the purchase and use of this machine before it, too, becomes a prominent and unregulated occupant of the medical commons?

MEDICAL PRACTICES FOR POTENTIALLY PREVENTABLE CONDITIONS

There are at present substantial claims on our resources that could be reduced appreciably on the basis of existing knowledge. The savings in lives, disability, and money resulting from polio vaccine are often and appropriately cited as evidence of a triumph of modern medical research. However, carelessness in prophylactic programs has recently led to a recrudescence of poliomyelitis. Another striking example was the increased incidence of measles that followed a decrease in distribution of measles vaccine (at least in part the result of decreased federal support). The annual number of reported cases of measles decreased from almost 500,000 in 1962 to 22,000 in 1968 (Landrigan and Conrad, 1971), but, with lessening of attention to control programs, rose again to a high of 75,000 in 1971. The incidence has since receded, but the need for constant attention is apparent. It has been estimated that the economic benefit of measles vaccine over a ten-year period exceeded $1.3 billion. The savings in terms of lives saved and cases of mental retardation averted (Barkin and Conrad, 1973) are even more important.

Fluoridation provides another example of how preventive measures can spare our resources. There is persuasive evidence that we could halve dental decay among children by fluoridation, at an annual cost of less than 20 cents per person. Nevertheless, less than 60 percent of the United States water supply was artificially fluoridated in 1972 (Maxwell, 1974).

Compensation paid last year in the United States by the Social Security Administration alone for victims of black lung exceeded $500 million. The physician, lacking specific treatment for this condition, is largely limited to treating complications and providing the emotional support required by patient and family. Although it is admittedly difficult to estimate the cost of preventing this condition, it seems likely that it would not begin to approach present costs in economic, let alone human, terms.

Although preventive medical care often has little effect where poor social conditions are allowed to persist (McDermott, Deuschle, and Barnett, 1972), this is not always the case (Alpert et al., 1968; Gordis, 1973). Gordis, for example, has shown that over a three-year period in an urban area with comprehensive medical care, rheumatic fever was about one third lower than in comparable parts of the same city without such care. The implications for reductions in valvular heart disease and nephritis are apparent, and the long-term economic effects would probably be highly beneficial.

There is, perhaps, even more evidence of how changes in social conditions can reduce demands on medical resources. For example, it is well known that, probably in large part because of improved nutrition, deaths from tuberculosis had fallen tenfold in Britain in the century before the first effective medical measures became available (McKeown and Lowe, 1974). Also highly relevant, although difficult to quantitate in terms of economic effects on the commons, are conclusions drawn from an examination of birth certificates for New York City for the year 1968. If a New York mother was white, native born, and a college graduate, her infant's chances of dying before his first birthday were nine per thousand. Corresponding chances for the infants of black, native born mothers with an elementary school education were fifty-one per thousand (Institute of Medicine, 1973).

Also difficult to deal with are conditions whose prevention requires changes in individual behavior. This year 70,000 American males will die of lung cancer—more than the total number of victims of the three next most common forms of cancer, well over 90 percent of all people with lung cancer, and approximately the same proportion killed by it more than twenty-five years ago. The admittedly impressive advances in cancer surgery, radiotherapy, chemotherapy, and anesthesia and in our understanding of certain aspects of carcinogenesis have had no effect on this or, in fact, on most prevalent forms of cancer. It is estimated that as much as 90 percent of all cancer in this country is the result of environmental factors. In lung cancer, cigarette smoking has unquestionably been implicated. How to respond to that information, thereby sparing the medical commons, remains a challenge. So far as other forms of cancer are concerned, has an adequate fraction of the massive resources committed to cancer programs been allocated to identifying carcinogens and to reducing exposure?

PROGRESS AND PROSPECTS IN HEALTH CARE DISTRIBUTION SYSTEMS

While we must draw further upon our resources to increase access to medical care for the people who are now underserved, the commons is clearly approaching depletion. This fact makes it the more urgent that new demands be limited to practices that have been conclusively demonstrated to meet well-defined needs. New practices must also be shown to be more important than whatever will be displaced as a result of their adoption.

McKeown (1973) points out that too often in medicine tasks are approached without any adequate survey of the nature of the most important problems. Now that there is generally successful management of infectious diseases, he emphasizes, the currently most pressing problems in Western societies are congenital disabilities, including mental defects, mental illness, and diseases of aging. Any approach designed to provide access to health care for an underserved population cannot purport to be comprehensive if it does not give serious attention to these problems. McKeown's list was neither offered as all-inclusive nor in fact was it intended to describe needs specific to the United States. In a study of children in a large urban American community, Kessner, Snow, and Singer (Institute of Medicine, 1974) found a shockingly high prevalence of all the conditions being investigated. More than one-fourth of children six months to three years old had anemia, and more than one-fourth of children four to eleven years of age failed a comprehensive vision screening examination. Twenty percent of all children had evidence of middle-ear disease, and 7 percent of those four to eleven years old had hearing loss in speech frequencies that could interfere with learning. Illustrating yet another kind of need, the studies of Brook et al. (1974) have shown that even by minimal criteria, only two-thirds of the patients discharged from a highly respected American teaching hospital had adequate follow-up care during the six months after discharge. For most of the other patients, any benefit derived from hospitalization had been lost by the time of the six-month evaluation interview. All these diverse needs point to the necessity of attention to deficiencies frequently found in planning the delivery of health care—deficiencies in collecting and evaluating information, in analyzing results, in determining costs, and in using valid data as a basis for action.

Admittedly, not all needs of an adequate medical care delivery system can be described in quantitative terms. One example in my view is the security implicit in the existence of an organized medical care system to which people can quickly and easily turn. There must be a telephone number that can be called at any time of day or night and that offers access to enlightened advice, and, if needed, entry into the system. The voice on the telephone need not be that of a physician; indeed, that would be wasteful. However, it is not too much to expect it to be that of a person who is concerned, compassionate, and informed, who has access to the caller's medical record, and who can offer practical and sensitive responses—that is, suggestions for effective action and reassurance appropriate to the problem. My own experience with a prepaid group practice left a strong impression that this service was as much appreciated as any other.

Like most contemporary medical dilemmas, assessing the quality of medical performance is easier to identify as a problem than to deal with. Economic as well as sociologic, psychologic, and other considerations suggest that medical care systems be arranged so that the skills of the medical care provider are matched to the job undertaken. Methods for continuing evaluation of performance would help to achieve this end and to promote flexibility as our capabilities improve.

Of course, medical care, no matter how well delivered, is not the sole solution to most of the health problems that confront us. Kessner's population was an urban one, and many of the deficiencies that he and his colleagues observed could be attributed more to the social, economic, or demographic characteristics of the children than to how or where they received medical care (Institute of Medicine, 1974). This is not an argument against the need for greater access to better medical care, for it would surely be possible to improve the medical situation described. Rather, it is a way to emphasize that changes in social factors—

housing, nutrition, education, etc.—are necessary in any comprehensive and effective approach to health problems.

The innovations that are needed or that are in prospect must be preceded by pilot tests. Not only is pretesting an integral part of any research endeavor, but as has been indicated, the difficulties of eliminating medical practices once they are widely disseminated make it imperative that there be rigorous evaluation.

WHO WILL PROTECT THE COMMONS?

It was not so long ago that the commons bore relatively few expensive practices, there were no well-defined limits, and the conscientious physician took from it what he deemed essential for his patient. Recently, however, we have witnessed major advances in expensive technology, greater complexity of medical problems, greater expertise in medical and health matters on the part of nonmedical professionals, and greater participation by consumers in dealing with major issues. These developments have all taken place in a short time and appear to be accelerating. Meanwhile, no well-conceived methodology for governing access to the medical commons has evolved, despite the ever increasing need for setting priorities, particularly as we approach the institution of national health insurance. Certainly, our failure to confront these very difficult problems has not meant that problems have not been dealt with. However, when we had relatively limited capabilities and seemingly unlimited resources, the consequences of a largely laissez-faire policy were not so visible and so painful as they now are. Unless safeguards not in view are conceived and applied, the priorities for use of the commons will continue to be set as they have been—at best by well intentioned policy makers with information of limited quantity and quality, and at worst in anarchic fashion.

How should priorities be set in the United States? Who should set them? How much should be allocated for health in toto? Of that total, how much should be allocated for medical care? How much for research, and in that category, how much for basic science and how much for applied? How much for medical education? How much for educating the public? Of each fraction, how should apportionments be made? And what, in each case, should be the quid pro quo? If a hypertension management program can receive only a limited sum, how should that money be optimally used? If renal dialysis cannot be universally available, who should qualify for treatment? What kinds of people should make these decisions? On what basis should their decisions be made?

Although there are no simple answers to these questions, let me first emphasize how I believe national priorities cannot and should not be set. It is surely not fair to ask the physician or other medical care provider to set them in the context of his or her own medical practice. A physician or other provider must do all that is permitted on behalf of his patient. In that sense the physician is and should be responsible, with his patient and the patient's family, for setting priorities for that patient's management, within the limits available. The patient and the physician want no less, and society should settle for no less. For example, if society has set no ground rules for the use of kidney dialysis other than medical ones, and if in a physician's judgment his eighty-year-old patient's overall condition warrants dialysis, everything must be done to see that he is so treated. On the other hand, the physician can, however reluctantly, accept society's constraints regarding eligibility requirements for kidney dialysis, even if he does not consider them to be in the best interests of his patient.

I believe it is as inappropriate to indict physicians for the depletion of resources on the commons as it is to expect physicians alone to determine priorities. The challenge for the medical profession is how to join with others in effective decision making. In this context, let us return to the three problem areas of the commons described earlier.

In the face of conflicts between the interests of the individual patient and of society, choices must be made concerning how much of (or whether) our resources should, for example, be spent for kidney dialysis and for heart transplants, and if so, who is eligible. Physicians must help gather and present as realistically and comprehensively as possible scientific and medical information about kidney dialysis and heart transplants, and then join with a variety of other professionals, including statisticians, epidemiologists, economists, policy analysts, lawyers and, ultimately, politicians and the public in setting priorities. Clearly, decisions will heavily depend on both the quality and the quantity of information provided by the medical profession.

To protect the commons from useless, prematurely introduced, or otherwise inappropriate practices, the physician must join statisticians, epidemiologists, and economists to ensure that no practice is widely adopted without prior evaluation. As reported by Cochrane (1974), the British National Health Service encourages examination of new diagnostic and therapeutic practices, often by randomized clinical trial, and then submits them for approval by an officially appointed board. (Thus, for example, at the time of Cochrane's presentation neither the carcinoembryonic antigen test for cancer nor coronary-artery bypass graft operations had yet been approved.) As Cochrane (1972) has stressed, clinical validation of a practice is not by itself adequate reason for its dissemination. It must be shown to be more effective than other practices available for the same medical problem. And even if this second requirement is satisfied, its value should be manifestly greater than that of those other practices that its adoption would displace.

It is in the third area, prevention, that long-term opportunities are greatest for protecting the resources of the commons. Here, too, the physician must join with others, including consumers, if programs are to be maximally effective. The example of the costs and our therapeutic limitations in the management of black lung was earlier stressed. Although the physician by himself can do little to prevent the condition, his effectiveness in prevention could be amplified many times if he were joined by the mine operator, the union official, the politician, the lawyer, the chemist, the engineer, and others. In addition, a more widespread understanding of the limitations of therapeutic medicine could generate greater attention to the need for campaigns directed at preventing black lung and the myriad other conditions for which we can now do so little.

It cannot be overemphasized that our successes in prevention of disease reflect in large part the fruits of research. If these successes are to be followed by the many others we and future generations so badly need, a substantial and predictable fraction of our resources must be set aside for basic scientific research, and for education of research scientists. In my view it is essential that society create mechanisms that separate the demands on the commons of research and of education from those of medical care, for these should not be forced to compete with each other on a continuing basis.

In conclusion, two points seem to me worthy of special emphasis. The first is that the critical question confronting the medical professions is not whether society will find ways to govern access to and control the use of the medical commons. (A people that was sufficiently aroused to create a Food and Drug Administration to control pharmaceutical preparations will surely find mechanisms for controlling medical and surgical procedures when the effects of inadequate restraints become more widely evident.) The question, rather, is how physicians will participate in the creation of control mechanisms in a manner that reflects both enlightened self-interest and the public interest. Physicians must join with educators and others to find ways to encourage the general public to understand more about not only their bodies but also the limitations and uncertainties of medical care, so that society's decision making can be as fully informed as possible. Indeed, only if physicians assume a major role can they contribute adequately to the protection of the public interest.

Secondly, it is essential that the process of decision making with respect to the medical commons be maximally flexible. Many technical approaches to medical care that were acceptable a decade ago are inadequate today; the same thing must be said about medical judgments and even ethical and moral decision making. Much of what we physicians and our fellow members of society agree is appropriate for 1975 will probably be inadequate for the conditions of 1980. Although it is unfortunately true that existing data are inadequate in most cases to permit fully enlightened decision making today, decision making must and does go on, nonetheless, sometimes by default. This fact makes it more urgent that the process undergo continuing review and revision, to permit us to deal with the issues that inevitably emerge from any reordering of priorities and from continuing progress.

REFERENCES

Alpert, J. J., et al. "Effective Use of Comprehensive Pediatric Care: Utilization of Health Resources." *American Journal of Diseases of Children* 116 (1968): 529-33.

Astvad, K., et al. "Mortality from Acute Myocardial Infarction Before and After Establishment of a Coronary Care Unit." *British Medical Journal* 1 (1974): 567-69.

Barkin, R. M., and Conrad, J. L. "Current Status of Measles in the United States." *Journal
of Infectious Diseases* 128 (1973): 353-56.

Brook, R. H., et al. "Effectiveness of Inpatient Follow-up Care." *New England Journal of
Medicine* 285 (1971): 1509-14.

Bunker, J. "Risks and Benefits of Surgery." *Benefits and Risks in Medical Care,* edited by D.
Taylor (a symposium held by the Office of Health Economics). Luton, England:
White Crescent Press, 1974.

Cochrane, A. L. *Effectiveness and Efficiency: Random Reflections on Health Services.*
London: Nuffield Provincial Hospitals Trust, 1972.

Cochrane, A. L. "The Feasibility of Relating Quality Control to Medical Outcomes: A Critical Appraisal." Presented at the fall meeting of the Institute of Medicine, National
Academy of Sciences, Washington, D.C. (November 6, 1974).

Committee for the Assessment of Biometric Aspects of Controlled Trials of Hypoglycemic
Agents. "Report." *Journal of the American Medical Association* 231 (1975):
583-608.

Gordis, L. "Effectiveness of Comprehensive-Care Programs in Preventing Rheumatic Fever."
New England Journal of Medicine 289 (1973): 331-35.

Griner, P. F. "Treatment of Acute Pulmonary Edema: Conventional or Intensive Care?" *Annals of Internal Medicine* 77 (1972): 501-06.

Hardin, G. "The Tragedy of the Commons." *Science* 162 (1968): 1243-48.

Institute of Medicine, Panel of Health Services Research. *Infant Death: An Analysis by Maternal Risk and Health Care (Contrasts in Health Status, vol. 1).* Washington, D.C.:
Institute of Medicine, National Academy of Sciences, 1973.

Institute of Medicine, Panel on Health Services Research. *Assessment of Medical Care for
Children (Contrasts in Health Status, vol. 3).* Washington, D.C.: Institute of Medicine,
National Academy of Sciences, 1974.

Jaffe, N., et al. "Adjuvant Methotrexate and Citrovorum-Factor Treatment of Osteogenic
Sarcoma." *New England Journal of Medicine* 291 (1974): 994-97.

Kinlen, L. J., and Doll, R. "Trends in Mortality from Cancer of the Uterus in Canada and in
England and Wales." *British Journal of Preventive and Social Medicine* 27 (1973):
146-49.

Knatterud, G. L., et al. "Effects of Hypoclycemic Agents on Vascular Complications in Patients with Adult-Onset Diabetes. IV. A Preliminary Report on Phenformin Results."
Journal of the American Medical Association 217 (1971): 777-84.

Landrigan, P. J., and Conrad, J. L. "Current Status of Measles in the United States." *Journal
of Infectious Diseases* 124 (1971): 620-22.

Liberthson, R. R., et al. "Prehospital Ventricular Defibrillation: Prognosis and Follow-up
Course." *New England Journal of Medicine* 291 (1974): 317-21.

Martin, S. P., et al. "Inputs into Coronary Care During 30 Years: A Cost Effectiveness
Study." *Annals of Internal Medicine* 81 (1974): 289-93.

Maxwell, R. J. *Health Care: The Growing Dilemma.* New York: McKinsey, 1974.

McDermott, W., Deuschle, K. W., and Barnett, C. R. "Health Care Experiment at Many
Farms." *Science* 175 (1972): 23-31.

McKeown, T. "A Conceptual Background for Research and Development in Medicine."
International Journal of Health Services 3 (1973): 17-28.

McKeown, T., and Lowe, C. R. *An Introduction to Social Medicine* (2nd ed.). Oxford:
Blackwell Scientific Publications, 1974.

Medical World News. "Does the U.S. Need 80,000 Coronary Angiograms a Day?" *Medical
World News* 15, no. 34 (1974): 14-16.

3

Mitchell, J. W. "Exfoliative Cytology in Screening for Cervical Cancer—A Critique." *Canadian Medical Association Journal* 105 (1971): 833-36.

Mitford, N. *The Sun King.* New York: Harper & Row, 1966.

University Group Diabetes Program. "A Study of the Effects of Hypoglycemic Agents on Vascular Complications in Patients with Adult-Onset Diabetes." *Diabetes* (Supplement) 19 (1970): 747-830.

Weinstein, M. C. "Allocation of Subjects in Medical Experiments." *New England Journal of Medicine* 291 (1974): 1278-85.

Wennberg, J., and Gittelsohn, A. "Small Area Variations in Health Care Delivery." *Science* 182 (1973): 1102-08.

Part III

Unresolved Issues

8

Control of Health Services

Selection by Roger M. Battistella and David B. Smith

Management science is used eclectically herein to refer to the body of ideas and techniques developed in support of increased rationality in decision making and which, increasingly, are perceived to be relevant in the treatment of applied economic problems of cost control, effectiveness, productivity, and efficiency, together with strengthening the role of central authority for policy, planning, and program coordination at the macro- and micro-level.

The influence of management science in the health sector has expanded considerably in recent years, implying a significant but subtle departure from conventional views of health care. An understanding of the implications of management science demands a careful critique that goes beyond the frequently facile rhetoric and overly ambitious claims of its advocates and the often naive objections of its detractors. This paper attempts to provide such a critique by exploring some of the major reasons underlying the growing power of management thinking. It then assesses its repercussions—intended and unintended— which are examined in light of the fragile, complex, and highly reactive nature of health services organization in a technologically advanced society.

Through explication of the underlying values and appraisal of the short- and long-run consequences, the position taken here is that, unless tempered with moderation, the drive for stronger management and attendant quantification in the health sector could lead to unanticipated deleterious results in the form of

Reprinted by permission from "Toward a Definition of Health Services Management: A Humanist Orientation," *International Journal of Health Services* 4, no. 4 (1974), pp. 701-21. Copyright 1975 by Baywood Publishing Co.

(a) further erosion of social cohesion already sizably weakened by industrial-urban processes; (b) additional increases in stresses and strains contributing to the emergence of mental-emotional illness as a major health problem of contemporary living; and (c) declining progress in efforts to achieve more favorable rates of economic growth. These possibilities could occur, either wholly or partially, through (a) the substitution of economic for ethical criteria at the point where services and patients meet; (b) the restructuring of hospitals and other health care institutions from normative to utilitarian and more bureaucratic forms of organization; (c) the subtle effects of language in shaping perception and guiding action; and (d) the biases, frequently unrecognized, of a new generation of experts in policy and program planning who, by virtue of their training and the conditions of employment, are typically insensitive to the moral, social, and political dimensions of problem solving in the social services sector.

MANAGEMENT SCIENCE IMPETUS

The Shift in Emphasis

The emphasis on scientific management in the United States is not a completely new development. Placing things in perspective, health care reformers have been advocating management and planning as a means of dealing with problems of access, continuity, comprehensiveness, and quality as long ago as the mid-1920s, in the dissemination of the Dawson Report from England which called for the regional restructuring of health services based on the principles of division of labor and standardization of production processes; and the completion in the U.S. in the early 1930s of the Report of the Committee on the Costs of Medical Care which recommended a restructuring of health services along coordinated corporate lines, and stimulated, among other things, the first successful continuously operating graduate training program in hospital administration at the University of Chicago.

In contrast to earlier attempts to establish management principles in the organization and delivery of health services where, because of a commitment to humanitarian ideals, the focus was on social reforms, the emphasis has shifted in recent years to economic aspects. This is apparent in the popularity in policy-making circles of words like efficiency, cost-effectiveness, and productivity. Such language signals the ascendency of economic-managerial values and a new style of decision making.

Underlying Causes of the Shift in Emphasis

Possibly more than any other cause, the impetus for management today stems from the mounting preoccupation of top government officials with health costs and expenditures which are perceived to be rising uncontrollably and impacting unfavorably on the national economy. To be sure, other considerations are involved, such as improved access and availability among underserviced low-income and geographically isolated populations and broader and more uniform standards of care, but they are for the most part secondary to finance and accounting priorities.

The fixation on economic matters is a reaction to the phenomenal expansion in health spending which, over a twelve-year span, more than tripled in size, increasing from $26 billion in 1960 to over $83 billion in 1972. In relation to the U.S. gross national product (GNP), the amount allocated for health shot up from 5.2 to 7.6 percent (Cooper and Worthington, 1973). Throughout much of this period outlays increased annually at a rate double that of economic growth, and it was predicted that unless slowed down health might consume as much as 10 percent of the GNP by 1980 (Rice and McGee, 1970). This figure taken by itself may not seem unreasonable from the standpoint of the quality of life standards possible in an affluent society like the United States, but health spending does not occur in isolation—it must compete with other demands and needs under conditions of perpetual insufficient resources. For example, educational expenditures have also been rising at a similar rate, with the likelihood that health and education together may consume 20 percent of the GNP by the end of the decade.

The difficulty of reconciling conflict due to competition for limited resources is especially acute, given that fiscal policy must cope with the frequently contradictory politics of spending, where voters pressure for more and better publicly supported services while simultaneously fighting to hold the line on taxes or lower them. In a democratic society, this inconsistency is both a cause of insecurity among elected officials and fuel for demagoguery in which aspirants to political office promise more than can be delivered, all the while encouraging taxpayers to believe that they can have their cake and eat it too. As witnessed by the current troubled state of the general economy, simultaneously high rates of public and private spending can be highly inflationary. Macroeconomic theory dictates that one must yield to the other.

The ongoing attempts of the federal government to slow down health spending is a consequence of the redirection of financing begun in the mid-1960s following passage of an unprecedented volume of new programs which gave the public sector a larger share of the fiscal responsibility for health services. In contrast to the forty-year period prior to 1966 when the public share of total spending remained fixed at about 25 percent, the percentage spiraled to 40 percent in the five-year period ending in 1971, due mainly to the enactment of Medicare and Medicaid programs which made government funds available for health service payments to the aged and to the poor (Cooper and Worthington, 1973). Although its proportional share of total spending has undergone little change since 1971, pressures are still escalating for government to take on an even larger role; there are a number of national health insurance proposals receiving serious attention by the Congress which could have the effect of extending some form of financial protection against health care costs to all population groups. For an analysis of the various proposals together with the sociopolitical forces shaping policy on national health insurance, see Battistella (1973) and Waldman (1974).

On balance, the results of increased public spending have been disappointing. In fiscal years 1966 through 1970, the government made available a total of $15.6 billion in new money for the purchase of hospital and physician care, only to find that for every dollar allocated as little as 25 percent went to additional services—the remainder was dissipated by inflation (Rice and Cooper, 1971). This experience is primarily what prompted the government in January 1973, following an eighteen-month trial with the stabilization program launched in August 1971 for dealing with problems in the general economy, to retain mandatory wage and price controls in the health services industry after lifting them for most other services. The importance of controls is mirrored in the fact that the 10.3 percent increase for health spending in 1972 represented the lowest annual increase in six years. Moreover, because the GNP showed the highest percentage gain in recent years (8.4 percent), health spending rose only slightly as a proportion of the GNP—from 7.5 to 7.6 percent (Cooper and Worthington, 1973).

Though hard to follow because of a crisis-like atmosphere provoking frequent changes of direction, the strategy for slowing down health expenditures covers a broad front and is multifaceted: to raise productivity through strengthened management and improved modes of delivery; to reshape supply to close the gap with demand and to introduce less costly substitutes for high-priced specialized services; to experiment with alternatives for effecting demand such as consumer health education and greater private responsibility for payment through deductibles and coinsurance; and, finally, to rationalize organization and delivery to replace the existing large number of small-sized producers with fewer large-sized entities to achieve economies of scale and improved coordination.

Another cause of the shift in management science from social to economic objectives is the high priority now assigned to economic growth as an instrument for resolving many of the domestic political conflicts emanating from consumer expectations which have outgrown the national resources and for strengthening and enlarging the nation's position in international trade. The technical requirements and psychological climate accompanying a planned program of expansion are, by and large, unfavorable to social services. Evaluated in terms of their contributions to the economy, labor intensive and highly personalized services like health do not compare well. Low-productivity health services are viewed as a dampening effect on growth by offsetting gains in other parts of the economy, and as a significant contributor to the inflation correlated with economic acceleration. In this climate the mixture of altruism and self-interest causing professionals to advocate larger budgets and an expansion of services formerly hailed as a form of social commitment is often derided as an extravagance and vested-interest politics.

Currently there is, moreover, the danger of an emotional backlash on the part of policy makers who, whether out of conviction or otherwise, accepted the premise of many health-spending advocates that public outlays would level off following initial steep increases once the backlog of the unmet needs of the aged and the poor had been satisfied. Failure to experience this leveling off in Medicare and Medicaid costs has caused many public officials to conclude that the demand for health services is infinite. Increasing at the rate of around 15 percent a year, these two programs now account for three-fifths of all government health expenditures: they constituted 75 percent of the $4 billion increase in public outlays in 1972 (Cooper and Worthington, 1973). Together with other programs entitling individuals and local government to specific benefits (social security, welfare, veteran's services, revenue sharing), Medicare and Medicaid are difficult to control. Although it is true in the strictly legal sense that what Congress has wrought it can undo, it is very difficult politically and morally speaking to take away from people benefits they have grown accustomed to. Spending for such programs is open-ended pretty much, growing automatically with increases in the eligible population, such as, for example, the number of people reaching retirement age or the size of the population with incomes falling below the officially set poverty line. Collectively referred to as "entitlement" programs, they account for 50 percent of the 1974 federal budget and are the most rapidly growing component of federal spending.

Because of other forms of fixed spending, such as debt and interest payments, only about 30 percent of the federal budget is considered to be discretionary today. Even this figure is somewhat misleading for not all programs in the discretionary category are equally manipulable; payroll for civilian and military personnel comprises three-fifths of the total and another one-fifth is spent for defense purposes. Of the remaining one-fifth in the discretionary category medical research and manpower training is the single largest component and this fact explains why so much emphasis is now being placed on reducing spending in these two areas (Dale, 1974). Exasperation at all this may lead to faith in the value of health services being replaced by skepticism. Indeed, there are signs to suggest that this is already happening.

The belief in the efficacy of biomedical research and technology dominant throughout most of the post-World War II period is being displaced by the attitude that scientific-technologically intensive services have reached the stage of diminishing marginal social benefit. Because of the large capital requirements of today's highly specialized services and the shift in disease problems toward chronic conditions and the care of the terminally ill, it is costing the nation increasingly more to accomplish increasingly less improvement of overall health levels. Apart from accidents and, to a lesser extent, cancers and suicides, there are now no significant causes of death before middle age. Thus money spent on health is regarded as being less an investment than a form of consumption, and the payoff to the individual is thought to be far greater than the return to society. For an elaboration of this conclusion, see Fuchs (1972).

The pressures for economy combined with the need to generate savings for financing investments in economic growth were no doubt an important consideration in the Nixon Administration's attempts to curtail drastically in the proposed 1974 budget spending for health and other social services falling within the category of controllable expenditures. These pressures also underlie the movement toward selectivity rather than principles of universalism in designing statutory benefit programs. An example of the consequence of these forces is the stratification of publicly financed medical payment programs by social class and age, and the persistent attempts to amend Medicare legislation to require the aged to assume a larger share of the costs of their hospital and physician care through imposition of more sizable deductible and coinsurance charges. The intent is illustrated in the following examples. In planning for the 1974 budget the Nixon Administration sought unsuccessfully to increase consumer use charges in Medicare which would result in an estimated reduction of federal expenditures by $500 million in 1974 and by $1.3 billion in 1975 (Fried et al., 1973). This strategy has not been abandoned, however. It has been retained as an essential element in the administration's national health insurance plan inherited by President Ford, which remains a leading contender among the many national health insurance proposals now awaiting congressional action.

In addition to separate schemes for the gainfully employed and the poor, the administration proposal calls for a number of improvements in the Medicare program, the most important one being a guaranteed protection against the large-sized cost of major illness. In return for security from catastrophic cost, the aged will be required, however, to pay out of pocket for a larger share of the cost of routine care. On the assumption that day-to-day care is for the most part either unnecessary or non-life-threatening, the idea is to get the aged to finance, through deductibles and coinsurance charges, roughly 15 percent of the cost of operating a liberalized Medicare program.

This approach seems justified if one can accept the conclusions reported by researchers from the prestigious Rand Corporation which has received government funds to carry out studies on the cost-reduction and utilization-behavior effects of coinsurance and deductibles (Newhouse, Phelps, and Schwartz, 1974). However, instead of being looked to as a model piece of applied economic analysis, this study may become better known as an exercise in propaganda and an illustration of the distortions which can result when research is dependent for survival on funding sources whose interests are affected by findings and their interpretation. It could also serve as an example of the limitations of analyses, to be described more fully in a later section, which concentrate too heavily on narrow managerial-economic efficiency criteria to the detriment of larger social concerns; and which attempt to influence policy with findings derived from theories which fail to capture reality adequately.

Among the many limitations of this study, simplifying generalizations are used, oftentimes implicitly, such as: most health services utilization is either frivolous or unnecessary or fails to result in any improved physical status; early initiation of health care is unrelated to the efficacy of treatment; and consumers are in a better position to judge whether utilization is proper or not than are physicians. Also questionable is the assumption that the primary cause of the inflation being experienced in the health sector is of the supply-demand type described in traditional market competition theory rather than the cost-push type resulting whenever powerful groups are allowed to pursue their self-interest in the absence of effective controls and accountability. The study, moreover, ignores the ethical and medical implications of the relationship between illness, income, and age.

Economic forces also fuel pertinacious efforts to eliminate problems through redefinition, as illustrated in the lowering of benefits for aged Medicare patients in long-term facilities now deemed to be receiving custodial rather than active medical treatment services. If funds are not reassigned from nursing home care to improved housing, and custodial and residential accommodations, a far greater share of the burden of paying for the cost of illness can be expected to fall on the aged and their families in future years.

The public, too, in a reversal of its former position, is becoming more critical of the value of health spending. It has both reasonably and emotionally faulted the entire community of health professionals for hypocrisy in pretending to be motivated more by altruism than self-interest, being imperious in dealings with its clients (the middle class as well as the poor), and being generally incapable of managing the nation's health resources responsibly.

LIMITATIONS OF MANAGEMENT SCIENCE

Much of the mystique of the power of medicine and the goodness of the medical profession is being stripped away by the combined assault of economic pressures and public opinion. While a certain amount of debunking is in order, the emotionalism generated by economic exigencies can be counterproductive. It generates polarization of issues, obscures clearheaded analysis, and encourages simple-minded solutions.

Substitution of Economic for Ethical Criteria in Health Service Exchanges

One of the more frequently mentioned solutions for mastering the health cost problem involves turning things over to the market and the acquisition of more business-type practices. To advocates of this approach, competition and techniques associated with profit-making activity are regarded as the panacea for monopolistic services grown overly complacent by too much security and inefficiency due to bureaucratic red tape. By no means confined to market ideologues, the tendency to look to the private sector for leadership is a reflection of core cultural values of individualism and the market in which private enterprise epitomizes efficiency and progress in contrast to public administration, which is equated with waste, malfeasance, and malevolence in its exercise of power. These values constitute what may be described as the "cult of the market."

The market cult phenomenon was manifest in the decision of the Nixon Administration to build profit making and competition into its health strategy as a means for speeding up organizational restructuring and efficiency. The Health Maintenance Organization Act of 1973 (PL 93-222) stands as testimony to the weight of such values. The Health Maintenance Organization (HMO) concept embodies efficiency principles drawn from the big business model and is directed at moving physicians from solo practice and retrospective modes of fee-for-service reimbursement to group practice and prospective modes of payment based on capitation and negotiated annual budgets. A much discussed feature of the HMO concept is the use of market-type incentives which allow medical groups to keep a share of any money in their budget unspent at the end of the year. The idea is for physicians to become more cost conscious in making their treatment decisions. The exercise of informal cost-benefit criteria in combination with motivation for economic self-gain is viewed as the key for stopping physicians from prescribing services of questionable efficacy and from consideration of the desirability of expensive care for persons who have few years of remaining life or for whom the probability of successful treatment is low. Another feature is the encouragement of competition for patients and profits among medical groups

which supporters are convinced will assure greater efficiency. Detailed information on the principles behind the HMO concept may be found in U.S. Department of Health, Education, and Welfare (1971) and *Health Maintenance Organizations* (1972).

At one extreme there are the market advocates whose ambition is to pattern health services after the comprehensive, balanced mechanical systems employed by large-scale corporations: (a) standardization of product; (b) continuous operation of production processes through automation; (c) reorganization of
structure in the form of comprehensive-integrated systems; and (d) improved decision making through centralization and assimilation of control techniques such
as cost accounting, capital budgeting, and computerized information flows. The
goal is to improve predictability and control through planning and efficiency
through the substitution, whenever possible, of mechanical for human means,
along with economies of scale. At the other extreme, private sector advocates
seek to remove rationing of health services from the public arena by restoring
the operation of free market pricing and the naturalistic force of the "invisible
hand" which, if not always just in dealing with humans wants, is considered to
be vastly more efficient than political and bureaucratic alternatives. To members
of this latter group, the insecurity of the classical atomistic-anarchical competitive market is the ultimate determinant of efficiency, and planning is anathema.
For illustrations of the continued hold which the classical market exercises in
influencing thinking and recommendations on health policy, see American
Enterprise Institute for Public Policy Research (1972).

It is difficult to follow just what pro-market supporters have in mind because of a confusing tendency on their part to intermix monopolistic with oli-
gopolistic and perfectly competitive types of markets. The language and symbols
they evoke are vestiges from the dreamy world of Adam Smith, which—if it ever
existed—was more the exception than the rule. It may be an indication of the
paradoxical influence of dogma that all market spokesmen see themselves as de-
fenders of the virtue of competition and survival of the fittest when few are
prepared to apply the law of uncertainty and risk taking to their own operations.
One is struck by the reluctant but rapid extension of government activity in
every sphere of the private sector as subsidizer of profits and regulator of
ruinous competition, most often at the behest of business and industrial interests, as illustrated most recently by the plight of the defense industry con-
tractors (Lockheed), the rail industry (Penn Central), and the airlines (Pan American World Airways).

It is ridiculous to proclaim that there are few things wrong in the health
sector that cannot be cured by a large dose of any form of competition, let alone
the market. The chaotic history of diploma-mill medical education at the turn of
the century and experience-rating private health insurance in the 1950s and

1960s is stark evidence of the social dysfunctionality of the profit-competition motive in the health field. The evidence suggests that even nonprofit competition is dysfunctional because of the large capital costs associated with the provision of modern medical services and the scale of organization required for efficient operations. It is misleading, if not irresponsible, to contend that the enlargement of the private sector and expansion of competition will bring more choice within the reach of consumers and raise efficiency levels when, in point of fact, the efficiency requirements of today's costly health care technology are causing society to centralize services and restrict choice through removal of costly overlapping and control of capital expansion based on certificate of need.

The types of efficiency incentives being proposed also strain credulity. Good medical care requires that the transaction between providers and patients not be impeded by considerations of economic gain. Instead of incentives for overservicing found in fee-for-service or those for underservicing contained in the HMO idea, the commanding motivation at the point of decision ought to be to provide care consistent with patient needs and with prevailing standards of acceptable practice.

The ahistoric invocation of the private sector and market mechanisms obscures the reason why society acted at an early date to insulate health services from the unbridled play of the competitive market. The emotional vulnerability of the sick and their potential for economic and other forms of exploitation account in part for the designation of medicine as a profession. In return for high status, prestige, and income, physicians are expected to place the interest of their patients ahead of their own when the two come in conflict, to treat all patients in accordance with prevailing standards of good medical care, to avoid partiality in dealings with patients, and to limit services provided to areas of achieved competence. The expectation that these unusually demanding obligations will be taken seriously is what has invested the profession with its historic sacerdotal powers and what accounts for the high public esteem it has traditionally commanded. In a matter so vital to community and individual welfare, normal rules of the market like "caveat emptor" and "sell at the highest price" have limited application. The obvious limitations on consumer sovereignty, because of the knowledge gap in diagnosis and treatment between lay persons and physicians, led society to restrict entry into the health market to qualified persons; the significance of illness and illness treatment to the public interest led it to administer prices at a range within reach of the general population. (These points are elaborated further in the well-known sociological work by Parsons (1951, pp. 428-79) and the work of the leading economist Arrow (1963).) Most recently, society (in response to rising consumer standards involving access to illness treatment services and the breakdown in rationing based on modified principles of ability to pay and charity) has gone significantly further in declaring that health care is a right. Health has been declared, in principle, a merit good which, because of the combination of externalities and importance for consumer satisfaction, does not lend itself easily to market rationing. It is therefore ironic, if not reactionary, that at a time when health is acquiring even stronger social connotations as a symbol of quality of life aspirations there is serious talk of returning to the market and a concept of management based on principles of competition and self-gain.

Restructuring of Health Care Institutions Along Utilitarian Lines

Whether rooted in the early industrial engineering teachings of Frederick Taylor or the "cult of the market," management science promotes major changes in the organization and management of health care institutions. Just as the market has become the remedy for the overall system of health finance and distribution, the classical management machine approach to organization is pictured as the optimal solution for boosting productivity in hospitals and related health facilities. The centralized structures of the large private corporations are to be imitated and idolized for their mastery of unit costs and efficiency. Yet despite whatever advantages it may possess, such an outlook is myopic in failing to perceive what is fundamental to the integration and effective functioning of health care organizations.

The basic problem all organizations face is how to hold together as a unit. The power or "social glue" used to bind may be predominantly normative, utilitarian, or coercive. While every organization utilizes a mixture of these, hospitals and other health care institutions historically have been essentially normative institutions. Patients comply with medical staff and nursing orders not so much from fear of punishment or economic sanctions, but presumably from values of shared social concerns for their health and that of other patients—values which tend to be shared by those comprising the health team. Indeed, in any smoothly running hospital such values shape the conduct of even the most unskilled employees. The prominence of social concern for health has acted as the basis for the separation of authority in hospitals between purely administrative and/or hotel-keeping functions from patient-care functions. Loss of administrative and economic efficiency due to the diffusion of managerial authority has been judged a small price to pay for preserving human and scientific values in the treatment and care of the ill. (The significance of normative values for the integration of health care organizations is described in Etzioni, 1961.) Yet one cannot help but notice the growing practice among hospital administrators to adopt new titles from business and industry such as president, vice president, and chief executive officer; the old title of hospital administrator is quickly disappearing. This suggests a preference for, and possibly a movement toward, hierarchical distributions of authority characteristic of the private sector in contrast to the familiar management triangle in hospitals which diffused authority between the board of trustees, the hospital administrator, and the medical staff.

This may imply a rejection, whether intentional or not, of other options more consistent with past practice and better suited for reconciling managerial-economic imperatives with primary goals of illness treatment and patient care (e.g., the collegial or team approach introduced recently in the English National Health Service where authority is shared among representatives of the major interests responsible for the smooth running of the hospital—central administration, medicine, nursing, and finance and accounting).

The dominance of patient welfare values is fundamental in hospitals and related facilities given the uncertainty and complexity surrounding patient care. It should never be forgotten that healing, which is the end objective of treatment, is vitally affected by the emotional state of sick individuals and that the purely subjective aspects of the physician-patient relationship—trust and faith—may be far more important for accomplishing the job than the quest for efficiency through classical management paradigms. Productivity and rigid adherence to proper procedures have taken a back seat to normative values in health organizations for good reason. Consequently, there is understandable apprehension over inroads being made by utilitarian-bureaucratic principles in performance evaluation and output; health services will always fall short due to their adherence to social and ethical standards rather than to economic-managerial standards of efficiency. The imposition in hospital management of industrial machine models facilitates the replacement of the patient service ethic by motivations which are much more calculating and economically self-serving.

The benefits of machine models when applied to normative organizations can be short-lived and self-defeating. As illustrated by recent developments in hospitals and medical practice, patients become suspicious of professionals' motives and malpractice suits skyrocket. This is met, in turn, by more defensive behavior by organizations and practitioners culminating in more extensive costly tests, enervating red tape, and reciprocal distrust. With individuals motivated by values of self-gain and rational calculation, it is no wonder that employees begin to organize to protect their economic interests and to narrowly restrict the scope of their responsibilities to patients and to the organization; unionization of professional and nonprofessional personnel is a predictable response. More time is spent worrying about the assignment of blame than trying to solve problems and take on additional duties until law suits and suspicion mount, and effective management of any form becomes impossible—this is already observable in many large urban hospitals.

Effects of Language

Language indisputably affects the perception of problems and behavior. It is obvious from the preceding discussion that much of the language accompanying management science activity addressed at raising the performance of health services planning and delivery is biased in favor of economics and depersonalized processes of production. Price elasticity of demand, cost-benefit study, input-output analysis, net revenue and cash-flow maximization, human capital maintenance, discounted future earnings, computerized information and control systems, cybernetics, human resources administration, and engineering for behavior modification are but a partial illustration of the centrality of material values in management science. In encouraging the interpretation of complicated social problems in terms of industrial-machine paradigms and in confusing the market value of the individual with right to welfare, the rhetoric of management science makes it easier to write off as a loss population groups like the aged, the disabled, and the poor, removed from the economic mainstream or contributing little to the process of private capital formation and the growth of the economy. Cost-benefit analysis is unlikely to justify spending money on these groups. The decision can only be made on grounds of social justice and equity. Nevertheless, policy at the federal level is being increasingly guided by calculations of the payoff to the national economy. There are serious efforts underway, as in the case of the HMO, to alter the physician-patient relationship so that the treatment decision is more heavily weighted by cost and payoff calculations, as contrasted with traditional humanitarian values and incentives.

The conditioning effect of language has made it easier to discuss publicly in the United States a number of previously restricted subjects including the wisdom of sustaining through costly technologic means the lives of terminally ill patients and the advisability of supporting in expensive institutions incurables falling into the "vegetable" category, such as the hopelessly mentally ill and retarded, nonfunctioning congenital defectives, and accident and stroke victims experiencing substantial neurologic damage. The reverence for life and respect for the uniqueness of the individual, long the moral mainstay for the care of the sick, are endangered by the latent consequences of management values and methods eschewing the intangible and the abstract as either impractical or a bad investment.

The subtle moral erosion that takes place through use of such language is perhaps more of a danger than its possible overt manipulation in support of socially distasteful decisions. The language can dull moral sensibilities and channel concentration more on technocratic means than on the underlying assumptions and purposes of decision making by introducing bias which leads to a false representation of reality and to faulty policy conclusions. Much of the bias in management science is difficult to discern due to its preference for mathematical symbols and equations which, no matter how useful for abstract model building, obscure the substantive features of applied social issues. While quantification efforts can be understood as an attempt by practitioners to improve their status by assuming the trappings of a science, it also represents an escape from having to admit to the shortcomings of objective analysis and a concealment of methodologic dead ends. Cost-benefit analysis and other techniques for assessing the value of services like health and the returns to individual welfare and collective well-being, services essentially ethical and subjective in nature, are a good example of the tendency in management science for elaborate attempts to objectify what is not and cannot be simply objective. By implying that it succeeds in doing so the language of management science creates a false sense of confidence in our understanding of complex problems and confuses narrow constructs of efficiency with the larger moral and political ends of social policy. (A more extensive discussion of bias in policy research may be found in Myrdal, 1969, pp. 43-62.) Moreover, in the hands of practitioners inundated in their day-to-day operations by constraints of time and other demands, a quantitative approach to problem solving can introduce a systematic bias against nonquantifiable programs on the grounds that qualitative justifications are impracticable if not "soft" and "muddleheaded." These insufficiencies notwithstanding, the influence of objective-quantitative analysis in government decision making appears to be growing larger.

The ill-defined way in which management science is proclaimed as the answer to problems within health services organization may reflect the complexity of health care problems today and the growing sense of public alarm over sharply rising costs and gaps in delivery. The absence of clear-cut solutions may cause politicians pressed with the need to demonstrate action to point to management as the answer. Invocation of the language of scientific management may be today's brand of conjuration and hagiography.

A New Generation of Experts

The imperatives of economic growth and cost saving have altered considerably the makeup of the body of advisory-analytical experts assisting policy makers in government. In place of the politically sensitive generalists of the past, consisting mainly of gifted amateurs and professionals schooled in public affairs and the law, the tendency now is to look to specially trained nonpolitical persons conversant in finance and budgeting, and proficient in the application of techniques useful for dealing with productivity and efficiency questions in areas such as resource allocation, organizational restructuring, program evaluation, and policy analysis.

Originating in the machine-man relationship of the industrial revolution (and promoted by the successes of military defense planning techniques in World War II), the new experts are characterized by a systems approach to problem solving involving a heavy application of quantitative methods drawn mainly from engineering and economic sources. The application of this approach to managerial and fiscal problems in government programs acquired considerable visibility in the early 1960s. As popularized by the Secretary of Defense during the Kennedy Administration, Robert McNamara, the purpose of systematic analysis was to assist in identification and justification of objectives, specification of available alternatives for the achievement of objectives, computation of the costs and benefits of alternatives, and the assessment of the chances of successful program implementation. Based on reports of its successes in the defense area, the systems approach has been extended to all agencies at all levels of government and has become an entrenched feature of bureaucratic existence. (The history, together with a pungent critique of the shortcomings of systems analysis and management science, may be found in Hoos, 1972. For a broader, more theoretical presentation in the context of developed economies, see Thoenes, 1966, pp. 169-214.)

In the course of its dissemination, the systems approach has helped to implant the notion "that what government affairs needed is better management, and the more scientific, the better at that" (American Enterprise Institute for Public Policy Research, 1972, p. 47). In the Nixon Administration, the notion of scientific management was modified somewhat to refer especially to techniques and practices of the business world and a scale of centralization of authority for program planning and coordination suggesting the concept of supermanagement. According to Hoos (1972, p. 96):

Scientific corroboration can be cited as a reason for attacking a problem not only across traditional bureaus and divisions but also outside jurisdictional units and boundaries. In effect here is a tool for circumventing traditional checks and balances and undermining, for better or worse, the bureaucratic structure.

In a related vein, management science in the name of objectivity and rationality can also be used to defuse politically charged issues and to remove them from the vicissitudes of public debate.

In developing the political role of managerial science, the tradeoff between expediency and democracy is seldom explicit; in many respects politics is beginning to resemble the management of technical efficiency. Techniques of rationality hold out the potential for circumventing conflict arising from democratic processes of political choice and value judgments. Because they tend to be regarded as an intrusion on the business of government, political problems are treated as administrative problems.

Because of the diversity of skills involved, expertise in the new management science is difficult to establish. The ranks of the specialists are staffed with accountants, economists, econometricians, systems engineers, and business analysts. Evidence of competency is based primarily on the successful completion of a Ph.D. dissertation in which cost-effectiveness or some other accepted technique is brought to bear on a policy problem and on one's reputation for demonstrated practicality through means of occasional employment as a consultant to public or private agencies.

The ultimate aim of management science (i.e., the explication of assumptions and systematic assessment of the cost and effectiveness of alternatives) unquestionably contributes to a better grade of decision making and an improvement in governmental operations; where it falls short is in the implementation stage. Too often analysis is dependent on abstract models and arbitrary assumptions divorced from the realities of the environment in which decisions must be applied. These limitations are compounded by the practitioners whose knowledge of the problem area is often superficial because of training in a narrow graduate study area or because of job pressures to move quickly from one problem to another. It remains doubtful whether these deficiencies can be ameliorated through construction of more accurate measures and proxy indices alone. Nevertheless, a number of distinguished economists have expressed reservations about the power of quantitative methods. Leontief (1968) feels the models used are deficient because "the lack of factual knowledge of conditions existing in the real world forces the model builder to base many if not all of his general conclusions on all kinds of a priori assumptions chosen for their convenience rather than for their correspondence to the observed facts." Likewise, Boulding (1966) has warned against the temptation to try to quantify essentially subjective phenomena into indices. Regardless of whether the attempted quantification is in terms of money or some more complicated measure of payoff, it "introduces elements of ethical danger into the decision-making process, simply because the clarity and apparent objectivity of quantitatively measurable subordinate goals can easily lead to failure to bear in mind that they are in fact subordinate." In short, such methods make no allowance for humane sentiments or moral judgments. They frequently promote reductionism to the point of absurdity and to the likely conclusion that we may be looking to the wrong experts for help.

Regardless of whether something as subjective as health can ever be operationalized successfully and whether the methodology is capable of handling the enormously complicated interaction patterns of the large number of variables constituting the reality of policy decisions, quantitative analysis conceals considerable bias beyond that mentioned earlier. While actively disclaiming the influence of values and ideology other than the search for objectivity, most quantitative analysts remain by way of their socialization and training in business schools and departments of economics the unconscious if not conscious apostles of the market and business. Their involvement in the policy-making machinery helps to stimulate and reinforce the tendency of harried public officials to accept simple answers to complex problems, like calling for substitution of the market for public leadership in the delivery of health services. Policy recommendations ostensibly rooted in objective analysis more often than not are offshoots of normative economic theory containing a number of archaic assumptions about how people ought to behave and the way power is organized and distributed in society; e.g., man is an essentially hedonistic creature driven by calculated self-interest; rational decision makers always seek to optimize utility at the margin; because power corrupts, the best government—given the absence of power in the competitive private sector—is minimal government; there is an inevitable harmony between private interests and public good; and the ultimate test of value lies in its exchange price. (The relationship of so-called objective analysis to normative theory is developed more thoroughly by Myrdal (1955). An insightful critique of the shortcomings of normatively based objective economic analysis in the study of health economics is provided by Berki (1972).) The propensity of market-oriented analysts is understandably to see health services as another class of market goods. Therefore they either ignore or consciously disclaim any special characteristics of health services extending beyond mere efficiency to encompass matters of justice and equity. There is also a temptation to superimpose orthodox market frames of reference like consumer sovereignty and supply-demand explanations of inflation, which are not only irrelevant to what is occurring in the health field, but inapplicable in the general economy as well.

It may be impossible to devise a perfect solution in practice, but informed and responsible policy making requires a process of multiple inputs and a range of alternative options. Though often condemned as inefficient, systemic dissonance arising from the orderly presentation of many views and interests has long been the cornerstone of enlightened public policy. The disproportionate inclusion of quantitative and pro-market analysts in the policy process and the prevalent attitude of dismissing as irrelevant the potential contributions of social scientists and persons interested in ethical dimensions is shortsighted. Unless balanced by social, political, and moral inputs, health policy may not only suffer from political myopia, but may fail entirely in relating to the wants of the people.

CONSEQUENCES

If health policy can no longer afford to ignore the troublesome questions of efficient resource allocation, it can less afford to lose sight of the qualitative-ethical facets essential to the promotion of individual and community welfare. Clearly, there is a need for a more comprehensive and better integrated approach.

Social Cohesion and Mental Health

Health services play a major role in keeping society together. Conventional functions include disease prevention, illness treatment, and care of the long-term sick. Health services also partially fill the emotional-spiritual void in today's highly developed society created by the breakup of family structure and other primary groups, the decline of religious faith, the trauma of accelerating rates of social and technologic change, the cultural uprootedness and emotional maladjustment associated with high rates of population mobility, the pressures of urban-industrial living, and the depersonalization of interpersonal relationships caused by bureaucratization. While these changes are firmly associated with progress in material comfort and individual freedom, they have exacted a heavy price in community disorganization and individual despondency. The alarming increase in acts of violence (such as murders, rapes, skyjackings, political confrontations, assassinations, and urban crimes) and the soaring incidence of mental illness, drug addiction, and alcoholism attest to the difficulty a highly developed society like the United States has in keeping its social and political relations intact.

The problems are in large measure reverberations of the cultural revolution accompanying industrial progress in which utilitarian values have replaced older community values. Utilitarian culture is the foundation stone of a market economy. In the name of efficiency it diminishes the individual by focusing on a side of his life that is significant not in its personal uniqueness but only in its usefulness to others. In the name of productivity it places a greater stress on performance (winning or losing, success or failure) than upon the character of the intentions and the motivations that shape a person's actions—propriety and adherence to moral standards are secondary to the exigencies of productivity. In this climate things are good or evil not in themselves, but in whether they produce agreeable outcomes, and the question of personal worth is resolved by exchange value. Man has no intrinsic worth, only that which can be priced and exchanged in the job market; only those things which make money are useful. (For a fuller discussion of the development and implications of utilitarian culture, see Gouldner, 1970, pp. 61-87.)

With the decline of the family, the neighborhood, and the church, health is the only remaining major social institution to which modern man can turn for the comfort and nourishment of deep-seated emotional and spiritual needs. Perhaps values of compassion, sympathy, understanding, charity, and individual dignity sound anachronistic, but together with responsibility to care for the sick they are a vital feature of civilized life and the philosophical hallmark of health services. That these values have survived so long in the health field notwithstanding the internal challenge from scientific-technologic medicine and the external assault of utilitarianism may be a measure of the depth of modern man's unfilled needs and the functional significance of humanitarian values in the machine-like culture of a market economy.

The relationship between health and advanced industrial society may be more complementary than imagined. In maintaining a link to the past, health services provide an important anchorage for individuals awash in an anomic sea. In responding to subjective needs, health services provide a refuge from the rigors of highly depersonalized living. In placing social and ethical criteria ahead of efficiency and productivity, health services provide a place of refuge. In terms of their functionality for encouraging unification of interests, health services contribute considerably to the maintenance of political stability and consensus. They are, in conjunction with other social services, an adaptive mechanism for social survival and tension management, and comprise one of the more enlightened ways by which societies maintain themselves and survive. Through their role in resource reallocation they ameliorate social conflict, make possible a measure of restitutive justice, and strengthen the bonds of social solidarity. They are a major force in denying the prediction of the inevitable collapse of capitalism and the industrial economy. (For an elaboration of the functionalist argument and other views of the role of social services, together with their theoretical antecedents, see Pinker, 1971.)

The chaotic contemporary urban-industrial scene reaffirms that, although many still strive for a better material standard of living, a growing number of others are trying to attain a better balancing of materialism with quality of life aspirations. Society may be approaching the state of diminishing marginal benefits in its use of material goods as an instrument for motivating and guiding individual behavior. In any event, it is difficult to imagine how people can be expected to accept the discipline of labor and productivity if they themselves feel expendable and insignificant.

Economic Growth

The assumption that health services spending conflicts with economic growth is questionable. In fact, little empirical research has been devoted to proving what is a highly abstract assumption. On balance, the widespread egalitarian reform in the post-World War II period in western and northern Europe has been correlated with higher rather than lower rates of progress. Many planners and politicians are beginning to realize what has long been accepted in Sweden, that health and welfare reforms, instead of being an impediment, actually may provide the floor for a strong and more vital economy (Myrdal, 1972). Significantly, for the ten-year period ending in 1966, total taxes expressed as a percentage of the GNP increased from 29.4 to 41 percent in Sweden, and in the United States increased from only 25.8 to 28.2 percent (First National City Bank of New York, 1968). In the decade 1959-1969, the GNP grew at an annual rate of nearly 5 percent in Sweden as compared with about 4 percent for the U.S. (Statistical Office of the European Communities, 1970, p. 24). Near the end of that period (1966-1968), public health expenditures (as distinct from total health expenditures) amounted to from 5 to 6 percent of the GNP in Sweden in contrast to from 2 to 2.5 percent of the GNP in the U.S. Even with the sharp increases associated with Medicare and Medicaid, public outlays for health in the U.S. have not, as recently as 1973, grown appreciably beyond 3 percent of the GNP (Simanis, 1970; Lindencrona, 1971; Skolnik and Dales, 1974).

Should it indeed be the case that public consumption cannot be increased without lowering the rate of increase of private consumption (if inflation is to be avoided), it does not necessarily follow that to act in favor of something so basic to human wants as health decrees a lower rate of increase in economic growth. Quite possibly in a society where people are reacting against the depersonalization of a market economy and the tiresome, if not boring, effects of machine methods of production and incessant competition, the opposite may be true.

In choosing between the two methods of health services management, it should be remembered that the taxes Americans pay are not out of line with those of persons living in countries in comparable stages of development. Actually, with the exceptions of Japan, where total taxes are substantially lower, and Canada, where the tax burden is about the same as that in the United States, the U.S. tax burden ranks at the bottom of the scale. Average total contributions for the period 1967-1969 equalled only 30 percent of the U.S. GNP as contrasted with 34.1 percent in Denmark, 34.2 percent in the United Kingdom, 35.1 percent in West Germany, 37 percent in France, 37.8 percent in the Netherlands, 38.7 percent in Norway, and 40.7 percent in Sweden. (It is true that, in personal income taxes, total direct taxes on households, and direct taxes on corporations, the U.S. ranks close to the top.)

A solution for obtaining additional revenues may lie in turning to largely untapped indirect forms of taxation and social security contributions. Unlike most highly developed nations where the practice is to lean more heavily on indirect sources rather than on direct taxes, the U.S. has opted for a policy of high rates of direct taxation and low rates of indirect taxation, so that while total taxes are low relative to other developed nations the volume of complaint is loud (Organization for Economic Cooperation and Development, 1972, p. 71). The trend, however, is toward placing greater reliance on indirect taxes for financing social programs. Payroll taxes for social security and related programs have been growing rapidly in recent decades and in 1975 they are planned to account for nearly 30 percent of all federal budget receipts, compared with 23 percent in 1970 and 16 percent in 1960. Throughout this period the federal budget receipts from individual income taxes have remained quite steady, varying only slightly in the range of 44 to 47 percent. Reliance on corporate income taxes has, however, diminished from 23 percent in 1960 to 17 percent in 1970 and 15 percent in 1975 (Bechman, Gramlich, and Hartman, 1974). This trend reflects the dilemma encountered in all advanced capitalist-democratic countries whenever faster economic growth is followed as an expedient alternative to potentially politically divisive and tension-producing schemes of income redistribution through the direct taxation of individuals. Lower taxes on business and industry are justified as necessary for financing investments that will produce faster growth rates enabling all interest groups to benefit, no matter how unevenly, without the appearance of having had anything taken away.

The consequence of insufficient government spending is predictable: retardation of the public infrastructure and social services. Publicly supported services in the U.S. in the form of housing, welfare, health, and social security benefits for unemployed, disabled, and retired workers rank among the least developed among advanced industrial nations of the world. The unprecedented high level of consumer comfort available to those who can afford it in the U.S. conflicts sharply with poverty, unemployment, and social misery—conditions perhaps greater in scope and intensity than any in the developed world. In a nation where it is assumed that every individual possesses the opportunity and means to provide for himself there is little provision for those who fail to make it or fall behind.

The progressivity in principle of a policy of resorting to direct taxes in the United States is weakened severely in practice by the loopholes which riddle the tax system and enable those who could and should pay more to pay far less than their fair share. Closing these loopholes and tax dodges enjoyed by the wealthy and the large corporations could significantly expand opportunities for further developing publicly supported health services in the U.S. Subsidies in the form of investment credits, foreign tax credits, and accelerated depreciation write-offs amount to some $50 to 60 billion annually—or about a quarter of the federal budget. It has been estimated that a more modest and realistically attainable closing of loopholes would produce at least $10 billion a year in additional revenues (Shanahan, 1973).

In light of the available options for raising revenues, the reluctance to expand funding of publicly supported health services merits reconsideration. The strategy with the best probability for successfully bringing the population of the country closer together and for maintaining a strong economy may well involve more health and social service spending, rather than less.

SUMMARY AND CONCLUSIONS

The idea has been advanced that the selection of priorities in health policy is based less on what is good and just in a moral sense than on what produces profit and saves money. Contrary to intent, such an approach may be counterproductive, resulting in harmful effects in terms of contributing to a mounting deterioration of human relations in modern society with a parallel exacerbation of sociopolitical unrest, to greater amounts of personal stress with correspondingly higher rates of mental illness, and to lower rather than higher rates of economic growth. Correcting our priorities requires a stronger financial base and a greater reliance on public rather than private consumption.

The current preoccupation with management in the health services may be an overreaction to the fears of many economists (mainly speculative) that objectives of economic growth and high rates of spending for social services are not compatible.

While supportive of some arguments for stronger management and welcoming the contributions it can make to the provision of a better organization and the distribution of health services at lower costs, one must urge caution, lest concern with efficiency and productivity backfire. By virtue of their roots in business-industrial applications, managerial techniques are, despite claims of objectivity and value neutrality, biased in favor of the selection of simplistic private sector solutions. By virtue of their emulation of science and its methods, they are biased in favor of the selection of quantifiable programs. By virtue of their foundation in normative theory they are highly reductionistic and unrepresentative of the realities of applied decision making. They also tend to be highly insensitive to the social, political, and moral dimensions of problem solving which are the cornerstone of social policy, and differentiate it from decision making in the private sector, where in the name of capital accumulation one need look at efficiency and productivity only in terms of rate of return on investments and what the contribution to profits will be.

Judiciously used with an understanding of both their limitations and their implicit biases, the techniques of management science can help to clarify policy choices within precisely circumscribed areas. However, in the milieu of contemporary policy making management science functions less as an analytic tool than as an ideology which obfuscates the inherently complicated social and ethical components of health services. This leads inevitably to the subservience of quality of life goals to narrowly defined means of technical and economic efficiency. At the levels of both analysis and ideology there is a need to complement the utilitarianism of management science with a stronger humanist orientation.

POSTSCRIPT

The bulk of this article was conceived and written as the Nixon Administration was entering its second term of office and as the major outlines of its effort to impose its will on the health sector were becoming more concrete. The events of Watergate have overtaken this initiative and the future of health policy is fluid. Certainly one of the messages of the Watergate affair is that the process by which decisions are made can be equally if not more important than the actual choices—a basic truism about democratic societies and the structuring of their institutions that seems to have been overlooked at times because of the rapture with managerial ideology in government which had its beginnings in the Kennedy Administration. There is a good deal of bipartisan rhetoric in the air presently focused on the "healing" of the nation. It remains to be determined whether concerns over "healing" will predominate for long over narrow preoccupations with economic values and the well entrenched but oftentimes hidden ideological blinders of management science in which technique is seen as a superior substitute for human judgment. The struggle over defining the ultimate nature of health care and the appropriate function of health services continues. Albeit guarded, there is, however, some cause for optimism. Recognition of the larger contributions described in this article which health services can make to social well-being may have influenced President Carter to urge the Congress to rank national health insurance among the nation's leading domestic legislative priorities.

REFERENCES

American Enterprise Institute for Public Policy Research. *Proceedings of the Conference on Health Planning, Certificate of Need, and Market Entry.* Washington, D.C.: The Institute, 1972.

Arrow, K. J. "Uncertainty and the Welfare Economics of Medical Care." *American Economic Review* 53 (1963): 941-72.

Battistella, R. M. "Towards National Health Insurance in the U.S.A.: An Examination of Leading Proposals." *Acta Hospitalia* 13 (1973): 3-22.

Bechman, B. M.; Gramlich, E. M.; and Hartman, R. W. *Setting National Priorities: The 1975 Budget.* Washington, D.C.: Brookings Institution, 1974.

Berki, S. *Hospital Economics.* Lexington, Mass.: Lexington Books, 1972.

Boulding, K. "The Ethics of Rational Decision." *Management Science* 12 (1966): B-165.

Cooper, B. S., and Worthington, N. L. "National Health Expenditures, 1929-1972." *Social Security Bulletin* 36 (1973): 3-19.

Dale, E. L., Jr. "Must the Budget Be Uncontrollable?" *Sunday New York Times* (September 1974): 2F.

Davis, K. *Medical Policies and Costs* (testimony before the Subcommittee on Consumer Economics of the Joint Economic Committee of the U.S., 93rd Congress, 1st Session). Washington, D.C.: Government Printing Office, 1973.

Etzioni, A. *A Comparative Analysis of Complex Organizations.* New York: Free Press, 1961.

First National City Bank of New York. *Monthly Economic Letter* (April 1968): 45.

Fried, E. R.; Rivlin, A. M.; Schultze, C. L.; and Teeters, N. H. *Setting National Priorities: The 1974 Budget.* Washington, D.C.: Brookings Institution, 1973.

Fuchs, V. R. "Health Care and the United States Economic System: An Essay in Abnormal Psychology." *Milbank Memorial Fund Quarterly* 50 (1972): 211-37.

Gouldner, A. W. *The Coming Crisis of Western Sociology.* New York: Basic Books, 1970.

Health Maintenance Organizations: The Statements of President Richard M. Nixon and Secretary Elliot L. Richardson of the U.S. Department of Health, Education, and Welfare. Washington, D.C.: Government Printing Office, 1972.

Hoos, I. R. *Systems Analysis in Public Policy: A Critique.* Berkeley: University of California Press, 1972.

Leontief, W. "Review of *Perspectives on Economic Growth.*" *New York Review* (October 10, 1968): 32.

Lindencrona, F. "The Organization of Health and Medical Services." *The Swedish Health Services System* (lectures from the American College of Hospital Administrators, 22nd Fellows Seminar, Stockholm, 1969). Chicago: American College of Hospital Administrators, 1971.

Myrdal, G. *The Political Element in the Development of Economic Theory.* Cambridge, Mass.: Harvard University Press, 1955.

Myrdal, G. *Objectivity in Social Research.* New York: Pantheon, 1969.

Myrdal, G. "The Place of Values in Social Policy." *Journal of Social Policy* 1 (1972): 1-14.

Newhouse, J. P.; Phelps, C. E.; and Schwartz, W. B. "Policy Options and the Impact of National Health Insurance." *New England Journal of Medicine* 290 (1974): 1345-59.

Organization for Economic Cooperation and Development. *Expenditure Trends in OECD Countries, 1960-1980.* Paris: OECD, 1972.

Parsons, T. *The Social System.* Glencoe, Ill.: Free Press, 1951.

Pinker, R. *Social Theory and Social Policy.* London: Heinemann Educational Books, 1971.

Rice, D., and Cooper, B. S. "National Health Expenditures, 1929-1970." *Social Security Bulletin* 34 (1971): 3-18.

Rice, D., and McGee, M. F. *Projections of National Health Expenditures, 1975 and 1980* (Research and Statistics Note no. 18). Washington, D.C.: Office of Research and Statistics, Social Security Administration, 1970.

Shanahan, E. "Mills Challenges Capital Gain Taxes on Some Investments as Hearings Open." *New York Times* (February 6, 1973): 24.

Simanis, J. G. "International Health Expenditures." *Social Security Bulletin* 33 (1970): 18-19.

Skolnik, A. M., and Dales, S. R. "Social Welfare Expenditures, 1972-1973." *Social Security Bulletin* 37 (1974): 3-18.

Statistical Office of the European Communities. *Basic Statistics of the Community* (10th ed.). Brussels: Office for Official Publications of the European Communities, 1970.

Thoenes, P. *The Elite in the Industrial State.* New York: Free Press, 1966.

U.S. Department of Health, Education, and Welfare. *Towards a Comprehensive Health Policy for the 1970s: A White Paper.* Washington, D.C.: HEW, 1971.

Waldman, S. *National Health Insurance Proposals* (Publication no. SSA 74-11920). Washington, D.C.: HEW, 1974.

Selection by Roger M. Battistella and Theodore E. Chester

The monitoring and evaluation of the efficacy and cost efficiency of medical services compelled by the Professional Standards Review Organization (PSRO) program represent a radical break with long-established principles of autonomy in medical practice. Notwithstanding the skepticism of critics, who either quarrel with the goals of the program or believe that they do not go far enough, this analysis concludes that the benefits are important enough to compensate for the many risks and limitations. Unrealistic short-term demands on the part of government may, however, stifle the program and endanger its survival. The cooperation of the medical profession is essential to the introduction and maintenance of changes in clinical practice which are responsive to political requirements for stronger and more uniform quality controls and sensitive to costs.

The significance of the PSRO program is not easy to grasp. Propaganda disseminated by competing interest groups clouds understanding of the reasons for its origin and solicits superficial analysis and interpretation. Illustrative of the confusion surrounding the program are (1) the claims by the American Medical Association that it is a sinister extension of "big brother government," when, in fact, the AMA was a prime mover in getting the Congress to approve the program in the first place; (2) the claims that government is "pouring new wine into old bottles" in an attempt to assuage the suspicions of medical practitioners

This selection, "The Professional Standards Review Organization Programs: A Political-Economic Assessment," was prepared especially for this volume.

219

about losses of clinical freedom which could erupt into resistance and non-cooperation; and (3) the complaints of political critics who believe that the government is "insensitive to social needs" and will, therefore, assign a higher priority to saving money than to improving the availability of high-quality services, notwithstanding repeated assurances that the two are interconnected and will be given comparable weight. (For an overview of these conflicting interpretations, see Turner, 1974; Hicks, 1973; American Medical Association, 1973. For more detail, see U.S. Congress, 1974a; Cohen, 1975.)

The purpose of this paper is twofold: to describe some of the economic and social forces guiding the evolution of the professional service organizations, and to assess the benefits and risks, including some of the consequential secondary effects, for government, providers, and consumers. The significance of the program for other highly developed countries experiencing similar pressures for cost containment and quality assurance is also discussed.

PROGRAM AIMS AND ORIGINS

The PSRO program was conceived by legislative sponsors as a twin-barreled strategy for containing the costs and raising the standard of services rendered to recipients of federally funded health care programs (i.e., Medicare, Medicaid, maternal and child health, and services for crippled children). It provides, through sanctions designed to appeal to the enlightened self-interest of the medical profession, for the monitoring and evaluation of the utilization of acute hospitals and long-term care facilities in accord with reasonable standards of acceptable medical practice.

Organizations under the domination of medical practitioners are entrusted with the responsibility of assuring the social accountability of physicians by rating their diagnostic and treatment decisions against locally established criteria and by advising them of deviations from criteria which may indicate that inpatient services are being used unnecessarily, or that the care given to patients is medically questionable or inappropriate. Penalties for violators include the withholding of payment for services, fines up to $5,000, and exclusion from further participation in Medicare and Medicaid.

Authorization for the PSRO program stems from the 1972 Amendments to the Social Security Act (U.S. Congress, 1972). Specifically, PSROs are empowered to carry out the following four functions: first, the determination of whether services provided are medically necessary and in accordance with prevailing areawide standards in ascertaining the eligibility of doctors and hospitals for reimbursement in federally funded programs; second, the development and use of alternatives to costly forms of treatment and institutionalization in hospitals and nursing homes; third, the establishment and regular review of statistical profiles of the services rendered by individual hospitals and medical practitioners; and, fourth, the analysis of the volume of unnecessary, substandard, and/or inappropriate services through the review of aggregated data of groups of hospitals and practitioners.

PROGRESS IN IMPLEMENTATION

A total of 203 agencies have been designated. On average, each service area will include thirty-five hospitals and a population of one million, counting nonrecipients of government-sponsored health services. (A concise summary of the legislative provisions and a status report on progress in implementation may be found in U.S. Department of Health, Education, and Welfare, 1977a.) The proportion of the U.S. population subject to PSRO controls is about one-fourth which, in turn, accounts for nearly one-third of the annual personal medical services consumption. The dimensions of the PSRO effort form a critical mass sufficient for the accumulation of the necessary experience, should lawmakers decide to make coverage universal.

The complexity of the PSRO undertaking, which is both politically daring and technically challenging, is mirrored in the unusually long lead-time of six years set originally to complete the implementation. Because the complications have been greater than foreseen, the program is not expected to be fully operational before the early 1980s.

The support of at least 25 percent of the physicians in active practice within the service area is required before an organization can win approval. Evidence of unhappiness among as few as 10 percent of the physicians in an area is sufficient to force a poll. Each PSRO is required also to complete a planning phase and a conditional period prior to receiving the federal government's full endorsement. The planning phase allows for the enrollment of physicians and a tooling up of procedures and organizational structure. The conditional stage runs for a minimum of two years and is designed to assure that each agency is capable of performing its mission before obtaining final approval. Full endorsement signifies that a PSRO is satisfactorily performing both short-term and long-term inpatient care review.

Progress to date in the implementation of the PSRO program has been slow but steady. The number of conditional organizations grew from eleven in 1974 to 108 in 1977. Government sources anticipate 183 conditional and twenty fully designated PSROs by the end of the 1978 fiscal year. The power reserved to the Secretary of the Department of Health, Education, and Welfare to allow other qualified organizations (e.g., health maintenance organizations and health departments) to execute PSRO functions has been a spur to cooperation among otherwise recalcitrant private medical practitioners.

The legislation provides for the establishment of advisory bodies to assist the Secretary of Health, Education, and Welfare on matters of implementation—the National Professional Standards Review Council and statewide Professional Standards Review councils. The National Council consists of eleven physicians appointed by the Secretary, who are recognized as experts in the field of quality assessment and who are, moreover, sensitive to the procedures and needs of private practice. The responsibilities of this body include: advising on policy matters, providing for the development and distribution of information to PSROs, reviewing and assessing the performance of PSROs, and submitting an annual report to the Secretary and to Congress on its activities and those of the PSROs. The primary duties of the statewide councils are to coordinate PSRO activities within their boundaries, to provide technical assistance, to assist in the evaluation of each PSRO's performance, and, if necessary, to assist the Secretary in finding a qualified replacement PSRO. Statewide councils are allowed only in states with three or more PSROs. To date, eighteen states have met the requirement. Membership on the councils is required to consist of at least four public representatives (i.e., persons knowledgeable about health care, of whom at least two are recommended by the governor) together with representatives from the state hospital association and state medical society. Each PSRO is entitled to a single member.

Each statewide council and each PSRO in states without a statewide council is required to have the advice and assistance of a seven- to eleven-member advisory group, representing nonmedical health professionals and hospitals and related health care facilities. The legislation also provides for the establishment of temporary statewide support centers to assist interested physicians' groups in completing the qualifying requirements for selection in the PSRO program. Support for this activity is scheduled to be phased out once the PSRO network is completed.

BENEFITS ASSESSMENT

One should not surmise that the PSRO program represents a one-sided victory of the federal government over a reactionary medical profession, steadfastly opposed to any encroachment upon traditional clinical freedoms. Surprising as it might appear, given the historic antipathy between the parties, the program is more of a partnership effort in which both the federal government and the AMA have made concessions in the expectation of receiving some valued returns. The immediate benefits of this association are substantial and probably will grow with time. They encompass consumers as well as government and providers. The scope of the PSRO mandate and the complexity of the relationships involved contain ingredients for the production of external effects which may outweigh in their consequences the outcomes intended by the program's sponsors.

Government

The pressures impinging on the federal government to control runaway spending for Medicare and Medicaid is the most common explanation of why PSROs were established. (The cost-containment aspects of the PSRO strategy are presented in Congressional Research Service, 1978.) Expenditures for these two programs have far surpassed the initial estimates. The open-ended arrangement whereby the government is required to reimburse providers for reasonable and customary charges inevitably has created pressures for intervention, because of its intrinsically inflationary nature.

The PSRO program builds on and expands earlier utilization review requirements introduced separately to control excess utilization of Medicare and Medicaid. To say that the results of the government's experience suggest that there is a great deal of room for improvement is to understate the enormity of the problems it has encountered. Evidence compiled by the federal government and other sources reveals a shockingly high incidence of questionable and often unnecessary medical procedures performed in hospitals. These procedures can waste lives as well as dollars. It is estimated that as much as 17 percent of the elective surgery performed would fail to be confirmed, if subjected to a second medical opinion. The consequences for Medicare and Medicaid are stupendous. "There were an estimated 2.4 million unnecessary surgeries performed in 1974, at a cost to the American public of almost $4 billion. These unnecessary surgeries led to 11,900 unnecessary deaths" (U.S. Congress, 1976, p. 39). It has also been estimated that as much as one-fourth of the surgeries performed in hospitals are simple enough to be done on an outpatient basis. Assuming that as little as $300 could be saved for each case of nonhospitalized surgery, the savings applicable to the Medicaid program alone are calculated to approximate $150 million annually (U.S. Congress, 1976, p. 32). Surplus bed capacity contributes to some of the unnecessary hospital costs. It is claimed that up to one-fifth of the existing capacity of hospitals could be eliminated with no harmful effects on the health of the population (Congressional Research Service, 1978, p. 23).

Adverse drug reactions are another risk confronting hospitalized patients. The literature suggests that the prevalence of adverse drug reactions among hospitalized medical patients ranges from 6 to 15 percent (Karch and Lasagna, 1975, p. 13). The dangers of hospitalization vary directly with increases in the numbers of complex procedures carried out and length of stay. White has cited data in Congressional testimony underscoring just how dangerous hospitals have become. "In at least one study, 20 percent of the patients experienced some hazardous episode and 7 percent died as a result" (U.S. Congress, 1974a, p. 116). It is doubtful whether more than one-fourth of all the tests, procedures, and therapeutic regimens imposed on patients are more beneficial and useful than harmful or useless (U.S. Congress, 1974a, p. 116). Parallel to this assertion, Blue Shield (1977) decided recently to discontinue routine payment for thirty diagnostic and surgical procedures of questionable value (e.g., basal metabolic rate; ballistocardiogram; angiocardiography, single or multiple plane, in conjunction with cineradiography; radical hemorrhoidectomy; hypogastric neurectomy; ligation of internal mammary arteries).

Conditions in long-term facilities are worse than those in acute hospitals.

From one-fourth to one-half of Medicaid expenditures for nusing home care is said to be for patients who could be cared for equally well and for less money in the home or in the community (U.S. Congress, 1971, p. 7). Evidence of substandard patient care is widespread, for example, insufficient medical and nursing attention, inadequate control of drugs, physical abuse, and exposure to unsanitary conditions and hazardous environments (U.S. Congress, 1974b). Studies of hospitalized mental patients reveal similarly deplorable conditions of improper placement, inadequate medical care, and abuse (see, for example, Fuller, 1974; Rosenhan, 1974, pp. 267-86).

Secondary benefits

It is predictable that the effect of the greater availability of more systematic and reliable data will be to provoke questions about whether differences in utilization patterns can be supported on medical grounds and to generate political pressures for reducing gaps among social groups and geographic areas (Caper, 1974). Despite the fact that their medical needs tend to be greater, members of minority groups receive fewer services than others. Facilities for the poor and minority groups are often located in settings suggesting the continuing presence of discrimination and other barriers to equal treatment. For example, whites use nursing homes and intermediate care services at a rate five times greater than minorities, whereas minorities are admitted to state and county mental hospitals at twice the rate for whites. The rate of blacks in mental institutions is slightly more than 50 percent greater than the rate for whites. For ambulatory services, racial minorities are twice as likely to use a clinic or an emergency room as whites. Compared to whites, racial minorities undertake greater travel time and experience longer office waiting times. Minorities are also less apt to receive preventive health services than whites. Major differences also may be found in Medicaid payments per recipient, which are 75 percent greater for whites than for members of minorities (U.S. Department of Health, Education, and Welfare, 1977b).

Medicare and Medicaid have been plagued from the start by large regional disparities in hospital admissions and lengths of stay. Among Medicare enrollees, for example, the admissions rate per 1,000 in 1973 averaged 321 for the nation as a whole, but ranged from a low of 241 in Maine to a high of 457 in North Dakota. While the national average length of stay was 11.7 days, it ran from a low of 8.0 in Virginia to a high of 15.5 in New York. Differences in the use of hospital and physician services account principally for the considerable variation in public outlays. Thus, in 1969 public spending for hospital care in the District of Columbia was roughly 3.5 times greater than the national average, whereas in Mississippi the amount was less than the average by nearly half. Spending for physician services in California was almost double the national average, while outlays in South Carolina were only half that for the country as a whole (U.S. Department of Health, Education, and Welfare, 1977c, pp. 79-100).

More uniform access to health services has implications for larger social goals. It would boost economic progress in underdeveloped regions of the country and help to lessen tensions among racial and other minorities. The responsibility of the National Professional Standards Review Council to review regional norms, and to approve all instances when local norms deviate widely from regional practices, provides powerful leverage for the leveling of differences within and across regions.

Taken on its own, the purpose of the PSRO program is deceptively straightforward—to restrict the reimbursement of providers participating in federally funded health programs to medically necessary and efficacious services given on a least-cost alternative basis. The implications telescope, however, when juxtaposed with cognate developments. Looked at as a whole, the multitude of cost-containment activities currently sponsored by the federal government compose a pattern of major change in the organization and delivery of health services. Together with programs in the areas of regional planning, health maintenance organizations, hospital reimbursement experiments, and attempts to cut back the supply of hospital beds and to affect the number and distribution of medical practitioners by specialty, PSROs are an important cog in the creation of a nationwide planning and management system capable of responding effectively to signals communicated from the center.

From the Nixon Administration onward, the White House has insisted that a system of workable controls over spending and standards of care is a precondition for national health insurance. A reluctance to incur a repeat performance of the explosive cost increases associated with Medicare and Medicaid lies at the bottom of this insistency (U.S. Congress, 1974a, 1977a, 1977b; U.S. Department of Health, Education, and Welfare, 1976, pp. 29-46). The future of national health insurance is tied, therefore, to what PSROs and related programs show can be done to assure economy and effectiveness in health services.

Organized Medicine

Amidst mounting doubt about the benevolence of a previously sacrosanct profession, the denigration of self-regulation as a euphemism for monopoly power has become fashionable. What was long the lonely terrain of frustrated reformers has become crowded with opportunists and curiosity seekers sensing the collapse of a once-inviolable mythology. Even government agencies formerly noted for keeping a reverential distance have joined in the attack. Organized medicine is now being challenged in the courts by the Justice Department and the Federal Trade Commission to show that it is not engaging in unfair restraint of competition. (These attacks are causing the AMA to modify slightly restrictions against competition and advertising; see, for example, American Medical Association, 1977.) And statements from the President's Council on Wage and Price Stability implicate the professional ethic as mere monopolistic license (see Shabecoff, 1978).

Against the backdrop of criticism signaling the imminent decline of professional prerogatives, the PSRO program offers organized medicine what may be a propitious opportunity to halt the flow of recent reversals to the practice of self-regulation vital to the continuation of a free and vigorous profession. Lawyers and dentists are also experiencing a sizable erosion of trust and faith among politicians, which may indicate the emergence of a general antiprofessional sentiment in national policy (Demkovich, 1976; *Wall Street Journal,* 1977; Kohlmeier, 1976). If so, the fate of the PSRO program could be a political bellwether for other professions, if for no other reason than the superior status and power commanded by medicine. (Some measure of the erosion of status previously enjoyed by the medical and legal professions may be found in Goodman, 1978, and the cover story on lawyers in the April 10, 1978 issue of *Time.*)

It is a sign of the changing times that management has penetrated deeply into the once exclusively medical domain of quality assurance. The participation of hospital administrators and trustees stirred by recent court rulings expanding liability for medical malpractice has been legitimized further by the accountability demands on payments which hospitals receive from public sources. Much to the chagrin of the medical profession, others also became involved. In order to determine the appropriateness of services ordered by doctors for Medicare and Medicaid patients, the government authorized the participation of insurance companies and public agencies associated with the administration of the programs. This was particularly resented by organized medicine, which objected loudly to the growing authority of insurance company clerks and bureaucrats in medical matters (Bauer, 1975; Goran et al., 1976).

In battling unrelentingly to restore the principle of peer review in the clinical arena, the AMA achieved notable success. Changes in PSRO regulations adopted in 1976 require that a determination of medical nonnecessity be restricted to physicians, and then only after careful consultation with the physician whose decision is being questioned. The role of nonmedical personnel is restricted mainly to monitoring standards established by physicians. Because of differences in treatment of the long-term ill, there are, however, provisions for nonmedical health professionals to participate in the setting of patient care standards for skilled and intermediate care nursing homes. (A review of AMA objections to the original PSRO mandate and the legal maneuvering resulting in changes acceptable to the medical profession may be found in *Federal Register,* 1976.)

Practitioners upset over how standardized treatment norms and formalized peer review might cramp their clinical freedom are not entirely without compensation. Physicians cooperating in good faith with PSRO requirements and procedures need not worry about not receiving payment for services provided to recipients of government programs. Those who comply are assured in advance of receiving full payment for their services and are thereby freed from worrying about bill collection.

Furthermore, the legislation implies strongly that some relief may be forthcoming in the malpractice area. The civil annuity provision states that no physician or other provider of health services shall be civilly liable for actions taken in reliance upon or in compliance with PSRO-developed standards, provided due care is exercised. The Congressional intent, clearly, is to give doctors an incentive to cooperate (U.S. Department of Health, Education, and Welfare, 1972, pp. 13-14). Although patients will continue to have the right to bring legal suit, the courts, entangled in a field in which they have neither expertise nor clear guidelines, may succumb to the idea that practice consistent with PSRO standards and norms is an acceptable test of quality and act accordingly to narrow the boundaries for litigation (Blum et al., 1977, pp. 166-67).

Malpractice is an especially serious problem for U.S. physicians (deLesseps, 1977, pp. 145-61). Due to increased litigation and a trend toward larger jury-awarded settlements, private companies underwriting malpractice insurance have sought to withdraw from the business or to hike premiums by as much as 300 percent. For practitioners in vulnerable surgical specialties (orthopedics, neurosurgery, etc.), the annual cost of malpractice insurance protection is as high as $40,000 in some states. Unhappiness over projected increases and dissatisfaction over the reluctance of government to provide a satisfactory remedy is what precipitated the widely reported walkouts and job slow-downs and a march on the state capitol by doctors in California in 1975. (A popularized presentation of the issues may be found in the June 9, 1975 issue of *Newsweek*; see also Bird, 1975.)

Enigmatic Opposition of Organized Medicine

The AMA's public opposition to the PSRO program is puzzling. It is not at all what one would expect, given that the legislation was introduced and steered through the Congress at the behest of the organization's leadership. (This is made clear in Senator Wallace Bennett's response, on the Senate floor, to AMA allegations about the deleterious effects of PSROs; see U.S. Congress, 1974a, pp. 534-39.) One explanation, deduced from the realpolitik of organizations compelled to adjust to rapid changes after periods of prolonged stability, is that the AMA leadership may be too far ahead of rank-and-file members who are either less well-informed of the issues or are true believers in the antigovernment catechism espoused by AMA officials over the past half century. That is to say, the AMA leadership may be a captive of its own rhetoric. Saying one thing publicly, while doing something else privately, may be the price for retaining membership support (see Hague, 1974). After nearly two years of vacillation and indecision, the AMA's House of Delegates, a representative body closely attuned to rank-and-file sentiment, decided to endorse rather than oppose the program, possibly in the hope of influencing the interpretation of objectives and future changes to suit the interests of the medical profession. Consequently, the AMA has interpreted the program as intending to provide the highest quality of care possible, in contrast to the legislative preamble which says that the aim is to foster cost-effectiveness as well as appropriateness of services (see the testimony of AMA officials in U.S. Congress, 1974a, pp. 59-73).

Another explanation derives from the behind-the-scenes tactical maneuvering accompanying the process of conflict, negotiation, and compromise, which is an indispenable part of policy making. Having obtained a number of substantial concessions as quid pro quo for its cooperation, the AMA leadership possibly sensed a chance to obtain additional concessions by projecting a tough bargaining stance in public. Threats of noncooperation are common tactics for keeping the door open to further negotiation and compromise. In this vein, the leadership of organized medicine was especially frustrated over its inability to convince even its staunchest supporters in government that responsibility for the administration of the PSROs should be assigned to state medical societies affiliated with the AMA. The Congress concluded that the societies are no longer sufficiently representative of active practitioners to meet the requirements for public accountability because of declining membership among doctors and their popular image as trade associations (see Bennett, 1974). Obviously, the delegation of administrative responsibility to state medical societies would be an important step for securing and consolidating the power of organized medicine over the conditions of practice. The AMA has worked unwaveringly toward this objective and succeeded in getting the Secretary of Health, Education, and Welfare to recognize and fund a role for state medical societies in the provision of technical assistance and continuing education services to regional PSROs within their boundaries (see Senator Bennett's rebuttal to AMA criticisms in U.S. Congress, 1974a, p. 64).

The AMA also succeeded in liberalizing restrictions against the designation of single statewide PSROs. Among the 203 agencies designated for the United States (including the District of Columbia, Puerto Rico, the Virgin Islands, and other territories), thirty-one are statewide agencies. This list soon may be expanded to include Texas and Minnesota, which have petitioned for a single PSRO, despite guidelines requiring that each PSRO be small enough to allow efficient and manageable operation, and the active participation of local physicians (U.S. Department of Health, Education, and Welfare, 1977a, p. 6).

Another important item for negotiation and compromise centered on the provision in early drafts of the legislation requiring that doctors not be allowed to admit patients directly to hospitals without first getting the approval of a review committee that the utilization is necessary and desirable. Such a requirement is not mandatory in the PSRO program presently, but it remains a real possibility. When former Secretary of Health, Education, and Welfare Weinberger attempted to initiate preadmission review in 1975 to contain costs for hospital care in Medicare and Medicaid, the AMA persevered in getting a court injunction and the offensive requirement was removed in a revision of the program regulations, making prospective review a voluntary option (*Federal Register*, 1976, p. 13452). To date, only a single PSRO has exercised this option (U.S. Department of Health, Education, and Welfare, 1977d, p. 14).

The AMA prevailed in obtaining yet other modifications of the legislation when it was in the draft stages, including (a) the deletion of national norms of patient care; (b) the deletion of federal ownership of PSRO records; (c) the requirement for a referendum of physicians to determine whether a PSRO represents them; and (d) the initial restriction of PSRO responsibility to institutional care. Perhaps the single most important concession was the requirement that within a PSRO only physicians can make final decisions regarding the professional conduct of another physician (Sullivan, 1974).

The restoration of peer review and the notion that only physicians are capable of judging the medical necessity of the treatment given to a patient by another physician unquestionably is the biggest victory won by organized medicine. These are cardinal requisites for professional autonomy and freedom, with important spillovers for status, income, and ability to influence public policy.

Secondary benefits

Organized medicine will gain more from the PSRO program than reported thus far. Beyond the benefits mentioned, the development of information systems containing profile data on the clinical performance of individual practitioners is conducive to the drawing of relevant comparisons which could become a constructive tool for continuing education and self-improvement (Jesse et al., 1975). Appropriately organized and used, such an approach would be vastly superior to present methods in the U.S. which, following graduation from medical school and licensure, emphasize such punitive sanctions as censure, suspension, and loss of the right to practice.

The popular reproach that seldom-used penalties for malpractice and unethical conduct are irrefutable evidence of the inability of professionals to regulate themselves is too simplistic (McCleery et al., 1971). Such methods undoubtedly do not work well because they are too negative. Punishments ranging from loss of self-esteem to professional disgrace and loss of livelihood are too severe to be applied commonly by colleagues who (in the light of the baffling complexity of medicine today and the subjective nature of treatment) fear that there, but for the grace of God, go I! It is doubtful whether even lay persons could bring themselves often to impose such severe penalties on errant physicians. The reluctance of jury members to bring in convictions in drunken driver cases illustrates a similar psychological dilemma.

The issue of whether negative sanctions could be made to work through more vigorous enforcement is largely academic, considering that advances in legal due process have made it cumbersome to impose stiff penalties threatening rights as fundamental as the pursuit of one's occupation. The protracted legal postponement of relief is a strong possibility, even for the worst cases of wrongdoing. The information systems accompanying PSRO development substitute more positive incentives for keeping practitioners up-to-date on medical advances and for raising the standard of their diagnostic and treatment ability (U.S. Department of Health, Education, and Welfare, 1974a).

In addition to establishing a suitable framework for continuing education, PSRO data will help to expand the objective foundation of medicine. Despite the image aroused by achievements in science and technology, much of medical practice remains bound by custom and faith. Often aggressive and irreversible procedures, such as coronary bypass surgery and radical mastectomies, are approved and adopted without carefully controlled studies of their cost, safety, and efficacy (Bunker et al., 1977; Cochrane, 1972).

Differences in the way specific illnesses are treated often have little or no clinical justifications. Hospital admissions and lengths of stay vary widely by diagnosis within and across geographic areas, and the type of treatment received by sick persons can differ profoundly, depending on the type of specialist visited. For example, family practitioners, internists, orthopedists, and urologists treat backache dissimilarly. Other examples of the ambiguity of medical practice can be cited: the treatment of urinary tract infection varies depending on whether a gynecologist, urologist, or internist is consulted. In the treatment of rheumatism, the orthopedist generally is more aggressive than the rheumatologist. Similar differences in aggression prevail for the treatment of tonsillitis, depending on whether a pediatrician or otolaryngologist is in charge; for the treatment of lumps in the thyroid, depending on whether an internist or surgeon is in charge; and for the treatment of certain neck and head tumors, depending on whether a radiotherapist or a surgeon is in charge. (For an insight into the many shadow areas of medicine, see Ingelfinger et al., 1974.)

Variability in diagnosis and treatment will fade on exposure to normative standards derived from consensus among participating physicians. Placing of the burden of proof on physicians whose practices deviate appreciably from local standards of reasonableness will also reduce variability. Whether this is good or bad is arguable. The worst fears conjure up a deadening effect on innovation, should standards become relegated to "cookbook" status, a blind obedience to defensive medicine, and too heavy an emphasis on the policing of errant behavior (see the testimony of Joseph E. Boyle in U.S. Congress, 1974a, pp. 96-119).

On the other hand, PSROs may constitute an invaluable network for the accumulation and transmission of the large numbers of cases necessary for statistically reliable studies of the natural history of disease and the cost, safety, and efficacy of treatment alternatives. Under the best of circumstances such a system would also allow sufficient decentralization and flexibility for clinical innovation and the availability of teaching material directly appealing to local physicians engaged in effective career-long learning. While it is true, as contended by skeptics, that in the short run the case load of individual hospitals is too limited to allow them to document adequately the four diagnostic-specified medical case evaluations (MCEs) required annually to comply with quality assurance requirements, the need to correct this shortcoming will facilitate the cooperation and sharing essential for statistical reliability. (Criticism of the value of MCEs may be found in Institute of Medicine, 1976, pp. 1-6; Brook and Avery, 1976, pp.

221-52.) Properly done, the results of such studies will serve as objective feed-back for the revision of utilization norms on the place, length, and type of treat-ment for diagnostic-specific conditions appropriately adjusted to reflect differ-ences in severity of illness and personal attributes conditioning the risks to the patient.

All physicians stand to benefit from the PSRO program, but some may benefit more than others. The public interest objectives of the program coalesce with a heightened protectionist mood within the surgical specialties to form a political compound portending a drastic curtailment of the clinical scope of non-certified practitioners in surgery and medicine (see American College of Sur-geons and American Surgical Association, 1975).

A serious shortcoming of American medicine is that, following licensure, physicians are free to take on any medical procedure, no matter how complex (Stroman, 1976, pp. 114-39). Many hospitals have voluntarily imposed restric-tions on admitting and surgical privileges, in an attempt to assure standards of medical care, but the practice is far from universal. The consequence is that near-ly one-half of all operations done in the U.S. are by noncertified surgeons (American College of Surgeons and American Surgical Association, 1975, p. 11). The dangers to patients from a system which grants medical privileges too freely surely will be crystallized by PSRO data and furnish impetus to political de-mands for better and more uniform standards of care, regionally and nationally.

The prohibition of general practitioners and other noncertified practi-tioners from performing procedures for which they are unqualified is long over-due. The access of general practitioners to hospitals and the liberal policy towards certification has been put forth in the U.S., paradoxically, as a means for promoting quality medicine, while most other highly developed nations acted long ago to limit hospital practice to qualified practitioners, on the same grounds (see, for example, Welch, 1976, p. 181). Unrestricted medical privileges remained largely unchallenged in an era of resource abundance marked by a sup-ply of manpower insufficient to meet rising demands in the wake of increases in consumer purchasing power and higher rates of public spending. Now that re-sources are scarce and rates of growth are declining, the argument for open hos-pital privileges is less persuasive. Trepidation among many certified practitioners about unwanted reductions in work and income, as the result of more stringent government measures to contain costs through cuts in the supply of hospital beds and controls over hospital admissions and lengths of stay, could trigger de-fensive measures hastening the restriction of hospital privileges to certified prac-titioners. The added worry within many specialty fields that laissez-faire policies have resulted in an oversupply of practitioners is a further incitement to protec-tionism.

The report of the Study of Surgical Services in the United States (SOSSUS), sponsored jointly by the American College of Surgeons and the American Surgical Association, points to the dilemmas underlying the swing towards protectionism. Among other things, the report states that operative workloads, on average, are too low to support both the income expectations and quality of work of surgical practitioners. The income of surgeons is directly correlated with the number of procedures performed because of the preponderant reliance on fee-for-service payment. Regardless of mode of payment, the performance of a minimum number of procedures is required routinely in order to maintain an acceptable level of skill, especially in the case of complex surgical procedures. The SOSSUS report states that many surgeons are not being kept busy enough. Operations performed at such low rates as 0.5 per 1,000 population include some of the most complex procedures for cancer, gall bladder, prostate, congenital anomalies, hip reconstruction, and cardiac problems. Generally speaking, the rate of successful outcomes in such complex procedures is directly related to the number of operations performed by surgeons (American College of Surgeons and American Surgical Association, 1975, pp. 81-82).

The self-interest of surgeons about the effect of an oversupply of practitioners on personal income are revealed in the results of interviews conducted by the SOSSUS: 47 percent of general surgeons in the U.S. believe there is an excess supply of manpower in their specialty, as contrasted with 41 percent of cardiac surgeons, 40 percent of thoracic surgeons, 31 percent of neurosurgeons, 22 percent of ophthalmologists, 20 percent of plastic surgeons, and 20 percent of obstetrician-gynecologists. Over half of all surgical specialists believe that there are too many general surgeons, signaling that the days of the generalist may be limited in surgery as well as in medicine (American College of Surgeons and American Surgical Association, 1975, p. 77). The motivation may not be praiseworthy, but the propensity of surgical specialties to limit hospital privileges may produce some highly favorable results in the end.

Consumers

Any improvement in quality standards certainly would be preferable to the prevailing laissez-faire environment which, as described earlier, allows for an unacceptably large volume of medically questionable, unnecessary, and harmful procedures. Much unnecessary surgery is thought to be due to a surplus supply of surgeons and to the lack of effective controls over what they are allowed to do. Physicians trained as surgeons, or seeing themselves as surgeons, are predisposed in accord with role imagery to prescribe more aggressive therapies. They are more likely to operate, whereas colleagues in medicine are more disposed to prescribe drugs. (These issues are amplified in Fuchs, 1974, pp. 60, 70-74, 95.) A comparison with England gives some basis for this conclusion. Surgical rates in England, adjusted for population differences, are approximately half those in the U.S. where, interestingly, there are nearly twice as many physicians practicing surgery. Controls limiting surgery to certified practitioners would, it is claimed, lower unjustifiably high U.S. rates by reducing the supply of surgeons to a number approaching the supply of surgeons in England (American College of Surgeons and American Surgical Association, 1975, pp. 32-36).

It is highly improbable that major alterations can be made in the structure of surgery without important ripple effects for nonsurgical specialties. Comparable problems of surplus manpower and declining demand will stimulate similar attempts to restrict access to medical beds. Consumers will be the chief beneficiaries of this struggle. With nowhere else to go, general practice, family practice, and possibly other types of practice within the primary care spectrum will concentrate more on health care problems which have not been receiving sufficient medical attention, due to the glamour and rewards of hospital-oriented treatment. The benefits of having a better balanced distribution of medical manpower by specialty and a clearer delineation between hospital-based and community-based medical practice will multiply, if primary care practice is decentralized to optimize accessibility for patients, and if controls on the staffing and equipping of practices result in more efficient and effective use of sophisticated and costly equipment and procedures.

Disassociated from acute hospitals, self-interest alone will steer primary care practitioners into assuming a larger role for hitherto neglected areas involving the care of the mentally ill and chronically sick aged, both in the community and in nursing homes and related facilities. The environment generally would be conducive to the fulfillment of the long-sought synthesis of prevention, treatment, and rehabilitation at the core of progressive concepts of primary care.

A lowering of hospital and nursing home utilization also will contribute to the development of community-based alternatives generally thought to be better for patients than institutional care. As stated earlier, hospitals and nursing homes are dangerous places. It is conservatively estimated that from 7 to 10 percent of acute patients suffer compensable injuries in the course of hospital treatment (Pocincki et al., 1973, pp. 50-64). In the area of long-term care there are the additional hazards of social dependency, physical atrophy, and emotional depression which mitigate against rehabilitation and return to normal living.

While PSROs are focusing initially on short-term hospital inpatient services, they are required eventually to review all institutional services. To date, fifteen PSROs have been designated to perform two-year demonstration projects in long-term review, indicating a high commitment to moving swiftly in this field in tandem with the growth of administrative capabilities. The broadening of PSRO responsibility from institutional care to services provided in physicians' offices, necessary for closing the holes in the protective net of quality assurance, does not appear far off either. Toward this end, the government has funded five PSROs to undertake demonstration studies of ambulatory care review and announced plans to double the number of projects (U.S. Department of Health, Education, and Welfare, 1977d, p. 49).

RISKS ASSESSMENT

The range of social change encompassed by the PSRO legislation and the political complexity of the issues, which must be reconciled if the program is to succeed, invite ambiguities of purpose and conflicts in administration which will have a major influence in shaping the evolution of the program. Internal stresses emanating from competing and often contradictory aims due to the political and economic differences intrinsic to the PSRO program may produce unanticipated consequences at odds with both the goals of vested interest groups and larger public welfare considerations.

Government

The policy decision taken by government to allow the medical profession an exclusive say in regulating the clinical decisions of its members strikes many persons as tantamount to appointing the proverbial fox to guard the chicken coop. If, as opponents claim, the medical profession has failed miserably in policing its members in the past, how can one accept that things now will be any better? (Stroman, 1976, pp. 114-39; Krause, 1975).

Individuals familiar with organized medicine's historical record in the field of quality control instinctively reject the wisdom of allowing it to have any monopoly powers whatsoever. They would agree with the admonitions of such sages as Adam Smith and George Bernard Shaw, who viewed all professional associations as conspiracies against the public. The small number of physicians who have been censured or suffered suspension or full loss of licensure by professional regulatory bodies, the spotty and often superficial nature of self-imposed hospital controls and voluntary accreditation, and the failure of the medical profession to develop satisfactory programs of continuing education are sustenance for pessimism. The evidence shows that severe sanctions are seldom imposed (Berlant, 1975, p. 79; Derbyshire, 1974). The AMA contends in rebuttal that discipline is being tightened in response to criticism. From 1971 to 1976, the number of disciplinary actions jumped nearly fourfold. The number of license revocations and probation actions is said to have increased threefold. Even so, the increase is dismissed by detractors as small, compared with the total number of physicians (*U.S. News and World Report,* 1977).

The repeated failures of the government's attempts to contain cost increases in publicly financed health programs for the aged and low-income populations through the establishment of utilization review committees in hospitals deepen skepticism about the feasibility of self-regulation. Hearings conducted by the Senate Finance Committee concluded that the utilization review machinery, which it imposed to curb cost increases in Medicare and Medicaid prior to the PSRO legislation, was more form than substance. It worked only when beds were in short supply. When beds were in surplus or occupancy rates were low, physicians on review committees were found to be reluctant to restrict hospital utilization to strictly clinical needs (U.S. Congress, 1974a, p. 519). No matter how tempting politically, facile explanations born of simple theories of professional monopoly powers are insufficient. Complex explanations are far more realistic since the motivations involved do not always fit neatly into the category of raw self-interest. There are more enlightening explanations.

Some problems are rooted in the economics and sociology of professional life (see, for example, Freidson, 1975). Given that both the income and quality of work done by physicians are related to volume of services performed, the decisions of practitioners serving on review committees are likely to be affected whenever underemployment is seen to be a problem. In addition to the motivation of self-interest, doctors on review committees will experience an understandable desire to help out colleagues whose workload is in danger of falling off. Dependence on an economically sound and expanding hospital to carry forward career interests actually may transcend the influence of fee-for-service income incentives.

Because the potential for influence is stronger in personalized rather than depersonalized situations, the whole process of peer review is highly susceptible to the pressures and expectations of colleagues. Individuals may be reluctant to make decisions detrimental to colleagues who are friends or who are members of networks for patient referral and for the conferring of professional honors and status.

The influence of the doctor-patient relationship must also be acknowledged. Hospital admission and length-of-stay decisions often are made to accommodate the convenience and social and emotional needs of patients, and cannot be supported on purely clinical grounds; they are, nevertheless, important to patient satisfaction, healing, and rehabilitation.

Considerations of financial solvency and organizational growth can cause hospitals to contribute to the undermining of the effectiveness of government-imposed controls. Utilization review committee members are susceptible to a combination of pressures which are related to the way in which hospitals and practitioners are paid. Payment of a per diem rate to hospitals and fee-for-service to doctors provides economic disincentives to restricting utilization to clinically justifiable cases when beds are in surplus, or occupancy rates are low. Whenever doctors' professional and economic welfare is inextricably tied to that of the hospital in which they hold staff appointments, medically appointed review committees are prone to err in favor of keeping hospital resources fully employed. Hospital administrators and trustees often are motivated to encourage and reinforce such sentiment.

In the absence of other criteria for judging performance, the maintenance of high occupancy is a prime factor in the performance evaluations of hospital administrators by boards of trustees. Fearful of the consequences of a fall in revenues for the hospital's ability to meet debts and other expenses, trustees also have an understandable desire to keep occupancy high—and one which has been intensified by the practice of government and insurance companies in recent years of pegging the rate of reimbursement to bed size and rates of occupancy. Low occupancy can result in a hospital being paid a lower rate designed for a smaller hospital.

Part of the blame for the failures of utilization review can be attributed to the inconsistencies and contradictions of federal and state government policies, which provide disincentives to cooperation. By sanctioning fee-for-service payment in Medicare and Medicaid, while at the same time striving through PSROs and other avenues to lower utilization of inpatient services, the federal government feeds the impression that the right hand does not know or care what the left hand is doing.

Another contradiction involves the reluctance of state officials to surrender independently developed machinery to control expenditures for medical services provided under Medicaid. New York State, for example, has insisted, with the tacit approval of the federal government, on continuing to run its own hospital utilization review program, despite the open competition with the PSRO mandate. The state's position is that the federally funded professional review organizations have failed to cut unnecessary surgery and hospital lengths of stay in comparison with a nearly 20 percent reduction by its own review program (Sullivan, 1977). By not acting to resolve this open confrontation the federal government feeds suspicions within the medical community about the sincerity of its commitment to peer review and discourages physicians and hospitals from taking PSROs seriously.

The dysfunctional conflict incorporated in the relationship between professional standards review and health maintenance organizations punctuates the need for greater coherence in health policy. Unless something is done to modify the situation, PSRO norms will interfere with innovations in patient care designed to enable HMOs to compete successfully with traditional forms of medical practice. Insofar as the PSROs are controlled mainly by physicians sensitive to orthodox forms of private practice (indeed, the legislation favors it), the vulnerability of HMOs is compounded (Gosfield, 1975, p. 91).

Secondary risks

Other stresses built into the PSRO structure may be more important in the long run—especially the delegation to hospitals of self-policing powers. Generally considered to be a constructive compromise to a bitter dispute over who should have the final say on quality, this arrangement could seriously handicap the ability of PSROs to discharge their responsibility (see Kinzer, 1976, pp. 105-31). The controversy producing the compromise is rooted in recent changes in the doctrine of liability for malpractice which, as previously described, caused hospitals to assume a more aggressive role in the field of quality assurance. In conjunction with the accountability requirements of publicly financed programs vital to hospital revenues, they underlie the growth of interest in the transfer of responsibility for manpower licensure from professional societies to hospitals. (These trends are described in Carlson, 1976; see also Yerby, 1975, pp. 84-101.)

The struggle between organized medicine and the hospitals precipitated by the above developments was evident in the political maneuverings preceding passage of the PSRO legislation. The American Hospital Association hesitated to relinquish its role in quality assurance to the medical profession for the reasons that it would compound their vulnerability to legal action and erode the authority of the hospital's administration and medical staff to decide vital questions of patient and service mix. To counter the AMA-sponsored PSRO initiative for nailing down the profession's monopoly over the assessment of quality, the American Hospital Association introduced its own quality assurance program (QAP) based on the experience of hospitals with internal review committees. The conflict abated following adoption of the compromise whereby, in return for recognition of the medical profession's exclusive claim to competence in quality assessment, the American Medical Association agreed that PSROs would allow hospitals to carry on their own internal reviews through use of QAP committees (see Brown and Sale, 1974; Turner, 1974). This relationship is acceptable to HEW so long as the QAPs can competently perform as PSRO surrogates (U.S. Department of Health, Education, and Welfare, 1977a, p. 29).

How long the *modus vivendi* between the hospitals and the medical profession will last is hard to predict. The outlook certainly will darken should hospitals, pressured by government to assume stronger controls over the production and quality of medical services, move in future years to constrain the presently flexible treatment privileges of generalists and noncertified practitioners, and act, moreover, to confine staff privileges to full-time salaried practitioners.

The crossfire pressures emanating from priorities for cost containment and quality assurance presage a precarious health policy role for hospitals, which may find themselves in a no-win situation. Should PSRO progress be interrupted by the resumption of the battle for control with organized medicine, hospitals will share in the blame. On the other hand, continuation of the alliance will invite the charge that it fragments responsibility. A more troublesome charge is that the stake hospitals have in keeping occupancy rates up, whether for purposes of economic security, prestige, or growth, renders them incapable of taking any truly effective cost-saving action. Another damaging criticism is that the constellation of vested high-technology interests in hospitals is predisposed to manipulate the redeployment of primary care for selfish reasons.

The prospects which PSROs pose for diminished reliance on inpatient services is an inducement for hospitals to influence the future direction of primary care. This could be done in at least two ways—first, by using the capabilities of hospitals in continuing education to promote a hospital orientation among medical and other health practitioners. Ironically, budget constraints and the indoctrination of most physicians in hospital medicine and conventional patterns of practice leads PSROs to be naturally sympathetic to hospital dominance in this area. If not always hospital-based, the chances are high that continuing education will originate in hospitals. In discharging their responsibility for the regional coordination of all educational programs, PSROs will tend, therefore, to sanction dependence on hospital care.

The second avenue involves the sponsorship and control of community-based primary care delivery systems. It can be anticipated that hospitals most vulnerable to diminished occupancy will be in the forefront of attempts in communities to increase the supply and availability of primary services. Control of the identification and referral of patients is paramount to the full employment of hospital specialists and other costly resources. The hospitals most vulnerable in this regard frequently are those offering a highly diversified mix of sophisticated and expensive services.

The commitment of many teaching hospitals to the training of nurse clinicians and physicians' assistants may rest partly on the expectation that substitute personnel will be more responsive in the screening and referral of patients to the needs of superspecialist medicine, awakened to the urgency of the issue of how to get sufficient patients in the right beds at the right time. Status differentials and the dependency of their livelihood on the patronage of medical practitioners make physicians' surrogates far more manageable, in principle, than independently licensed medical primary care practitioners whose relationships with hospital-based medicine are aligned to become more antagonistic in future years.

Providers

The quid pro quo whereby the medical profession has reacquired the exclusive right to regulate, monitor, and evaluate patient care quality in return for limiting the clinical freedom of the individual physician to treat each patient as he or she sees fit will be resisted by practitioners dreading the diminution of material and professional rewards. The political life of organized medicine is destined for a period of instability, unless rank-and-file members come to better appreciate and accept the sociopolitical realities buffeting the profession.

Turmoil will spring from changes in the relationship between generalists and specialists and the awarding of hospital staff privileges. Apprehension among primary care practitioners about being closed out of hospitals is an important source of dissension. General surgeons are no less likely to accept passively attempts to limit their clinical freedoms. A sense of increased class consciousness on the part of primary care practitioners displaced from hospitals will spark deep resentments over any attempt by hospitals to protect against declining admissions by seeking to influence the organization of first-contact services and patient referrals.

Conflict also will arise from interest differences among practitioners addressing utilization and quality review from a community-regional standpoint and those viewing things from the vantage point of individual hospitals. The implications for full-time salaried hospital doctors are difficult to predict, since there are so few in the U.S. Regardless of private practice versus employee distinctions, doctors will tend to identify more closely with hospitals where they have appointments than with the regional PSRO, thereby exacerbating divisions within the profession.

Secondary risks

The possible long-run effects of excessive controls over the freedom of practitioners to make clinical judgments are disquieting. Given the emotional anxieties accompanying illness, the sick characteristically prefer doctors who will look after them as individuals and who, moreover, will do what professional judgment deems best, subject to the resources available. The patient may therefore be put off by a doctor who feels bound excessively by PSRO directives and red tape which inhibits the freedom to make clinical decisions. Although assurances have been made by HEW that PSROs should not become involved in assessing and controlling individual clinical decisions, but concentrate instead on statistical profiles and descriptive averages, the mandate is sufficiently vague that the potential for such detailed interference does exist (see U.S. Congress, 1974a, pp. 835-38). The temptation to monitor practitioners more closely will intensify as consumers and elected officials become more knowledgeable about the large range for error in modern medicine.

If the best safeguard against narrow administration and overly zealous regulation hinges on the ability to recruit and keep good staff, the prognosis for enlightened PSRO leadership and enforcement is not good. Because of the overwhelmingly pro-business and free enterprise cultural bias, the best and brightest young men and women are not attracted to the public sector in the U.S. The stereotype is that only dupes, sloths, and incompetents enter and remain in civil service employment, since the government is seen as the employer of last resort for persons of limited ambition and ability. While it is possible to live with bad law if administration is in the hands of good people, the prospects are bleak, indeed, whenever authority and responsibility are given to the wrong people. In light of the growing antigovernment sentiment among U.S. citizens, and the commonplace assertion among candidates running for elective office that federal and state government bureaucracies are antagonistic to accountability and efficiency and have been allowed to grow too strong and must be cut back, there is proper cause to fret that PSROs may be run badly.

In addition to weakening patient confidence and trust in the doctor-patient relationship, which is inherently therapeutic in its own right, excessive monitoring and regulation could do more to promote mediocrity than excellence. Also, as enforcement of norms derived from the best existing practice is based on past experience, innovation and progress may suffer because of bad administration; for, to paraphrase George Bernard Shaw, it is the unreasonable people who make progress—that is, those who dare to question conventional wisdom. Bad administration will encourage practitioners to adhere to what is safe. It may also discourage talented young people from going into medicine.

These dire possibilities raise the question of who watches the watchers. Accountability and administration depend ultimately on trust. It may be useful, therefore, to recall that a profession is not just an organization; it is a collection of people who, in addition to the mundane motivation of self-gain, share a common vision based on values of service to the sick and scientific and technological excellence. Unless medicine can continue to collect its fair share of good people, it will decline. When all is said and done, the best assurance for high quality medicine may depend more upon maintaining among practitioners a strong sense of professional values and life-long education than upon oppressive supervision and policing.

A breakdown in public confidence and trust toward the medical profession, combined with an adversarial relationship between clinicians and regulatory officials, could easily produce a form of paralysis by inviting a high rate of appeal of PSRO decisions. Lengthy legal maneuvering before administrative appeal bodies, from local and state levels to HEW, and judicial bodies, from civil courts to the Supreme Court, would not only handicap decision making, but effectively transfer it from trained specialists to judges who, because of differences in training and experiences, are not known for their ability to make good administrative decisions.

Consumers

Consumer protection groups find three chief faults with the PSRO program. First, proponents of the right of patients to sue for damages in the event of malpractice despair that litigation may become more difficult should the courts, as intended by Congressional sponsors of the legislation, accept good faith compliance with PSRO norms as an acceptable test of quality (see U.S. Department of Health, Education, and Welfare, 1974b, pp. 4, 9). Gosfield (1975, p. 36) contends, however, that, taken at face value, PSRO legislation will have little effect on what the common law already requires, except that incorrect choice of treatment method may become less admissible in malpractice suits than previously. Whether any curtailment of liability would be good or bad depends partially on the weight assigned to the costs, which can be quite high. For example, the added cost of hospitalization for an average stay, to cover malpractice insurance, is reputed to be more than $50. It is said that the annual cost for insurance per hospital bed in teaching hospitals would soon soar upward tenfold or more from present rates of roughly $100 (Stroman, 1976, p. 163). The problem may get worse, since only a small proportion (5 to 10 percent) of all compensable medical charges are now brought to the attention of lawyers and the courts, because of the reluctance of patients to sue formally (Pocincki et al., 1973, p. 12).

Some of the practical dimensions of the problems attributed to excessive litigation and the unpredictability of jury awards in the assignment of damages are visible in the trend toward no-fault automobile insurance, in which about half of the state governments prohibit court action for damages below a minimum ceiling ranging from $200 to $5,000. Pressures are mounting for a similar denouement to the medical malpractice problem. Other alternatives include compulsory mediation, the placement of ceilings on what lawyers can charge, and a shift away from punitive measures toward continuing education (Somers and Somers, 1977, pp. 288-305).

The corrosive fallout of a high volume of litigation on public confidence is something to ponder, also. The present fad for the demystification of medicine conceals a perplexing ambiguity. If pressures for greater accountability endorse the debunking of the medical mystique for the reason that one cannot bring demigods to account, the emotional impact and fears associated with illness lead erstwhile critics when they fall sick to ascribe superhuman properties to doctors. Medical educators often are similarly gripped with ambiguity. Proponents of science and technology find the mysterious aspects of medicine an embarrassing reminder of the limits of modern medicine, but, nevertheless, are forced to confess that medicine remains part art, and that the irrational component (faith, the power of suggestion and laying on of hands, etc.) contributes importantly to healing and recovery.

The second complaint of consumer groups focuses on the preclusion of consumers on PSRO governing boards (U.S. Congress, 1974a, pp. 151-57). There are some legal loopholes which could provide for limited consumer participation on statewide and local organizations, but it is unlikely they can be manipulated sufficiently to assure an effective voice for consumers (Gosfield, 1975, pp. 200-08).

The third complaint deals with objectionable rules and regulations barring public disclosure of information critical of individual practitioners and institutions (Gosfield, 1975, pp. 183-200). While one can be persuaded of the necessity of confidentiality for obtaining the cooperation of individual providers and for maintaining a more effective system of continuing education grounded in positive reinforcement, restrictions against the disclosure of aggregated data reflecting standards of care by groups of doctors and hospitals, broken down by specialty and geographic location, appear less convincing.

The drawing of comparisons between comparable communities is a useful tool in the hands of consumer groups, elected officials, and provider associations, for raising overall standards of care and for more effective resource allocation and planning for community health services within the context of the newly established regional comprehensive health systems agencies. The confidentiality of summary data is overly defensive and inimical to the goals of health planning. Data on utilization and quality are fundamental to intelligent planning.

The powerlessness of planning agencies to limit reimbursement when deficiencies occur makes cooperation more important. The obstacles to coordination between planning agencies and PSROs resulting from the dissimilarity of service areas are far less ominous than the withholding of information because of suspicion as to its eventual use.

The requirement for consumer majorities on planning agency boards undoubtedly deepens the distrust of the medical profession about potential misuse of PSRO data (see U.S. Department of Health, Education, and Welfare, 1977d, p. 149; Institute of Medicine, 1976, p. 8). The reservations are not totally ill-founded. No matter how strong the convictions that consumer accountability is a positive force for medical accountability, there remains a paucity of reliable information on what consumers can contribute to the upgrading of care. The results may prove paradoxical in practice. Physicians may find, surprisingly, that consumer participation is less threatening than imagined. As well as concentrating too much on the personal, rather than the technical, aspects of care, consumers may be highly deferential to medical authority. (On the need for more research, see Kelman, 1976.)

Secondary risks

The unhappy specter that PSROs may be pressured into paying more attention to cost-saving measures detrimental to good patient care is already materializing. Government officials, frustrated by their inability to bring spending for hospital services under control, have issued PSROs an ultimatum to demonstrate that they can be effective in lowering inpatient utilization or face elimination (U.S. Department of Health, Education, and Welfare, 1977d; see also Holcomb, 1978). The danger herein is that too heavy an emphasis on overutilization could result in the withholding of necessary services or the premature discharge of patients.

The preoccupation with overutilization is an offshoot of the "deinstitutionalization strategy" now being followed in a number of developed Western countries, in which the assumption is made that patients can be cared for equally well in the community for less cost. Originally limited to mental institutions, this view has spread to include chronic care hospitals and nursing homes for the aged, as well as acute hospitals. Admittedly there are large numbers of patients who, in principle, either would be better off or no worse off if they were treated outside of the hospital, but the principle of deinstitutionalization is a function of implicit, if not explicit, assumptions which may be incorrect—notably, that appropriate treatment capabilities exist in the community and that patients receive proper follow-up. Failure to meet these assumptions can be costly both to society and the individual. Inadequate follow-up in the community has been shown to result in patient neglect and a substantial undoing of the costly benefits of hospitalization. Too often, deinstitutionalization is a code word for the reinstitutionalization of patients in facilities where the standards of care are poorer than the inpatient services previously provided (see Bassuk and Gerson, 1978; Brook et al., 1971; Santiesteven, 1975). There are, moreover, serious doubts about whether community care is cheaper than institutional care, once all the costs to government and families are accounted for (Comptroller General of the United States, 1977, pp. 5-6).

Differences in training and employment make it difficult under the best of circumstances to coordinate hospital-based and community-based health services (e.g., hospital and home nursing, specialist and family practitioner), but the problems are multiplied in the case of the chronically ill aged, mentally ill, mentally disabled, and physically handicapped, because of the lack of a clear division of responsibility between health and social services. Further problems arise from the fact that publicly supported health and social services are the administrative and financial responsibility of different levels of government in the U.S. Social services typically are the responsibility of lower levels of government, whose smaller tax bases make it difficult to keep up financially with the increased demand for social services in community care programs.

The expense of community care is larger if services are staffed with professionals, rather than nonprofessionals. Not only are the salaries of professionals high, but their productivity is much lower in the community than in the hospital where, because of centralization, more patients can be seen per unit of time. Dependence upon the family for the provision of social services is illusory, given the erosion it has experienced as the result of industrialization and modernization. Not only is the modern family smaller and more mobile, but there has been a marked decline in the willingness of adult offspring to care for aged and chronically ill dependents in the home.

Deinstitutionalization is an idea more appealing in theory than in practice. The strong measures taken by government recently to push PSROs to show their cost-saving capabilities by emptying hospital beds will further complicate the public policy dilemmas, which could make community care a solution far worse than the problem. The strong pressures to empty beds reduce hope that the neglect of patients released from hospitals will be corrected through better discharge planning—which it was once thought PSROs would encourage (see, for example, Goran et al., 1976, p. 81). There can be no doubt that a greater sensitivity to the interrelationship between the medical, emotional, and social components of medicine is essential if the government is to avoid pushing PSROs into a stance inimical to good patient care.

SIGNIFICANCE FOR OTHER DEVELOPED COUNTRIES

The PSRO initiative possesses a significance for health professionals in other countries which surpasses conventional understanding. More important than any underscoring of the limitations of free enterprise health services proclaimed by proponents of public financing and ownership, the changes occurring in the U.S. signal a fundamental shift in health policy which transcends traditional capitalist and socialist alternatives in highly developed countries.

Differences in the financing and organization of health services notwithstanding, governments typically have granted medical practitioners considerable leeway in decisions affecting patient care—whether for reasons of inability to cope with the esoteric aspects of medicine, the political power of the medical profession, fear of the life-or-death consequences of a wrong decision, or some combination thereof. Freedom from interference in clinical decision making and other privileges typically have been justified as requisite for maintaining the morale and productivity of professionals entrusted with awesome moral and scientific responsibilities for the treatment and care of the sick and dying. This relationship between government and medical practice may be changing, however, because of stresses from simultaneous developments in the medical sector and the general economy supporting an expansion of managerial and planning controls.

Regardless of the scale of involvement in the financing of health services, the combination of increased costs of modern technology, rising public expectations, and inflation are imposing a steadily heavier burden on public financing. Inflation is a particularly serious problem with respect to the hospital-based services—expenditures for which have been growing in most developed countries at a rate of roughly 15 to 20 percent annually over the past decade. Rates of increase for health services are among the largest in the components of government budgets (see, for example, Maxwell, 1975, pp. 17-30).

The aging of the population and growth in the importance of chronic illness and congenital abnormalities have created a situation throughout the highly developed world where it is costing more and more to accomplish less and less. This realization is at the core of the movement towards closer evaluation of the cost, safety, and efficacy of expensive technologies and health services, and the generally more skeptical attitudes about the relationship between health spending and health status. Indeed, increasing open talk of the diminishing social benefit of health services (especially the hospital-based high-technology services) encourages governments to investigate whether investments in health services may have reached upper limits.

Largely on the assumption that there were sizable payoffs to be had from expanded hospital-based services which were undercapitalized, many governments, beginning in the 1950s, undertook massive spending programs aimed at upgrading the scientific and technological base of medicine and at making hospital and specialist care more readily available. The wisdom of continuing this investment policy is being re-examined, often within an environment of pungent antimedical criticism and propaganda denigrating the traditional status and privileges of the medical profession as a medieval ecclesiastic vestige, inappropriate to highly educated societies in which consumers are expected to play a more responsible part in health promotion and illness treatment (Starr, 1976). The consequences of this development are partly visible in the efforts in many countries to promote health education and to substitute less costly forms of community care for hospital-based services (Maxwell, 1975, pp. 41-52).

Among policy makers impressed by the idea that each new medical graduate is responsible through a working career for diagnostic and treatment decisions totalling approximately $300,000 yearly, few will accept that the divergent pressures for services expansion and cost containment can be harmonized without benefit of controls over what physicians are allowed to do.* The restructuring of medical practice from solo to bureaucratic-hierarchical arrangements and the substitution of capitation and salary for fee-for-service modes of reimbursement do not go far enough. The fact that over three-fourths of health services consumption is induced by physicians must also be acknowledged. Recognition of the gatekeeper function of practitioners in affecting utilization patterns and costs accounts for the growth of interest in limiting the supply of manpower through planning of aggregate and specialty output, and in normative measures for utilization review and quality assessment (see Wolman, 1976; McLachlan, 1976; Rhodes, 1976, pp. 122-40).

It may appear odd that a country which has lagged so far behind other developed countries in the restructuring of health services financing and organization should assume the lead in implementing a program so radical on the surface as the monitoring and evaluation of clinical decision making. Ironically, the United States may have more flexibility in this regard, simply because it has lagged so far behind. Because it is not as locked in politically as other countries which have pursued more active interventionist policies in the health sector, the United States government has more latitude to pursue options in a period when the role and value of health services is less clear and the need for economy and efficacy is intensifying parallel to the growing understanding that resources are less plentiful in highly advanced economies than commonly believed previously. Also, the stresses for cost containment and quality assurance may be more intensive in the United States, if for no other reason than its leadership position in the development of biomedical research and the proliferation of costly high-technology services made possible by laissez-faire policies and the absence of organizational controls in a system of fee-for-service remuneration which provides the underwriting for the performance of many questionable and possibly unnecessary procedures.

SUMMARY AND CONCLUSIONS

The nature and intensity of the policy disputes affecting the speed and direction of change compose a mixed forecast for the future of the PSRO pro-

---

*This figure is arrived at crudely by dividing total spending for health services by the number of doctors actively providing patient care, on the assumption that roughly 80 percent of utilization is the result of decisions made by doctors on behalf of patients.

gram. The answer to whether it warrants approval and support no doubt will vary, depending upon one's assessment of the tradeoffs. The position assumed here is that the expected primary and secondary benefits are substantial enough to compensate for the identifiable shortcomings and risks.

A major risk, both for consumers and government, is that providers may be driven by retrenchment and redundancy worries to manipulate PSROs for self-protection purposes. In order to assure the full utilization of excess capacity in beds and services, the program may be reduced to a tool for referring to hospitals the desired supply of the right sort of patients in response to the commands of hospital-oriented specialty interests. Consumers will also have to contend with the possibility that a government with its back to the wall financially may be pressured to cut hospital and nursing home utilization too severely, mindless of the longer-run costs from delays in treatment, failure to allow for sufficient convalescent time, and the unavailability of necessary follow-up services in the community. Cost-efficiency studies derived from PSRO data systems should, however, elucidate the false economies of crisis-motivated short-term solutions which contribute to greater disability or render futile costly forms of institutional treatment.

The sociopolitical realities suggest that the government will find that PSROs are not an effective device for combatting spending for hospital and nursing home care. The interlocking relationships between hospitals and doctors portend continuing heavy demands for costly institutional services. In addition, there are important limits to what can be done to control medical decision making. Even under the most tightly designed and aggressively administered controls, doctors will continue to hold the upper hand, if for no other reason than the artistic component of medicine. Because of the uncertainties of diagnosis and treatment and the role of emotions in healing and recovery, it is neither possible nor desirable to totally eliminate the autonomy of physicians in patient care. Measures which hazard undermining the invaluable contributions of the doctor-patient relationship to social and individual well-being, are irresponsibly short-sighted, especially since more prudent approaches to cost containment are available, including centralized budgeting, hospital and manpower planning, and closer scrutiny of the value and diffusion of new technologies in cost, safety, and efficacy.

Economic benefits can be expected from a reduction in the volume of medically questionable and unnecessary procedures due to the application of uniform treatment standards regionally and nationally, but they will not necessarily translate into lower aggregate spending—even if, following a tightening of the bed supply, utilization review committees behave as predicted to restrict access and lengths of stay. By all odds the opposite will occur, since the net effect will be to increase the case severity mix of hospitals and nursing homes. While beds will be used more selectively, the greater intensity of services will drive up the costs per day—possibly to the level of intensive care which runs roughly three times above the cost of ordinary care. The admission to hospitals of only the more seriously ill is unlikely, moreover, to shorten lengths of stay.

The PSRO effect on costs could be even worse, depending on the choice of method in quality assurance studies. Compared to outcome studies, process studies may inflate costs unnecessarily if the criteria selected are not rooted in scientifically controlled trials of the outcome of alternative treatment modes. The exposure of patients to iatrogenic illness would further defeat the economic objectives. The removal of the methodological options PSROs now have and the substitution of requirements for evaluations based on treatment outcomes is the most direct solution to the problem.

The chances are much sounder that peer review will do more to help identify and correct clinical and administrative deficiencies in the quality of care than to produce any great *cost* savings. The government's attempts to bludgeon PSROs into proving their worth in cost-savings terms seem, therefore, feckless and counterproductive (*Washington Developments,* 1977).

The strongest feature of the PSRO program by far is the opportunity it gives government to improve the standard of publicly financed medical services in line with higher expectations for quality assurance and social and territorial justice.

Some of the strongest objections to the PSRO program come from dissenters who have renounced the ability of the medical profession to police itself. Adherence to this position is most dogmatic among critics who believe that medicine has, whether through a paradox of progress or other means, reached the stage where it does far more harm than good to people. The charge, as articulated foremost by Illich, is that medically inflicted damages to health are a serious and growing menace, due to the side effects of increasingly powerful therapeutics and the fragmentation of medical knowledge and services (Illich, 1976). Even more devastating is the indictment that the medical profession's monopoly control of health services has the subtle effect of robbing individuals of their ability to take responsibility for their health and for dulling their senses to the social and environmental conditions that are mainly responsible for many of today's health problems. The hypnotic lure of currently fashionable assaults on the value of medicine and the integrity of the service ethic entices emulation without reflection of the consequences to patient care and community welfare.

It is a curiosity of the antimedicine doctrine that persons of strong liberal and humanitarian persuasions who join in the chorus to defrock the medical profession may become the partners of political adversaries who view health services in largely utilitarian terms. Much of the cost containment rhetoric promulgated by government today is discordant with professional values sanctifying life and the right to treatment, regardless of ability to pay. No matter how persuasive the pragmatic short-term arguments for abridging the service ethic, it is difficult to see how the interest of society and patients can withstand a system of medical care, in the long run, in which the profession is condemned as the enemy of the people and one's personal physician is suspect as a cost-benefit agent, indifferent to individual wants and needs. The social disorganization attributed to the diminished influence of church and community influences in modern living may pale in comparison with the costs of myopic strategies in which the overthrow of the medical profession is looked upon as the key to efficiency in the health sector.

The antimedicine fervor now in vogue obscures some potentially outstanding features of the PSRO program. Consumers will benefit from reductions in the volume of questionable, unnecessary, and harmful procedures. The introduction of professionally determined norms for the treatment of illness will hasten the developing trend to restrict the performance of complex medical and surgical procedures to properly qualified practitioners. Physicians disaffiliated from acute hospitals, finding nowhere else to turn, could become the nucleus of a rejuvenated system of primary care better attuned to first-contact medicine, the care of the chronically ill in the community, and the care of the elderly confined to nursing homes.

Both medical practitioners and consumers stand to gain enormously from the opportunities for effective lifetime learning and continuing education made easier by PSRO information systems. And the application of systematic monitoring and evaluation of clinical decisions will do much to raise the objective base of medical practice through the substitution of carefully tested therapies for procedures of unproven safety and efficacy.

Because systematic monitoring and evaluation represent a major break with the past, health providers are understandably nervous about the implications of PSROs—a state of mind compounded by the growing doubts of politicians about the value of medical care. It does not seem likely that the medical profession could accept and assimilate additional large changes at this time. Once, however, the PSRO program stabilizes and the profession's self-confidence is restored, conditions may become more favorable. In particular, it is to be hoped that it will soon be possible to soften present restrictions against public officials and consumer representatives on boards. What is now anathema may become more acceptable, as physicians grow to appreciate better the value of consumer participation for maintaining and strengthening public confidence indispensable to the survival of a self-governing and economically sound profession.

REFERENCES

American College of Surgeons and American Surgical Association. *Surgery in the United States.* Chicago: The College and the Association, 1975.

American Medical Association. "Senator Hits PSRO 'Panic.' " *American Medical Association News* 16 (November 19, 1973): 1.

American Medical Association. "AMA Urges FTC to Drop MD Ad Suit." *American Medical Association News* 20 (January 24, 1977): 1.

Bassuk, E. L., and Gerson, S. "Deinstitutionalization and Mental Health Services." *Scientific American* 238 (February 1978): 46-53.

Bauer, W. "A Profile of the PSRO Program." *Journal of the American Podiatry Association* 65 (December 1975): 12-18.

Bennett, W. F. "Education Is PSRO Goal." *Hospitals* 48 (March 1, 1974): 53-58.

Berlant, J. B. *Profession and Monopoly.* Berkeley: University of California Press, 1975.

Bird, D. "Malpractice Insurance: A Crisis in Health Care." *New York Times* (January 19, 1975): 1.

Blue Shield. "Medical Necessity Program: Inappropriate Procedures Identified" and "Rates To Be Discontinued for the Following Procedures." *Blue Shield News* 13 (June 1977): 1, 3.

Blum, J. D.; Gertman, P. M.; and Rabinow, J. *PSROs and the Law.* Germantown, Md.: Aspen, 1977.

Brook, R. H., and Avery, A. D. "Quality Assurance Mechanisms in the United States: From There to Where?" *A Question of Quality?,* edited by G. McLachlan. London: Nuffield Provincial Hospitals Trust, 1976.

Brook, R. H., et al. "Effectiveness of Inpatient Follow-up Care." *New England Journal of Medicine* 285 (December 30, 1971): 1509-14.

Brown, M. B., and Sale, W. B. "QAP: The AHA's Program." *Hospitals* 48 (March 1974): 59.

Bunker, J. P.; Barnes, B. A.; and Mosteller, F. (eds.). *Costs, Risks, and Benefits of Surgery.* New York: Oxford University Press, 1977.

Caper, P. "The Meaning of Quality in Medical Care." *New England Journal of Medicine* 291 (November 21, 1974): 1136-37.

Carlson, R. "Alternative Legislative Strategies for Licensure: Licensure and Health." *Quality Assurance in Health Care,* edited by R. H. Egdahl and P. M. Gertman. Germantown, Md.: Aspen, 1976.

Cochrane, A. L. *Effectiveness and Efficiency.* London: Nuffield Provincial Hospitals Trust, 1972.

Cohen, H. S. "Regulatory Politics and American Medicine." *American Behavioral Scientist* 19 (September/October 1975): 122-35.

Comptroller General of the United States. *Returning the Mentally Disabled to the Community: Government Needs To Do More* (Publication no. HRD 76-152). Washington, D.C.: General Accounting Office, 1977.

Congressional Research Service. *Health Care Expenditures and Their Controls* (2nd ed.). Washington, D.C.: Library of Congress, 1978.

deLesseps, S. "Malpractice Insurance Crunch." *Editorial Research Reports on National Health Issues.* Washington, D.C.: Congressional Quarterly, 1977.

Demkovich, L. E. "Doctors and Lawyers Fight the Madison Avenue Route." *National Journal* 8 (August 14, 1976): 1144-48.

Derbyshire, R. C. "Medical Ethics and Discipline." *Journal of the American Medical Association* 228 (April 1974): 59-62.

Federal Register. "Department of Health, Education, and Welfare, Social Rehabilitation Service and Social Security Administration: Utilization Review." *Register* (March 30, 1976): 13452-53.

Freidson, E. *Doctoring Together.* New York: Elsevier, 1975.

Fuchs, V. R. *Who Shall Live?* New York: Basic Books, 1974.

Fuller, T. E. *The Death of Psychiatry.* Radmor, Penn.: Chilton, 1974.

Goodman, E. "Rx for a Better Patient-MD Link." *Boston Globe* (April 11, 1978): 23.

Goran, M. J.; Roberts, J. S.; and Rodak, J., Jr. "Regulating the Quality of Hospital Care: An

Analysis of the Issues Pertinent to National Health Insurance." *Quality Assurance in Health Care,* edited by R. H. Egdahl and P. M. Gertman. Germantown, Md.: Aspen, 1976.

Gosfield, A. *PSROs: The Law and the Health Consumer.* Cambridge, Mass.: Ballinger, 1975.

Hague, J. E. "AMA Takes Amend and Cooperate Position on PSROs." *Hospitals* 48 (August 1, 1974): 19-21.

Hicks, N. "Nation's Doctors Move to Police Medical Care." *New York Times* (October 28, 1973): 1.

Holcomb, B. "Feds Reverse Decision Eliminating PSRO Funds." *Health Care Week* 1 (January 16, 1978): 1.

Illich, I. *Medical Nemesis: The Expropriation of Health.* New York: Pantheon, 1976.

Ingelfinger, F. J., et al. (eds.). *Controversy in Internal Medicine: II.* Philadelphia: W. B. Saunders, 1974.

Institute of Medicine. *Assessing Quality in Health Care: An Evaluation.* Washington, D.C.: National Academy of Sciences, 1976.

Jesse, W. F., et al. "PSRO: An Educational Tool for Improving Quality of Care." *New England Journal of Medicine* 292 (March 27, 1975): 668-75.

Karch, F., and Lasagna, L. *Adverse Drug Reactions in the United States.* Washington, D.C.: Medicine in the Public Interest, 1975.

Kelman, H. R. "Evaluation of Health Care Quality by Consumers." *International Journal of Health Services* 6, no. 3 (1976): 431-42.

Kinzer, D. "Inpatient Quality Assurance Activities: Coordination of Federal, State and Private Roles—The Hospital's Views." *Quality Assurance in Health Care,* edited by R. H. Egdahl and P. M. Gertman. Germantown, Md.: Aspen, 1976.

Kohlmeier, L. M. "Making the Professions Compete." *National Journal* 8 (January 3, 1976): 26.

Krause, E. A. "The Political Context of Health Service Regulation." *International Journal of Health Services* 5, no. 4 (1975): 593-607.

Maxwell, R. *Health Care: The Growing Dilemma, Needs vs. Resources in Western Europe, the US, and the USSR.* New York: McKinsey, 1975.

McCleery, R. S., et al. *One Life—One Physician, An Inquiry into the Medical Profession's Performance in Self-Regulation.* Washington, D.C.: Public Affairs Press, 1971.

McLachlan, G. (ed.). "A Question of Quality?" *Roads to Assurance in Medical Care.* London: Nuffield Provincial Hospitals Trust, 1976.

Pocincki, L. S.; Dogger, S. J.; and Schwartz, B. P. "The Incidence of Iatrogenic Illness." *Report of the Secretary's Commission on Medical Malpractice, Appendix* (Publication no. OS 73-89). Washington, D.C.: HEW, 1973.

Rhodes, P. *The Value of Medicine.* London: George Allen & Unwin, 1976.

Rosenhan, D. L. "On Being Sane in Insane Places." *Health and the Social Environment,* edited by P. M. Insell and R. H. Moos. Lexington, Mass.: Lexington Books, 1974.

Santiestevan, H. *Out of Their Beds and into the Streets.* Washington, D.C.: American Federation of State, County, and Municipal Employees, 1975.

Shabecoff, P. "Doctors Fees Rising at Fastest U.S. Rate." *New York Times* (March 23, 1978): 1.

Somers, A. R., and Somers, H. M. *Health and Health Care: Policies in Perspective.* Germantown, Md.: Aspen, 1977.

Starr, P. "The Politics of Therapeutic Nihilism." *Hastings Center Report* 6 (October 1976): 24-30.

Stroman, D. F. *The Medical Establishment and Social Responsibility.* Port Washington, N.Y.: National University Publications, 1976.

Sullivan, F. "Professional Standards Review Organizations: The Current Scene." *American Journal of Psychiatry* 131 (December 1974): 1354-58.

Sullivan, R. "2 Hospital Monitors Stir Growing Discord." *New York Times* (October 2, 1977): 22-23.

Turner, J. A. "Health Report/HEW Begins Medical Review; AMA, Hospitals Mount Opposition." *National Journal Reports* 6 (January 19, 1974): 90-102.

U.S. Congress. Special Committee on Aging. *Alternatives to Nursing Home Care: A Proposal* (92nd Congress, 1st session, 1971).

U.S. Congress. *The Social Security Amendments of 1972, Public Law 92-603* (92nd Congress, 2nd session, 1972).

U.S. Congress. Subcommittee on Health of the Committee on Finance. *Hearings on the Implementation of PSRO Legislation* (93rd Congress, 2nd session, 1974a).

U.S. Congress. Subcommittee on Long-Term Care of the Special Committee on Aging. *Nursing Home Care in the United States: Failure in Public Policy* (93rd Congress, 2nd session, 1974b).

U.S. Congress. Subcommittee on Oversight and Investigations of the Committee on Interstate and Foreign Commerce. *Report on the Cost and Quality of Health Care: Unnecessary Surgery* (94th Congress, 2nd session, 1976).

U.S. Congress. *Expenditures for Health Care: Federal Programs and Their Effects.* Washington, D.C.: Government Printing Office, 1977a.

U.S. Congress. "Controlling Health Costs." *Editorial Research Reports: National Health Issues.* Washington, D.C.: Congressional Quarterly, 1977b.

U.S. Department of Health, Education, and Welfare. *Legislative History of Professional Standards Review Organization Provisions of the Social Security Act Amendments.* Washington, D.C.: HEW, 1972.

U.S. Department of Health, Education, and Welfare. "PSRO: An Educational Force for Improving Quality of Care." *PSRO Transmittal no. 7.* Washington, D.C.: HEW, 1974a.

U.S. Department of Health, Education, and Welfare. *PSROs and Medical Information: Safeguards and Privacy.* Washington, D.C.: HEW, 1974b.

U.S. Department of Health, Education, and Welfare. "Theme: Preparing for National Health Insurance." *Forward Plan for Health, FY 1978-82* (Publication no. OS 76-50046). Washington, D.C.: HEW, 1976.

U.S. Department of Health, Education, and Welfare. *PSRO Fact Book.* Washington, D.C.: HEW, 1977a.

U.S. Department of Health, Education, and Welfare. *Health of the Disadvantaged Chart Book* (Publication no. HRA 77-628). Hyattsville, Md.: HEW, 1977b.

U.S. Department of Health, Education, and Welfare. *Papers on the National Health Guidelines: Baselines for Setting Health Goals and Standards* (Publication no. HRA 77-640). Washington, D.C.: HEW, 1977c.

U.S. Department of Health, Education, and Welfare. *PSRO: An Evaluation of the Professional Standards Review Organization, Vol. 1: Executive Summary.* Washington, D.C.: HEW, 1977d.

U.S. News and World Report. "America's Doctors/A Profession in Trouble." *News* 83 (October 17, 1977): 50.

Wall Street Journal. "Dental Group Is Target of FTC in Drive Against Codes It Says Limit Competition." *Journal* (January 17, 1977): 9.

Washington Developments. "PSRO Program Threatened with Loss of Federal Aid." *Developments* 6 (December 28, 1977): 1.

Welch, C. E. "Professional Licensure and Hospital Delineation of Clinical Privileges: Relationship to Quality Assurance." *Quality Assurance in Health Care,* edited by R. H. Egdahl and P. M. Gertman. Germantown, Md.: Aspen, 1976.

Wolman, D. M. "Quality Control and the Community Physician in England: An American Perspective." *International Journal of Health Services* 6, no. 1 (1976): 79-102.

Yerby, A. S. "Regulation of Health Manpower." *Controls on Health Care.* Washington, D.C.: National Academy of Sciences, 1975.

9

Social Justice

Selection by David Mechanic

Innumerable studies have demonstrated that the poor have a greater prevalence of illness, disability, chronicity, and restriction of activity because of health problems than those of higher status, and that they have less accessibility to many types of health services and receive lower quality care (Mechanic, 1968; Kosa, Antonovsky, and Zola, 1969; Norman, 1969; Medical and Health Research Association of New York, 1967; Dohrenwend and Dohrenwend, 1969; National Center for Health Statistics, 1970a, 1970b; Ferman, Kornbluh, and Haber, 1968). There are, of course, distinctions to be made, since the "poor" include a variety of persons and groups, different health and disease conditions are associated with varying causal factors, and failures in maintaining a good level of health and having access to necessary services are the product of a variety of sociocultural and environmental circumstances. Yet, it is a widely known fact that the environmental resources that influence the maintenance of health, the prevention of illness, and the amelioration of disease and disability are distributed in society in relation to the abilities of various groups to economically command them.

In this essay I shall focus on the poor as a special group, since it is clear that the prevalence of disease and levels of health are not related to socioeconomic status in a simple linear fashion. Most existing data suggest, in contrast, that particularly poor health levels and a high vulnerability to disease and

Reprinted by permission from "Inequality, Health Status, and the Delivery of Health Services in the United States," *Public Expectations and Health Care* (New York: John Wiley & Sons, 1972), pp. 80-101.

disability predominate in the poverty group, and that after a minimum income level is reached such differences tend to be more modest relative to differences in economic status. There are several factors that contribute toward this trend. Old people make up a disproportionate number of low income persons, and they also suffer from greater illness and disability. Furthermore, persons with physical difficulties and disabilities are frequently limited in employment possibilities which result in low socioeconomic status. Moreover, given the existing health insurance situation, once a person reaches a certain income level the probability is high that he will have some minimum insurance coverage to deal with serious episodes of illness requiring hospitalization. Although such insurance may be less than optimal, it will usually provide services in cases that involve emergencies or serious illness. Although level of income may determine the amount and quality of services that persons can afford beyond the minimum that typical insurance policies provide, these probably have only limited effect on health status and resulting disability. I do not mean to suggest that middle income persons do not face difficulties in finding adequate medical services at a price they regard as reasonable, and certainly most of the population would face profound difficulties in the face of such catastrophic conditions as chronic uremia. I focus on the poor, however, because I believe that it is particularly this group that faces the most serious consequences relative to illness and inadequate health care and that their problems are most difficult to resolve from the standpoint of public policy.

Social programs to ameliorate the consequences of illness, disability, and poverty have evolved slowly in the United States, and they have been typified by strong moral overtones and a tight hold on the purse strings (Handler, 1972). Throughout most of our early history, a strong sense of social Darwinism prevailed, and poverty was viewed as the outcome of natural selection which brought to the bottom those who were defective, lazy, or otherwise held in contempt. With time, there was a growing appreciation that chronic illness and disability were unpredictable, and public subsidy for the poor developed to supplement charity made available by religious and philanthropic groups. Public aid was always provided penuriously and frequently with the implication that those who required help did so because of their own personal failures or their unwillingness to make the necessary effort to look after their own needs. As social programs developed, they increasingly made distinctions between the deserving poor, those whose poverty was the consequence of unpredictable life events—such as the blind, the aged, the permanently disabled, and children—and the undeserving poor who were frequently seen as unwilling to work. With the depression and the unemployment of vast numbers of "respectable" able-bodied workers, the view of the deserving needy was extended to the temporarily unemployed, and social programs were developed to aid them. But general assistance in this country, and in the tradition of the English poor laws, has always been grudgingly provided with a conviction on the part of many that those on welfare or receiving other social benefits are undeserving and must be policed, supervised, or otherwise discouraged from becoming too dependent on the tax-payer.

In the area of health services, similar attitudes have prevailed. Although there have been many areas of the country, particularly in large cities, where the poor have been able to obtain health services from municipal or university hospitals, such services have often been characterized by fragmentation and impersonality and have frequently affronted patients' human dignity. Moreover, the *quid pro quo* was that since the patient was receiving free care, hospital personnel could use him as they wished to promote their teaching and research efforts, and a very different style of medical care prevailed on the public as compared with the private services (Duff and Hollingshead, 1968). By whatever criterion one wishes to adopt, whether it be the availability of services, the accessibility of most specialized personnel, or the courtesy and thoughtfulness with which services are rendered, it is clear and unequivocal that these aspects of care have been and continue to be directly related to the socioeconomic status of the patient.

Implicit in the criticism of the current state of affairs is a value judgment that health care services are more important than other consumer goods, and that their availability should be determined on a basis other than the ability to economically command them. Some dispute such "importance," but the fact that health services may not be as crucial to life as many believe is less important than the fact that people regard them so (Mechanic, 1968). Given the nature of our social and economic system, there is little reason to believe that if health resources are scarce the poor can substantially improve their access. Indeed, if we are to make a commitment in this country to provide a reasonable level of care to all Americans irrespective of their socioeconomic circumstances, a general expansion of the health sector must continue to take place, and there must be further development of health personnel, facilities, and services.

It is ironic that some economists and manpower experts, such as Eli Ginzberg of Columbia University, who recognize the role of the market in distributing health services, and who defend market mechanisms, are precisely those same economists who have opposed substantial increases in the provision of physicians and other services (McNerney, 1970; Ginzberg, 1966). It seems fairly evident that even if financing is made available for the poor to compete in the purchase of care, the more aggressive, demanding, and knowledgeable affluent will have major advantages in a marketplace of scarce personnel and resources. As Ginzberg (1969) argues:

Large-scale governmental financing can shift the relative position of various groups in their access to medical services, but there is little or no prospect—no matter how much money government invests—of equalizing the claims of all citizens so that need, rather than income determines the services rendered to each individual . . . any serious proposal to establish a more equitable system of medical care within our present society has no prospect of success unless profound structural alterations occur in our free-market economy. . . . With none of these changes even remotely possible, augmented purchasing power in the hands of the poor cannot effect any significant redistribution of medical services.

Following Ginzberg's reasoning, a condition for providing better care, barring profound structural changes, would involve some relief in the competition for scarce supply. At this point, Ginzberg shifts his argument and maintains that we already have enough doctors; what we need is greater doctor productivity and a more efficient health services system. But Ginzberg, in another context, has already recognized that profound structural changes are unlikely, and the kind of efficiency he is talking about is no more realistic. It is obvious that the efficiency of the health services system must be improved, but it is also reasonably certain that health progress for the poor will not be a product of improved efficiency in health organization alone.

In discussing social inequality and health, we cannot neglect the fact that stratification in health care is based not only on income, ethnicity, and race, but also on a variety of other implicit value systems that order the availability of care in terms of the character of the disorder, the age of those affected, the degree of chronicity and disability, and the like.* Differential attitudes in the delivery of health services persist in relation to patients with irreversible chronic diseases, geriatric patients, alcoholics, drug addicts and psychotics, and other patients who require intensive rehabilitation services (Mechanic, 1969a). Many of these categories of need tend to be associated as well with low income and minority status, but they pose more general problems.

Also, medical and other health priorities reflect the ethos of the society. A recent analysis, for example, illustrated that research in sickle-cell anemia, a problem concentrated among black Americans, received only a small fraction of the support and interest given to many other diseases causing less overall morbidity but which affect the more affluent.[†] Since then, the federal government has initiated a more significant program. The previous failure to develop a reasonable program in this area had little to do with the potential researchability of the field or the promise of new developments. In the past decade, the concentrated efforts and attention devoted to attacking paralytic polio, in contrast to feeble efforts in closing gaps in infant mortality, must be understood within the context that the incidence of polio was higher in the middle classes than in the lower classes (Simmons, 1958). The areas receiving official recognition and

---

*The impact of such influences on the care of the dying patient is described by Lasagna (1970). Similar observations were made by Sudnow (1969).

[†]"Sickle cell anemia occurs about one in 500 Negro births and median survival is still only twenty years of age. In 1967, there were an estimated 1,155 new cases of SCA, 1,206 of cystic fibrosis, 813 of muscular dystrophy, and 350 of phenylketonuria. Yet, volunteer organizations raised $1.9 million for cystic fibrosis, $7.9 million for muscular dystrophy, but less than $100,000 for SCA" (Scott, 1970).

attention depend, in large part, on the ability of affected groups to make their needs known and to organize in order to stimulate official response. In this context, the problems that most affect the poor have less public visibility and less impact on political and administrative processes. Clearly, we must give more attention to considering how social priorities are determined and how the needs of those less vocal or sophisticated can be properly weighed against the claims of other groups.

SOME ASPECTS OF THE RELATIONSHIP BETWEEN SOCIAL INEQUALITY AND HEALTH

Inequalities in health and health care develop in a variety of ways. I can appreciate that when the needs are so pressing, one becomes impatient with subtle distinctions in theory and concept. Such distinctions, however, are helpful and it is necessary to understand them in effectively closing the gaps in accessibility to health care and differential health status. Whatever our aspirations might be, there are no indications that in the near future we will experience a radical transformation in our values, our economic system, or in the distribution of wealth; and thus we must anticipate attacking the problems of health in an arena of scarce resources. The resources that become available must be used effectively in closing the gaps that we know exist and in preventing the further occurrence of differentials in areas where preventive intervention has some possibilities for success.

It is widely appreciated that the relationship between poverty and health status is part of a vicious cycle. Illness and disability are major causes of dependency and low socioeconomic status (Lawrence, 1958), and traditionally the lower income of the poor has limited their opportunities to receive services to increase their functional capacities and, indirectly, their income potential. Although in recent years the Medicaid program has improved the medical care situation of many poor persons, it is generally true that rehabilitation of the functional capacity of the ill and disabled is an underdeveloped aspect of our entire health care system, and frequently adequate services are just not available. In addition, persons who are seriously disabled and visibly handicapped are exposed to various forms of discrimination in employment as well as in other life areas, and often cannot use the skills and education they have because of arbitrary exclusion from the work force. Much social legislation for health services in the United States is oriented toward the irreversibly disabled (the deserving unfortunate), and frequently persons who are rehabilitable cannot receive public support for rehabilitation without first becoming indigent. Thus, social legislation often produces incentives against rehabilitation and gainful employment, and our social ethos defines the ill and disabled as lesser citizens.

Although the literature is uncertain concerning the relationships between the occurrence of disease and socioeconomic status—and, of course, this varies from disease to disease—it is clear and unequivocal that when the poor become ill, they suffer consequences more serious than those experienced by more affluent classes. The poor are less likely to receive adequate treatment, are more likely to come into treatment during more advanced stages of their illness, and are more likely to experience persistent morbidity and disability (Hollingshead and Redlich, 1958; Howard, 1965).* Moreover, the social position of the poor exposes them to lesser social protection for themselves and their families in that their jobs are generally less secure, they have less income to tide them through a serious illness, they are less protected by sick leave and other social arrangements, their illness is more likely to impinge on the performance of their work, and their living environment is less conducive to recovery and freedom from worry. The consequences of illness for the poor make illness a more frightening and disruptive experience, and probably encourage denial of illness and reluctance to enter treatment during its less evident stages of development (Koos, 1954).

I raise these issues, in part, because the problems characteristic of the cultural orientations and inclinations of the poor-sick for receiving medical care must be understood within the existential situation they face. When some segments of the poor come into contact with large medical bureaucracies, professionals often define their behavior as ill-adapted, and complain of the difficulties of delivering necessary health services to the poor. The poor, of course, are in no sense monolithic, and it is dangerous and misleading to offer generalizations about them as a special class. Yet a variety of studies have shown that one more frequently finds among the poor tendencies which make them less receptive to preventive care, less likely to conform to medical regimen, less informed about health matters, and the like (Rosenstock, 1969; Mechanic, 1969b; Green, 1970). To some extent, such responses reflect limited education, cultural and social deprivation, apathy and neglect, and fear. The responses also indicate the experience of the poor with impersonal medical institutions, inconsiderate personnel, and resulting humiliation. But such tendencies also reflect a problem of fit between social institutions developed by middle class Americans with middle class concepts that are not adaptive or sensitive to the special difficulties the poor may have in accommodating to such forms of delivery of health care (Strauss,

*This conclusion has as its basis a wide variety of studies which demonstrate greater chronicity and disability among the poor. Although it is difficult to find studies that compare the poor and more affluent on chronicity who have suffered from similar morbidity incidents, the general consistency in the literature supports the overall conclusion. There is evidence, however, that government programs in recent years have significantly increased the access of the physician for the poor, and as access to health services improves among the poor, we might anticipate some reduction in disability days. Bice and Eichhorn (1971), in reviewing utilization trends, have found that average use of physician services among those with lowest incomes has increased in recent years. Recent data on access to more specialized services or the quality of care are not available.

1969). In agreeing that there is a great deal more that can be done in structuring preventive and other services so that those in need of them find them more compatible with their orientations and understandings, we must also recognize that there are significant differences in the manner in which populations orient themselves to health and health institutions, and that such differences cannot all be explained by the lack of commitment, interest, or other limitations of health personnel.* The poor have special needs and problems that must be taken into account, but in any situation of scarcity of personnel and other resources, health facilities similarly face serious operational difficulties. We know that many medical and social programs oriented toward the poor and disabled frequently end up servicing those with lesser need. Such programs can be structured so that they are more responsive to the hard-core poor and disabled, but it is unlikely that the problems of providing access and service can be remedied if we underestimate the degree to which the client's orientations and reactions may be an important barrier to bringing about some reasonable fit. It is only when we recognize such facts that we begin to develop programs and procedures that overcome them.

INEQUALITY AND MORTALITY

The reduction of mortality, improvement of longevity, and the maintenance of a high level of health status is largely the result of improvements in nutrition, housing, sanitation, and the quality of life (Mechanic, 1968; McKeown, 1965). At the present time, the major causes of mortality and morbidity in the population—such problems as heart disease, cancer, stroke, accidents, mental disorders, and the like—are not impressively affected by medicine as it is practiced, and much of the medical care provided is ameliorative and supportive. Such care is important and should not be disparaged, but a realistic attack on the problem of health must recognize the true potentialities and limitations of medical practice. Similarly, major problems of health among the disadvantaged young—such as drug addiction—have not been easily amenable to medical control, and much of the solution to these problems may lie outside the traditional practice of medicine. Moreover, the unhappiness and the despair of the old, abandoned in their later years without function or status, or the alienation of the young depend more on social values and conditions generally than on the activities of health workers. I raise these issues because many of the problems of health related to inequality will not be simply responsive to the expansion of services, but require a more profound recasting of social values, practices,

---

*There is a rather vigorous dispute in the behavioral sciences as to the existence of a "culture of poverty." Existing evidence would suggest that although some poor tend to have orientations that exacerbate their condition and interfere with successful coping, the argument is frequently overstated. For a middle position, see Parker and Kleiner (1970).

and priorities. This will demand efforts more pervasive than those that can be mustered by the health sector alone.

In this essay, I shall restrict my attention to efforts possible through the health sector as it is traditionally seen with the understanding that health does not operate in a vacuum, but is responsive to the larger forces that shape society and people's lives.

The most persistent and impressive inequality in the health care area is the disparity between white and nonwhite infant mortality in the United States. Such differences are extremely large; the nonwhite rate has been almost double the white rate for some years, and although both whites and nonwhites have made progress in recent decades, the gap itself has persisted and has even given evidence of increasing. In 1968 the nonwhite rate was 34.5 deaths per 1,000 live births in contrast to a rate of 19.2 among whites.* Even the white rate is considerably higher than the prevailing rate in several other highly developed industrialized countries, and excluding nonwhites from the total would not change our position substantially. Thus, although the factors leading to infant death in America are exaggerated among nonwhites, they exist generally and contribute to what might be regarded as an excessive rate of infant death.

The factors affecting infant mortality are intertwined in a complex web, and it is not easy to isolate one or another factor as a major determinant. The opportunity of a new infant to survive is affected by the stature and health of the mother, which is in turn affected by her early nutrition and development, which may be a product of her social background, the economic status of her family, and so on (Illsley, 1967). Similarly, socioeconomic status is associated with the rate of illegitimate births, parity of the mother, age at the time of childbearing, quality of medical care received, and the like. Much of the data on which national trends are ascertained are collected in a fashion that does not allow for a detailed description of the manner in which these variables relate to one another, but further information is obtained from studies restricted to more limited populations.

The best predictor of infant survival is the birth weight of the infant which is correlated with the period of gestation, but there are significant variations in average weight at any gestation stage. The rate of infant mortality among infants weighing five and a half pounds or less at birth is seventeen times the rate among infants with higher weights at birth. In the first four weeks, the ratio is thirty to one. The experience of low-weight infants who survive the early period following birth continues to involve high risk. Low-weight infants who survive also have a high risk of such disorders as mental retardation, cerebral palsy, and epilepsy (Birch and Gusson, 1970; Chase, 1970).

Low-weight infants are more likely to be born to mothers who are under

*Estimates by the National Center for Health Statistics for 1969 and 1970 indicate white rates of 18.4 and 17.4 and nonwhite rates of 31.6 and 31.4. See Public Health Service, *Monthly Vital Statistics Report* (September 1971) and *Annual Summary for the United States* (1970).

fifteen years of age, nonwhite, of lower socioeconomic status, of less education, and among those who smoke. Current statistics suggest that low-weight non-white infants have a slightly better chance of survival than white infants of comparable weight (Shapiro, Schlesinger, and Nesbitt, 1968), but it is not clear whether this is a true advantage or whether it is a product of classification variations or differences in gestation of infants at comparable weight. In any case, it is reasonably clear that low-weight infants who constitute less than 10 percent of all births are a group at special risk, and it is imperative that this population receive effective prenatal and postnatal care and other types of health services. It is not clear, however, how this group can be most effectively identified.

There are a variety of other factors correlated with the occurrence of infant mortality, but none of these has an effect as large as birth weight. These factors include race, parity, maternal age, socioeconomic status, and illegitimacy. Although maternal age and parity are important, the combination of the limited influence of such variables, and the limited extent to which extreme values on these variables are characteristic of birth, results in a very small total impact on the overall rate of infant mortality (Chase, 1970). It seems unlikely that a coherent public policy can be built around such risks.

The situation is somewhat different among nonwhites, the poor, and illegitimate births and, of course, these three categories are associated with one another. Among both whites and nonwhites, the absence of a father recorded on the birth certificate is associated with a marked increase in rates of infant mortality and, similarly, one finds among both whites and nonwhites highest infant mortality in the lowest occupational groups. This social status effect is not uniform or clearcut, and it is apparent that certain cultural patterns and behavior can support a low infant mortality rate even in relatively impoverished circumstances (Anderson, 1958). The crucial point, however, is that extreme poverty is often associated with a pattern of living and orientations that involve extremely high risks of infant mortality, and this argues very strongly for particular attention to such high risk areas which ensure the development of adequate patterns of prenatal, maternal, and child care.

It is reasonably clear that well-organized public health efforts, associated with improvement in the overall life conditions of the poorest segments of our population, can result in a substantial decrease in the magnitude of infant mortality in the United States. It is extremely difficult to estimate specifically what constitutes a reasonable reduction in infant mortality given the tremendous variations characteristic of the living environments and cultures of the United States. Speaking relatively conservatively, I see no good reason why the national rate cannot in the coming years be reduced to a level of 15 or 16 deaths per 1,000 live births, which is higher than the present rate in Sweden.*

*In 1967, the United States ranked fourteenth in the world in favorable infant mortality experience with an overall rate of 22.4. The rate in Sweden was 12.9. There are many

The low rate of infant mortality, characteristic of the Scandinavian countries, is probably attributable to a variety of factors: the relatively limited variations in the social status of the population, biological characteristics of the population, the cultural homogeneity and development of the countries involved, the well-organized social services, and particularly those in relation to child and maternal care. These countries place a high value on child and maternal health, and have well-developed public programs to ensure a satisfactory outcome of pregnancy.

Although the experience of other countries is instructive and useful, there are usually wide gaps in culture and traditions from one society to the next, and it is particularly instructive to seek evidence from situations that are as comparable as possible to the circumstances for which one wishes to design programs. Although there is not a great deal of carefully collected data relevant to the issue at hand, we have some evidence from the United States relevant to the relationship between infant mortality and the delivery of health services.

Some valuable data result from a study comparing rates of mortality among subscribers to the Health Insurance Plan of New York (HIP), a large prepaid group practice program in New York City (Shapiro, Weiner, and Densen, 1958; Shapiro et al., 1960).* This study involving live births, fetal deaths, and infant deaths from 1955 to 1957 was executed carefully and with considerable attention to possible intervening factors that could affect the results. The investigators found that a higher proportion of the women in HIP initiated their prenatal care in the first trimester of pregnancy and that prematurity and perinatal mortality rates were lower than in New York City as a whole. When the New York City comparison sample was restricted to women delivered in a hospital by a private doctor, the difference in proportions of women seeking prenatal care was eliminated. HIP still retained a small advantage in respect to prematurity and perinatal mortality rates. This analysis took account of differences in demographic characteristics between HIP women and women in the city as a whole and other possible biasing factors.

The HIP study is suggestive, but one might reasonably suspect that persons choosing to obtain their care from a prepaid group, regardless of economic status, are somewhat more interested in their health, more knowledgeable about health matters, and the like, and thus it is difficult to generalize from this study to particularly high risk subgroups of the population. The HIP study did show

---

who are skeptical about statistics from other countries. One, however, need look no further than variations within the United States. Communities vary widely, some as low as Sweden; other communities in the same states have rates three or four times as high.

*Similar findings on improved outcomes for the indigent aged are reported by Shapiro et al. (1967). For a general review of such end result measurement studies, see Shapiro (1967).

clearly that among both whites and nonwhites, women using general ward services did considerably worse than women using either HIP or private physicians in New York City. These results are attributable probably to a variety of factors: selective factors both in terms of socioeconomic status and health risk among those using ward services, differing degrees of health consciousness in this group, and the fragmented and ineffective character of the New York City ward services relative to the problem. In New York City as a whole, at the time, 61 percent of white women were found to obtain prenatal care, primarily from private physicians. Among nonwhites and Puerto Ricans, the comparable statistics were 16 percent and 13 percent. Although the use of such services among white women increased only slightly within HIP, very large improvements took place among nonwhite and Puerto Rican women in HIP. The nonwhite percentage went from 16 percent to 55 percent, and the Puerto Rican percentage increased from 13 percent to 48 percent. Although these data are suggestive, we have no way of ascertaining how representative nonwhite and Puerto Rican women in HIP were of all nonwhite and Puerto Rican women.

Some very suggestive data are available from the City of Denver, Colorado, where in the period from 1964 to 1969 the Department of Health and Hospitals has developed a coordinated system of health services for the poorest areas of the city to attempt to meet the health needs of this population. Among the services provided were a neighborhood health center, conveniently located health stations, and more specialized clinic and hospital facilities. The program utilized specially trained nurses to assist physicians as well as a variety of workers from the areas serviced who received special training. Data are available comparing Denver's twenty-five lower socioeconomic ranked census tracts served by these new programs with the remaining census tracts in the city. In 1964 the twenty-five lowest tracts had an infant mortality rate of 34.2 as compared with a rate of 23.5 in the remaining tracts. In the twenty-five lowest tracts, the infant mortality rate decreased from 34.2 in 1964 to 21.5 in 1969. Rates of postneonatal mortality decreased from 11.3 in 1964 to 7.3 in 1969. Among the remaining tracts, infant deaths declined from 23.5 in 1964 to 19.7 in 1969. By 1969 infant mortality differences between the least favored socioeconomic tracts and other tracts had been largely eliminated (information received from the Denver Department of Health and Hospitals). Although we would want to know a great deal more about other changes that took place in these census tracts and the specific relationships between changes in services and reductions in infant mortality, these gross data suggest that it is possible to significantly reduce infant mortality. Similar findings have been reported by O.E.O. neighborhood health centers established in poor underserviced areas.

Mortality among adults also varies significantly by race and socioeconomic status. At almost every age, nonwhites and the poor suffer a higher risk of mortality; and, overall, adult rates of mortality in the United States lag behind other nations as well (Anderson, 1972). Although the trends are approximately similar to the situation described relevant to infant mortality, it is more difficult to provide evidence that these differentials can be markedly influenced by changes in the organization of medical care rather than more basic changes in the life circumstances of the poor.

There are no doubt circumstances where, for example, the lack of availability of medical facilities decreases the longevity of nonwhites and the poor relative to whites and those better off—for example, such as access to good medical care following a heart attack—but much of the differential is a product of more embracing life disadvantages the poor must face. Just as it is difficult to specify precisely the effects of medical care in general relative to other life forces, so it is difficult to specify how much specific gain can be achieved through better medical services as compared with a decent job, adequate housing, and a neighborhood free of the pathologies of drug addiction, alcoholism, and alienation. Improved access to medical care for all does not necessarily depend on any particular assessment of impact but can be based on a concept of social justice. Medical care is an important right as much because people see it as such as it is because of its specific impacts on the health of the population.

SOME NOTES ON FORMS OF HEALTH CARE DELIVERY AND THE POOR

Much of the problem of bringing health care services to the poor involves eliminating economic barriers to care and providing the required manpower and facilities for providing adequate care. There is evidence that suggests that major gaps in care can be closed if such conditions are fulfilled in a reasonable way.* The utilization of health services, of course, will also depend on social and cultural orientation toward the types of care provided, the manner in which care is organized, and the responsiveness of health personnel to medical consumers. Access to medical care decreases as costs increase, and costs must be measured not only in money terms, but also in terms of time, inconvenience, distance, embarrassment, or whatever.

Traditionally the poor, particularly in large cities, have depended very heavily on public clinics and outpatient departments for their care. Data collected during the interval of July 1965 to June 1967 indicate that physician visits in the United States no longer show any large variation by socioeconomic

*In general, there is evidence that systems that eliminate economic barriers to care are able to close the gap in medical utilization between the poor and the more affluent (Cartwright, 1967). Making available comprehensive services apparently leads to a higher level of utilization which cannot be accounted for by trivial and unnecessary uses of services (Darsky, Sinai, and Axelrod, 1958). A recent study of the Tufts-Columbia Point Health Center in Boston found that when economic barriers were removed, and attractive and convenient services were provided, the average rate of utilization of low income persons was considerably higher than for the population as a whole (Bellin and Geiger, 1970).

status, although nonwhites continue to have a lower level of utilization than whites among both men and women (age-adjusted data). Also, the children of the more affluent receive more physician services than those in families with more modest incomes (National Center for Health Statistics, 1968, 1969, 1970b). Overall, the change in the trend suggests that new programs for the medically indigent have had some impact on their rate of utilization of services which in the period from July 1965 to June 1967 resembled the level characteristic of the nation as a whole, but major gaps in access to medical care appear in many places, as the data on white-nonwhite differences suggest. There is also evidence that differences in the basic pattern of use of services continue to persist. While approximately 8 percent of whites received their medical care at emergency rooms or hospital clinics, more than one-quarter of nonwhites received their care in such locations. Nonwhites with incomes of $7,000 or more, however, were more likely than other nonwhites to see the physician in his office (National Center for Health Statistics, 1969). The medical significance of this varying pattern of care is in dispute, with some experts suggesting that the pattern of care available in large outpatient departments of teaching hospitals is superior to that available from private physicians in their offices. There may be some merit to this view but, as Duff and Hollingshead (1968) have so dramatically indicated, the potentialities for good technical medical care are not the same as high quality health care.[†]

Those with less knowledge and sophistication in particular, but probably all of us as well, require more than the episodic and fragmented care characteristic of the large hospital outpatient clinics. Although the well-educated and sophisticated consumers of medical care complain about the growing impersonality of care and the lack of responsiveness of medical personnel, such persons are often able to exploit existing resources through their aggressiveness, their ability to obtain information, and their demands for respect and courtesy. Those who are less sophisticated and assertive, because of lack of education or cultural orientations, are frequently confused and intimidated by the vastness and complexity of the large medical bureaucracy, and by the interchangeability of people and roles. The poor family with multiple difficulties, in particular, must deal with a variety of agencies and personnel to obtain needed care involving great time, patience, and initiative. Not only is the location of such care fragmented and

---

[*]In the period from July 1966 to June 1967, among children under age seventeen, whites averaged 3.9 physician visits a year and nonwhites averaged 2.0 visits a year. Among children with family incomes of less than $3,000 the average was 2.5 visits, while among those with $7,000 or more the average was 4.1 visits. Data collected for the period from July 1963 to June 1964, indicate that 66 percent of nonwhite children under seventeen had never seen a dentist, and 62 percent of those with family incomes of less than $3,000 were in a similar situation. The comparable figure among white children was 39 percent.

[†]This pattern is not unique to the United States (Cartwright, 1964; Forsyth and Logan, 1968).

confused but, frequently, no serious attempt is made to coordinate services or to deal with the array of health problems in its family context or in any relationship to one another. No matter how good any particular service may appear, when poorly coordinated, the overall pattern of care may be inferior and poorly fitted to the needs or social conditions of the persons involved.

THE CRISIS IN HEALTH CARE AND ITS RELATIONSHIP TO THE PROBLEMS OF THE POOR

The present crisis in health care stems from the inability of the health sector to accommodate effectively to the developments in medical knowledge and technology, the growth of more specialized activity, resulting failures in providing comprehensive and coordinated care, and rising aspirations for more and better health care. As the medical product becomes more valuable, and as the population becomes more sophisticated, more people seek services; and those who have been traditionally without equal access feel the lack of availability of services more acutely. Thus the crisis results from internal changes in the health sector, changing demographic and social aspects of the population, a redefinition of the role of medical care and its relevance on the part of the population, and the resulting increased demand, problems of cost and financing, and inflation in the medical care sector.

The growing sense of crisis is the product of various forces that have differentially affected varying interest groups in the population. Those in the urban ghettos and rural areas acutely feel their lack of access to physicians and other health services and demand change so that their needs can be met. Government officials, representatives of insurance companies, labor, and management are all alarmed at the growing escalation of medical care costs and the difficulties in stemming the inflationary tide that affect their programs and have financial implications for them. The providers—the hospitals, medical schools, clinics, and the like—are similarly concerned with growing costs, and particularly seek greater reimbursement or other more attractive financial arrangements. The average person is increasingly concerned about changing patterns of practice characterized by impersonality and bureaucracy, the difficulty of finding a personal physician who is responsive to his concerns, and alarm at the growing difficulty of obtaining a reasonable level of service at a price he can afford.

Although one might wish that the movement toward reorganization of medical services and national health insurance were based on a growing consciousness of social justice and an increased compassion for the plight of the poor, the fact is that this is only a subsidiary theme in what most centrally is a concern with costs and efficiency. As health care prices have risen, and as demands for care on the manpower pool have become more intense, federal and state officials have been concerned with establishing a ceiling on the uncontrollable costs of medical care within the programs they finance. Similarly, various third parties find that they must persistently increase their premiums to meet expenses resulting in continuing criticism from the public. It is this type of generalized concern that has stimulated much of the apparent activity, and if one considers the types of solutions being seriously entertained it is fairly apparent that they apply to the needs of traditional interest groups as much, if not more, than the special health needs of the poor.

PROBLEMS OF FINANCING HEALTH CARE

Although existing problems have been recognized for some time, they have been highlighted in the past few years. Few public commentators anticipated the inflationary impact of Medicare and Medicaid on the health services sector, nor was it appreciated to what extent rising costs under these programs in the context of other public expenditures would strain federal and state budgets encouraging re-examination of the entire issue of medical care. To some extent the growing costs reflected the buildup of need among the aged and the poor for medical services but, more acutely, it demonstrated that to invest in medical care without attempting to rationalize and organize health services delivery would be costly and only marginally successful. Attention has now moved from the earlier focus on providing assistance to special needy groups to means of providing health care in a more efficient and structured way.

THE PHYSICIAN SHORTAGE AND THE CRISIS OF MANPOWER

A prerequisite for effective health care is a reasonable quantity and distribution of facilities and manpower. The need for facilities and manpower is dependent, of course, on a variety of factors: how well they are distributed in the population, the patterns of need existing, the patterns of health service utilization in the population, and the like. Although the usual indicator of availability of manpower is the number available relative to some unit in the population, such figures can be highly deceptive since they often mask the factors described above. Moreover, such figures do not take into account such crucial matters as the types of tasks performed, relative efficiency in performing them, and the distribution of activities generally. Manpower shortages may result from too few professionals, from uneven distribution of professionals from one area to another, from uneven task allocation among professionals, and between professionals and ancillary workers, or from any combination of these factors.

In recent years there has been a slight increase in the number of physicians available relative to the size of the American population. For example, from 1950 to 1960 there were approximately 150 doctors per 100,000 population including doctors in nonpatient care activities. By 1967 this figure had risen to 158 (National Center for Health Statistics, 1970c). The increase has been sustained by some growth in the number of medical school graduates, but it is also the product of significantly relying on manpower trained by foreign medical schools who may often have significant handicaps in their medical training, the understanding of English, and appreciation of the patient's cultural patterns. If physicians not delivering patient care are excluded from these totals, then there were 132 physicians per 100,000 population in the United States in 1967. Even using such large aggregates as states, one finds enormous variation from one unit to another, ranging from 320 nonfederal physicians providing patient care per 100,000 population in Washington, D.C., and 203 in New York state to 69 in Mississippi and 75 in Alabama (National Center for Health Statistics, 1970c).

Such aggregates, however, are highly misleading since doctors tend to concentrate in metropolitan areas and in suburbs. There are, for example, almost four times as many doctors in metropolitan areas per unit population as there are in isolated rural areas. If one considers more meaningful units, more closely fitted to the distances within which people can reasonably seek medical care, such discrepancies become enormous. For example, in urban ghettos such as East Garfield, Chicago, there are thirteen physicians for 63,000 residents while in Kenwood-Oakland, Chicago, five physicians serve 45,400 blacks (Ferguson, 1970). A similar situation exists relative to many rural communities. Even these data do not reflect the magnitude of the problem in that doctors in ghettos and rural areas tend to be older than the average, and it is clear that even the few that exist are not being replaced when they die or retire.

Similar problems exist relative to most other health personnel, although the rates of such personnel are more easily enlarged. A notable exception is dentistry, where the dentist-patient ratio has not changed in the past two decades, being fifty-seven in 1950, and fifty-six in 1967. In considering these ratios, it is important to recognize that dentistry is usually given relatively low priority compared to other health services, and that it is only recently that we have begun to be concerned with inadequacies in the distribution of dental care. As people become more affluent, they are more able to afford dental care and more likely to seek it, yet it is ironic that a commensurate increase in the number of dentists has not accompanied growing demand for dental care. Dentists have learned to practice with greater efficiency in recent years, many making use of dental assistants, and thus the situation may not be quite as bleak as it appears—but it is bleak nevertheless. National data show that many Americans receive very poor dental care, and the pattern of dental care is clearly and substantially related to race and socioeconomic status (National Center for Health Statistics, 1965, 1966).

The basic problems of distribution of health manpower in general are similar to those involving doctors. Although there were 313 employed registered nurses in the United States per 100,000 population in 1967, these rates varied from 157 in Mississippi to 536 in Connecticut (National Center for Health Statistics, 1970c). Many types of health personnel are largely hospital-based in their activities, and their pattern of distribution follows the pattern of location of hospitals. But even when hospitals exist, they often face problems in recruiting doctors, nurses, and other highly skilled manpower when they are in urban ghettos and more isolated areas.

The physical location of doctors and other personnel is only part of the distribution difficulties. A major aspect of the problem, which has been creating increasing dissatisfaction in recent years, has been the manner in which health tasks have been distributed between doctors and among the health professions in general. Although the total pool of doctors relative to the population has been increasing, the number and proportion of doctors delivering primary medical care have been steadily decreasing. General practitioners are increasingly becoming defunct, and now constitute less than one-quarter of all doctors. A more realistic estimate of the availability of primary care physicians is to consider not only general practitioners but also internists and pediatricians, the latter taking considerable responsibility for primary health services. But even these figures are discouraging. In 1931 there were ninety-four primary care physicians per 100,000 population. This rate has shown a continuing trend downward to eighty-nine in 1940, seven-five in 1949, sixty in 1957, and fifty in 1965 (Fein, 1967). The downward trend is probably continuing.

It is somewhat surprising to find that the largest component of the medical profession is in the surgical specialties, and their size relative to the rest has been increasing, now accounting for approximately one-third of all specialists (Stevens, 1971; American Medical Association, 1970). The largest group among the surgeons is the general surgeons, and they are in competition as well with general practitioners and others who also perform some surgery. One overall effect of this concentration of surgically inclined doctors is the completion of a high rate of surgical activity relative to other health care activities (Bunker, 1970; Lewis, 1969).

PROVIDING HEALTH SERVICES FOR THE POOR

More recently, there has been an outpouring of analyses on the health care crisis. The typical discussion concludes with the recommendation that the solution to these problems lies in the development of widespread prepaid group practice, preventive care and health maintenance, and the use of a variety of new paramedical personnel as well as more effective use of those already in evidence. I do not wish to belittle these recommendations for there is much in their favor. But we should be aware that the central feature in current discussions of health care has continued to be the growing cost of services. As such costs have risen, they have put pressure on many different interest groups who together make up a powerful force in political affairs. As government through an incremental process has assumed payment for a greater proportion of the costs of medical care for the old and the poor, resulting inflation in the health care area and higher taxes has aroused many middle class consumers and has put considerable financial pressures on state finances as well as on the federal treasury.

Although the health problems of the poor are of concern to governmental and other groups, these interests are only part of the larger set of interests which are coalescing and forming a countervailing force against more traditional interests in the health field. It is not at all clear from current discussions how well the poor will do within the context of the types of reforms generally being advocated, but it is reasonably clear that in the absence of general reforms of our health care system, which bring benefits to many segments of the American population, the benefits provided to the poor will be unequal to the scope of the problems they face. It is already clear from the Medicaid program that coverage for the poor or near-poor will be fragmentary and uneven from area to area if the approach is a categorical one and if it is heavily dependent on tax support from the states and localities.

In the last analysis, we must recognize that the health care problems of the poor are a product of the larger sociopolitical system and of the more general organization of health care services in America. As long as these problems are seen as nothing more than slight maladjustments of what is basically a constructive approach to meeting the health needs of the country, it is unlikely that an adequate solution will be found. The poor are not a sufficiently powerful interest group to effectively compete in the establishment of priorities or in the distribution of available facilities, manpower, and services. Moreover, the problems of health care are only one part of a more complex pattern of social, economic, and environmental difficulties. It appears then that the health care needs of the poor can most constructively be met within a larger and more basic reconstruction of health care institutions in America, which ensure access to medical care for all and which establish a minimal level of health service available irrespective of social status or geographic area. It is doubtful that this can be achieved without greater direction over professional behavior. Access to care for all is available elsewhere in the world and under social and economic circumstances that pose greater pressure on national resources. The fact that the United States has still failed to achieve such modest goals is shameful. But even when we do, we will have hardly begun to face the underlying conditions that make the plight of the poor so difficult and their pathologies so prevalent. These problems will require a more frontal attack on our national values, our priorities, and our system of social stratification itself.

REFERENCES

American Medical Association. *Distribution of Physicians, Hospitals, and Hospital Beds in the United States* (vol. 1). Chicago: Department of Survey Research, 1970.

Anderson, O. "Infant Mortality and Social and Cultural Factors: Historical Trends and Current Patterns." *Patients, Physicians, and Illness,* edited by E. G. Jaco. New York: Free Press, 1958.

Anderson, O. *Health Care: Can There Be Equity? The United States, Sweden and England.* New York: Wiley-Interscience, 1972.

Bellin, S., and Geiger, H. J. "Actual Public Acceptance of the Neighborhood Health Center by the Urban Poor." *Journal of the American Medical Association* 214 (1970): 2147-53.

Bice, T. W., and Eichorn, R. L. "Socioeconomic Status and the Use of Physicians' Services." Paper presented to the American Public Health Association (Minneapolis, 1971).

Birch, H., and Gussow, J. *Disadvantaged Children: Health, Nutrition and School Failure.* New York: Harcourt, Brace & World, 1970.

Bunker, J. P. "Surgical Manpower: A Comparison of Operations of Surgeons in the United States and England and Wales." *New England Journal of Medicine* 282 (1970): 135-44.

Cartwright, A. *Human Relations and Hospital Care.* London: Routledge & Kegan Paul, 1964.

Cartwright, A. *Patients and Their Doctors: A Study of General Practice.* London: Routledge & Kegan Paul, 1967.

Chase, H. "Influence of Selected Demographic, Sociologic, and Biologic Factors on Infant Mortality." Unpublished report prepared for the Board on Medicine, National Academy of Science (1970).

Darsky, B.; Sinai, N.; and Axelrod, S. "Problem in Voluntary Insurance: Some Answers from the Windsor Experience." *American Journal of Public Health* 48 (1958): 971-78.

Dohrenwend, B., and Dohrenwend, B. *Social Status and Psychological Disorder.* New York: John Wiley & Sons, 1969.

Duff, R., and Hollingshead, A. *Sickness and Society.* New York: Harper, 1968.

Fein, R. *The Doctor Shortage: An Economic Analysis.* Washington, D.C.: Brookings Institution, 1967.

Ferguson, L. A. "What Has Been Accomplished in Chicago?" *Medicine in the Ghetto,* edited by J. C. Norman. New York: Appleton, Century, Crofts, 1970.

Ferman, L.; Kornbluh, J.; and Haber, A. (eds.). *Poverty in America* (revised ed.). Ann Arbor: University of Michigan Press, 1968.

Forsyth, G., and Logan, F. L. *Gateway or Dividing Line: A Study of Hospital Out-Patients in the 1960's.* New York: Oxford University Press, 1968.

Ginzberg, E. "Physician Shortage Reconsidered." *New England Journal of Medicine* 275 (1966): 85-87.

Ginzberg, E. *Men, Money, and Medicine.* New York: Columbia University Press, 1969.

Green, L. *Status Identity and Preventive Health Behavior* (Public Health Education Reports, vol. 1). Berkeley and Honolulu: Schools of Public Health, University of California and University of Hawaii, 1970.

Handler, J. *Reforming the Poor: Welfare Policy, Federalism, and Morality.* New York: Basic Books, 1972.

Hollingshead, A., and Redlich, F. *Social Class and Mental Illness.* New York: John Wiley & Sons, 1958.

Howard, J. "Race Differences in Hypertension Mortality Trends: Differential Drug Exposure as a Theory." *Milbank Memorial Fund Quarterly* 43 (1965): 202-18.

Illsley, R. "The Sociological Study of Reproduction and Its Outcome." *Childbearing: Social and Psychological Aspects,* edited by S. Richardson and A. Guttmacher. Baltimore: Williams & Wilkins, 1967.

Koos, E. *The Health of Regionsville: What the People Thought and Did About It.* New York: Columbia University Press, 1954.

Kosa, J.; Antonovsky, A.; and Zola, I. (eds.). *Poverty and Health: A Sociological Analysis.* Cambridge, Mass.: Harvard University Press, 1969.

Lasagne, L. "Physicians' Behavior Toward the Dying Patient." *The Dying Patient,* edited by

O. Brim, Jr., H. Freeman, S. Levine, and N. Scotch. New York: Russell Sage Foundation, 1970.

Lawrence, P. S. "Chronic Illness and Socio-Economic Status." *Patients, Physicians, and Illness,* edited by E. G. Jaco. New York: Free Press, 1958.

Lewis, C. "Variations in the Incidence of Surgery." *New England Journal of Medicine* 281 (1969): 880-84.

McKeown, T. *Medicine in Modern Society.* London: Allen & Unwin, 1965.

McNerney, W. "Why Does Medical Care Cost So Much?" *New England Journal of Medicine* 282 (1970): 1458-66.

Mechanic, D. *Medical Sociology: A Selective View.* New York: Free Press, 1968.

Mechanic, D. *Mental Health and Social Policy.* Englewood Cliffs, N.J.: Prentice-Hall, 1969a.

Mechanic, D. "Illness and Cure." *Poverty and Health: A Sociological Analysis,* edited by J. Kosa, A. Antonovsky, and I. Zola. Cambridge, Mass.: Harvard University Press, 1969b.

Medical and Health Research Association of New York. *Poverty and Health in the United States: A Bibliography with Abstracts.* New York: The Association, 1967.

National Center for Health Statistics. *Volume of Dental Visits: U.S.–July 1963-June 1964* (PHS Series 10). Washington, D.C.: Government Printing Office, 1965.

National Center for Health Statistics. *Dental Visits: Time Interval Since Last Visit: U.S.– July 1964-June 1965* (PHS Series 10). Washington, D.C.: Government Printing Office, 1966.

National Center for Health Statistics. *Volume of Physicians: U.S.–July 1966-June 1967* (PHS Series 10, no. 49). Washington, D.C.: Government Printing Office, 1968.

National Center for Health Statistics. *Differentials in Health Characteristics by Color: U.S.– July 1965-June 1967* (PHS Series 10, no. 56). Washington, D.C.: Government Printing Office, 1969.

National Center for Health Statistics. *Annotated Bibliography on Vital and Health Statistics* (PHS Publication no. 2094). Washington, D.C.: Government Printing Office, 1970a.

National Center for Health Statistics. *The Health of Children–1970* (PHS Publication no. 2121). Washington, D.C.: Government Printing Office, 1970b.

National Center for Health Statistics. *Health Resource Statistics: Health Manpower and Health Facilities* (PHS Publication no. 1509). Washington, D.C.: Government Printing Office, 1970c.

Norman, J. C. (ed.). *Medicine in the Ghetto.* New York: Appleton, Century, Crofts, 1969.

Parker, S., and Kleiner, R. J. "The Culture of Poverty: An Adjustive Dimension." *American Anthropologist* 72 (1970): 516-27.

Rosenstock, I. "Prevention of Illness and Maintenance of Health." *Poverty and Health: A Sociological Analysis,* edited by J. Kosa, A. Antonovsky, and I. Zola. Cambridge, Mass.: Harvard University Press, 1969.

Scott, R. B. "Health Care Priority and Sickle Cell Anemia." *Journal of the American Medical Association* 214 (1970): 731-34.

Shapiro, S. "End Result Measurements of Quality Medical Care." *Milbank Memorial Fund Quarterly* 45 (1967): 7-30.

Shapiro, S., et al. "Patterns of Medical Use by the Indigent Aged Under Two Systems of Medical Care." *American Journal of Public Health* 57 (1967): 784-90.

Shapiro, S.; Jacobziner, H.; Densen, P. M.; and Weiner, L. "Further Observations on Prematurity and Perinatal Mortality in a General Population and in the Population of a Prepaid Group Practice Medical Care Plan." *American Journal of Public Health* 50 (1960): 1304-17.

Shapiro, S.; Schlesinger, E.; and Nesbitt, R. L., Jr. *Infant, Perinatal, and Childhood Mortality in the United States.* Cambridge, Mass.: Harvard University Press, 1968.

Shapiro, S.; Weiner, L.; and Densen, P. M. "Comparison of Prematurity and Perinatal Mortality in a General Population and in the Population of a Prepaid Group Practice Medical Care Plan." *American Journal of Public Health* 48 (1958): 170-87.

Simmons, O. G. "Social Status and Public Health." Social Science Research Council Pamphlet no. 13.

Stevens, R. "Trends in Medical Specialization in the United States." *Inquiry* 8 (1971): 9-19.

Strauss, A. "Medical Organization, Medical Care, and Lower Income Groups." *Social Science and Medicine* 3 (1969): 143-77.

Sudnow, D. *Passing On: The Social Organization of Dying.* Englewood Cliffs, N.J.: Prentice-Hall, 1967.

10

Disease Prevention and Health Education

Selection by Roger M. Battistella

The purpose of this paper is to clarify the issues, evaluate the arguments, and identify potential value conflicts in the area of disease prevention and health education. A perspective is provided for the shift in health policy from illness treatment to health promotion, and the prospects for short- and long-term results are assessed. Because individual behavior change is put forward increasingly as a way to reduce health expenditures, particular emphasis is given to the potential of health education.

POLICY BACKDROP

The attention given to disease prevention and health promotion at the level of national policy during the past several years represents a reaffirmation of public health teaching so unexpected as to surprise even the most steadfast critics of postwar governmental priorities. Until recently, resources were concentrated onesidedly on the development of services for the treatment of acute-episodic illness, while providing only token sums for programs aimed at health promotion and other health needs. The aura surrounding the sudden rise in the status of preventive medicine approaches glamorous dimensions and is a marked contrast to the marginal role and dubious respectability it has commanded throughout the postwar period. The reasons for this turnabout no doubt are

This selection, "Individual Responsibility for Disease Prevention and Health Maintenance: Potential for Productive Interventions," was prepared especially for this volume.

many and complex. The timing suggests, however, the influence of economics and a growing awareness of the scarcity of health resources.

Exigencies of Cost Containment

The upsurge of interest in disease prevention and health education coincides with the reaction against the cost of health services observable in many recent health policy documents published by the government and other sources (see, for example, U.S. Department of Health, Education, and Welfare, 1976a; Council on Wage and Price Stability, 1976a; National Leadership Conference, 1977; Schultze, 1976, pp. 323-69). Together with provoking questions of how much of the national wealth should go to other uses, the size of the health sector, both in relation to the general economy and the federal budget, causes policy makers to ponder whether the results are worthwhile and to search for less costly alternatives.

Unless present rates of increase are arrested, it has been estimated that health services may account for as much as 12 percent of the Gross National Product by 1990 (contrasted with 8.6 percent in 1976). Due to a sharp rise in expectations of what government should provide for its citizens, the role of the public sector in the financing of health services has doubled since 1966 and it is under considerable pressure to provide more than its present two-fifths share of total spending. The trend within the public sector, moreover, is toward greater reliance on the federal government. Its share of public spending jumped from 3 percent to one-third between 1966 and 1976, and it now allocates 12 percent of its budget for health care. (These data on health care expenditures and the dilemmas posed for government may be found in U.S. Congressional Budget Office, 1977.)

The stagnation of economic growth, in conjunction with unusually high rates of inflation and the political unpopularity of tax increases, deepens whatever interest government officials and politicians have in economy and efficiency. The knowledge that over half of the increased spending for health care since 1950 can be attributed to price increases must be disturbing both to policy makers who care primarily about economy, and to those who endorse additional spending in the belief that it will lead directly to improvements in the quantity and quality of services. The uncontrollable growth of expenditures in Medicare and Medicaid surely adds to the consternation of believers in the value of spending more for health care. The high rates of increase handicap the efforts of government to maintain or start other costly health programs during a period of resource scarcity and rising public expectations. The annual rate of increase for Medicare and Medicaid is roughly double the amount of money spent on all other federal health programs combined.

The concern aroused within government by the cost problem approaches panic proportions. This is evident in the multiple and contradictory solutions now being followed. The gross disparities, ranging from the restoration of market competition to regulation and planning and the imposition of wage and price controls, communicate elements of desperation and chaos in health policy. (The range of responses is illustrated in U.S. Congressional Budget Office, 1977, pp. 31-60; Kinzer, 1977.)

Disillusionment with Curative Services

Hospitals generally are singled out as a major reason for the cost explosion, since they have grown in the postwar period to become the biggest and most inflationary component of the personal health care economy. About 40 percent of the money spent goes to hospitals today, compared with 25 percent in 1940, and the annual rate of increase in cost per patient day since 1965 has doubled over what it was in the preceding fifteen years (U.S. Congressional Budget Office, 1977, pp. 19-20).

Evidence that as much as one-half of the inflation in total health costs can be attributed to a combination of unnecessary overlap and duplication of hospital services, the spread of technologies whose worth has not been proven to be cost-effective or efficacious (e.g., coronary care units, cardiac bypass surgery, anticoagulant therapy), and the performance of a large volume of unnecessary and often harmful medical and surgical procedures, engenders a backlash against both hospitals and medicine in general. Consciousness of the limitations of modern medicine is made more intense by the broadening sentiment among policy makers that spending for acute-episodic illness treatment services has reached the point of diminishing returns due to the aging of the population and growth in importance of chronic-degenerative illness for which medicine cannot affect a cure. (Related data on the economics of hospital care and the dilemmas posed by changes in population structure and illness-treatment technologies may be found in U.S. Department of Health, Education, and Welfare, 1976b; see also Fuchs, 1974, pp. 79-104.) Faith in the efficacy of curative medicine is weakened further by critics who hold that life expectancy and health status are influenced less by health services than by nutrition, housing, education, environmental quality, and other factors determining living standards (see, for example, Carlson, 1975; Powles, 1973; McKeown, 1976).

Recognition of Role of Individual Choice

Ambiguity about the value of modern medicine is compounded by the parallel recognition that many of today's most important health problems are either self-induced due to the pursuit of hazardous life styles, or the result of congenital defects which could be prevented through better prenatal care, genetic counseling, family planning, and abortions. (A convenient summary of the importance of life style may be found in Knowles, 1977.) The antimedicine swing of the pendulum is not without irony. Medicine often is victimized by its successes in extending the survival of persons born with serious congenital defects (e.g., mongolism, spina bifuda) and elderly persons with serious illness. The cost of necessary supportive health and social services is now perceived to be a sizable burden, precipitating additional questions about the quality of survival and the cost-efficiency of illness treatment (on this point, see, for example, Gruenberg, 1977).

POLITICS OF DISEASE PREVENTION
AND HEALTH EDUCATION

The difficulty of having to match scarce resources with inflationary demands for health services spending predisposes policy makers to accept at face value solutions which promise to control expenditures, particularly if they do not appear to diminish the government's commitment to health services enjoying strong public support. The underlying motivations vary. For some decision makers the objective may be to reduce spending for popular but questionable illness treatment programs in order to free money for less popular but important treatment and preventive services. Others (e.g., nonbelievers in the value of modern medicine and ideological opponents of government support of health services apart from communicable disease control) may see an opportunity to save money and reduce the role of government by shifting responsibility back to individuals and families, where it was prior to the acceptance in the mid-sixties of the idea that health care is a right.

Regardless of the intentions, the pressures impinging on policy makers contribute to a climate in which it becomes expedient to blame the victims. Any reprehension for doing so is lessened by the fashionableness of assertions debunking the value of scientific medicine. Thus, while death rates have been dropping noticeably since 1970 following a fifteen-year lull, the reasons most commonly mentioned are nonmedical in nature, e.g., the lowering of speed limits for automobiles necessitated by fuel shortages; lowered tar and nicotine levels in popular cigarette brands; keener public consciousness of the benefits of regular exercise and other preventive health habits; and the legalization of abortion, the decline in the birth rate, and increased family planning (see, for example, Kristen, Arnold, and Wynder, 1977; Knowles, 1977).

Additional, if not more persuasive, justification for "victim blaming" stems from the extensive publicity given to a recently completed study which suggests that the single most effective and inexpensive way to improve life expectancy and health status involves getting individuals to practice some old-fashioned commonsense rules for good living (i.e., three meals daily at regular times and no snacking, moderate exercise two or three times a week, seven to eight hours of sleep a night, no smoking, moderate weight, and moderate use of alcohol). Adherence to these rules presumably would add from seven to eleven years to life expectancy. And the health status of elderly persons following all the rules would be equivalent to that of persons thirty years younger flaunting them (Belloc and Breslow, 1972). That the study is widely cited as definitive, notwithstanding the need for more carefully controlled long-term evaluations, underscores the element of expediency in health policy today. For practical but different reasons, to be elaborated below, both the government and the American Public Health Association have found it hard to resist the temptation to trumpet the study as the "second coming of public health."

Whatever benefits are possible from preventive medicine, the indications are that they can be achieved more effectively by changing social institutions rather than individual behavior. The realities suggest, however, that the latter approach will predominate initially, if for no other reason than the magnitude of the political and economic impediments to institutional reform.

Tradeoffs

The practical appeal of having individuals assume greater responsibility for health is hard to resist. Among other things, it can help to buy the time necessary for the incremental removal of obstacles to change in environmental areas. A health education strategy reduces the demands on government to instigate and sustain costly and controversial confrontations with powerful vested interests, in both the public and private sectors, for whom the manufacture of illness and disability often is an unintended or unavoidable byproduct of other objectives. Apart from the ability of such interests to influence elections and the actions of elected and appointed officials, the choices frequently are unattractive to both government and citizens.

There is no gainsaying that the scope of regulatory power to intervene in the environment has grown sizably in recent years for the purpose of providing a safer working and living climate for the population. Examples of recent legislation include the Occupational Safety and Health Act of 1970, the Consumer Product Safety Act of 1972, and the Safe Water Act of 1974, as well as other new controls for dealing with tobacco hazards, air quality, pesticides, solid waste disposal, lead-based paint poisoning, and others. But the predicament of having to choose between jobs and health promotion during times of high unemployment invariably dampens enthusiasm for the strong enforcement of existing programs and contributes to delays in the enactment of tougher controls. (For an elaboration of this point, see Somers and Somers, 1977, pp. 15-20.)

The choice is even more difficult for individuals living at the margin, especially those with family responsibilities. The choices are not always clear cut. Deference to economic priorities is made easier in instances where the effects of exposure to harmful environmental and occupational pollutants often do not become visible for as long as twenty to thirty years, thereby compounding the difficulty of pinpointing cause-and-effect relationships.

Direct conflicts of interest are an additional complication. The dependence of government on taxes intended originally to discourage harmful practices such as smoking and alcohol provides an example. The pragmatic rationale to circumvent opposition to direct taxation precludes the abandonment of taxes on "sinful activities" even when they have been shown to be unsuccessful in deterring consumption. The political ease with which such revenues can be raised causes some nationally respected health authorities to propose that taxes on harmful forms of consumption be expanded and earmarked to support research in health education and disease prevention (see, for example, Knowles, 1977, p. 78).

The confluence of interests among the private sector, government, and the public portends a cautious and unsteady approach to environmental controls and institutional reform. Unsurprisingly, in this context, the Congress has been debating for eight years the need for compulsory passive restraints in the manufacture of automobiles, despite evidence that fewer than 20 percent of drivers fasten their seatbelts (Holsendolph, 1977). The federal government has also been moving slowly in the field of occupational health, despite evidence that fewer than 5 percent of the places where people work have adequate safety and prevention programs and that nearly one million workers are being exposed to carcinogenic substances (Burnham, 1977a). Similarly, the government has moved slowly to implement mandates enacted in 1962 to eliminate the manufacture and sale of nonefficacious pharmaceuticals. It has delayed attempts to tighten and modernize drug safety requirements, notwithstanding estimates that as many as six million persons suffer adverse reactions each year. Prescription sales are big business—estimated at $7 billion in 1976. Doctors now write 1.5 billion prescriptions yearly, or an average of 5.7 per capita, in contrast to the situation in 1968 when only 820 million prescriptions were written. The drug industry is said to spend roughly $4,000 annually for each practicing physician to promote new products and to encourage the writing of more prescriptions (Burnham, 1977b).

Unclear Mandate for Intervention

The efforts of government to promote health are constrained further by the lack of a clear and coherent policy in the environmental area. Not only is competition for jurisdiction with state government often a problem, but federal policies frequently suffer inconsistencies which undermine public confidence and credibility. For example, the federal government bans the introduction of carcinogens in foods while allowing their introduction into air and water supplies. Tobacco smoking is discouraged by required package warnings and mass media announcements, while other agencies of government provide subsidies and other assistance to tobacco growers and manufacturers. And, while proclaiming the significance of disease prevention on the one hand, the government prohibits reimbursement for preventive care by Medicare on the other. (These inconsistencies are described in more detail in National Institutes of Health and the American College of Preventive Medicine, 1976, pp. 22-24.)

Unlike many other highly developed countries where political power is more highly centralized, the United States system of checks and balances fragments and diffuses responsibility. This not only impedes the formation of consensus essential for effective policy and program implementation, but inclines decision makers to opt for strategies aimed at changing individual behavior rather than social institutions. The bias intrinsic to the structure of political power is reinforced by traditional American values exalting the individual and freedom of choice to engage in any behavior that does not directly affect the safety and well-being of others.

Political ideology and the fragmentation of power help to explain why the federal government has been either unable or unwilling to adopt controls limiting the processing and sale of foods containing unacceptably high levels of harmful elements, such as sugars and animal fats. Despite indications that diet is the key to atherosclerotic processes accounting for nearly one-half of all deaths annually, the government continues to stress changes in individual behavior, rather than changes in food manufacturing. (For a highly informed and concise presentation of the issues and choices, see Winikoff, 1977.) The political constraints also help to explain the nonexistence of an effective national immunization program and why immunization levels among American children are among the lowest in the developed world. The question of why vigorous measures have not been taken to control the annual carnage on highways attributed to drunken drivers is also better understood in this light. (For a convenient overview of these and related preventable causes of disability and death, see Lazarus, Schorr, and Weitz, 1977, pp. 85-97; Holtzman, 1977, pp. 107-32.)

Cost-Effectiveness of Early Disease Detection and Treatment

The swing in recent years from faith to uncertainty and disbelief in the value of early disease detection and illness treatment (i.e., secondary prevention) is another reason to expect that individual behavior change will bear the brunt of the disease prevention campaign. Not only are most forms of screening for chronic-degenerative diseases, which are today's major health problems, considered questionable in cost-effectiveness terms, but many are now recognized to be harmful because of unwarranted exposure to radiation and unnecessary medical and surgical treatment tied to errors in diagnosis (The following references are illustrative of the declining belief in the value of early diagnosis and treatment: Kristen and Wynder, 1977; Bergman, 1977; Greenberg and Randal, 1977; Holland, 1975; Rushmer, 1975, pp. 61-65.) This criticism is not to be confused, however, with screening in prenatal care, in infancy and childhood, and for infectious disease which has been demonstrated to be effective. (For a balanced and competent assessment of the value of screening for acute infectious and chronic-degenerative forms of illness, see European Public Health Committee, 1974.)

It is a distressing manifestation of the unclear mandate for disease prevention that present programs for immunization and early detection for disease and disability among infants and children are so poorly developed in the United States. The shambled state of affairs surrounding the unsuccessful attempts to implement fully periodic screening for early diagnosis and treatment among low-income children provides stark testimony for this conclusion (Foltz, 1973).

Simultaneously with the decline of confidence in the value of secondary prevention for chronic illness, resistance to consumer use charges is softening. In contrast to the long-prevailing assertion in health education about the undesirability of barriers to early diagnosis and treatment, deductibles and coinsurance are put forward increasingly as a practical way to contain costs by discouraging "frivolous" utilization. Because the effects of treatment delays have not been studied sufficiently in patient outcome terms, fashion exercises a large influence on policy. More information is required about the interplay between out-of-pocket charges and income in decisions to initiate medical care for specific symptoms and complaints if cost-benefit assessments of early diagnosis and treatment are to be a responsible and worthwhile aid to decision making. Over long periods of time the costs of undue delay and self-medication may outweigh considerably any short-term savings. Intelligent policy requires closer study of the tradeoff between early initiation and delay. (Additional discussion of this point may be found in Office of Health Economics, 1974, pp. 33-35.)

Coalition for Individual Responsibility for Health Care

The elements of expediency and opportunism behind the revival of health education is not restricted to government alone. The prevailing policy climate makes for strange bedfellows. Business and industry surely grasp the advantages of encouraging greater employee responsibility in contrast to programs aimed at changing the work environment. Furthermore, the large contribution of payroll taxes to the financing of personal health services induces the private sector to support low-cost solutions to the problem of rising costs. (This conclusion derives from such recent publications as Washington Business Group on Health, 1977; Council on Wage and Price Stability, 1976b.) High-technology interests (e.g., hospitals, medical schools, and the medical research community), put on the defensive by the drive in government for cost containment, are understandably drawn to health education for the opportunity it provides for diffusing criticism for cost increases, while maintaining a political environment favorable to high-technology spending. (A review of recent actions taken by high-technology interests may be found in National Institutes of Health and the American College of Preventive Medicine, 1976, pp. 14-16.) Blue Cross' sponsorship of full-page ads in national magazines, such as *Time,* which chastise the "workoholic" male as an antisocial contributor to family disorganization and the hospital cost problem, advances the theme in an especially clever way. Radicals critical of the contribution of medicine to dependency and social control in advanced industrial societies look at health education as a liberating device for restoring autonomy to individuals and families (see, for example, Illich, 1976; a more balanced perspective is provided by Fox, 1977). And teachers of preventive medicine, long frustrated by the limited resources available to them in medical schools and by the gap in American medicine between prevention and treatment services in primary care, have not been slow to grasp the opportunity to change things in support of their viewpoint (see, for example, National Institutes of Health and the American College of Preventive Medicine, 1976).

The opportunistic temptations will be especially difficult for the public health community to ignore. Demoralized by the extensive reassignment of responsibilities for environmental control, policy, planning, and regulation to other agencies, and by the diminution of status and power it has experienced in recent decades, public health is poised for a comeback. Health education offers the chance to recapture some of its earlier status stemming from turn-of-the-century successes in communicable disease control and maternal and child health. (The scope and depth of interest in the revival of health education is manifest in the abstracts of the American Public Health Association, 1977a.) In spite of the magnitude of more recent successes against poliomyletis, rubella, and measles, public health has lost much of its momentum and become a backwater to mainstream developments in high-technology medicine.

Health Education Legislation

The National Consumer Health Information and Health Practices Act of 1976 (Title I of PL 94-317) was enacted to meet the growing concern about spending and the effect of health services on health status. Based on a working definition of health education as a process for closing the gap between information and practice and for motivating changes in behavior destructive to health maintenance, the legislation gives the Secretary of Health, Education, and Welfare broad powers to formulate national goals and strategies for health information, health promotion, preventive health services, and education on the appropriate use of health care. The emphasis assigned to individual responsibility for disease prevention and for the treatment of routine illness not requiring the attention of a physician is a conspicuous feature of the mandate, suggesting a major preoccupation with cost containment and economy. (These aims reinforce the priority for health education provided in the National Health Planning and Resources Development Act of 1974 (PL 93-641). For a convenient summary, see U.S. Department of Health, Education, and Welfare, 1977, pp. vi-vii.)

CAN HEALTH EDUCATION DELIVER?

The rhetoric of government officials proclaiming the strategic significance of prevention is grossly disproportionate to the money available. Spending for disease prevention and health education represents 3 percent or less of total health outlays (2 to 2.5 percent for prevention and control measures, and 0.5 percent for health education; see Knowles, 1977, p. 65). Federal budget allocations for health education increased from one-quarter of one percent in 1973 to 2 percent in 1977 and outlays for disease prevention and control are said to equal about 3 percent of the budget (Executive Office of the President, 1977, p.

202). These amounts remain far short of the 5 to 10 percent of total public and private spending which health education advocates claim is necessary for an effective national campaign (*Health Promotion and Consumer Health Education,* p. 58). The prospects for capturing a larger share of the budgetary pie are not good. During a period of limited growth and stable budgets it can only be done by taking money away from more glamorous and better-established competing programs. Over 70 percent of the money spent for personal health services in the U.S. is for treatment after the occurrence of illness; and over half of what remains is funneled into biomedical research aimed at getting a technological fix on illness. In a period of scarce resources, professional elan and ethics may be seen as a convenient substitute for money. Indeed, these values, belittled in recent years as the relics of outdated romanticism within the professions, are now seen to possess some practical utility. Government officials speaking at the 1977 meeting of the American Public Health Association exhorted public health professionals to show what they could do in the field of health education with existing resources and little promise of future help. The message throughout was that a rededication to service ideals would compensate for material shortages.

Another basic problem with health education stems from the omnibus way it is employed in practice to cover multiple and widely different objectives, for example: (1) inform people about health, illness, and disability and the ways they can improve and protect their own health, including more efficient use of the delivery system; (2) motivate people to want to change to more healthful practices; (3) help individuals to learn the necessary skills to adopt and maintain healthful practices and life styles; (4) foster teaching and communication skills in all those engaged in educating consumers about health; (5) advocate changes in the environment that will facilitate healthful conditions and healthful behavior; and (6) add to knowledge through research and evaluation concerning the most effective ways of achieving these objectives (see, for example, U.S. Department of Health, Education, and Welfare, 1973, pp. 17-22).

If "health education" is not to be misused as a code phase for "cost containment and resource reallocation," greater precision is necessary. To succeed, health education needs, at the minimum, to be target-specific in application and programs should provide for systematic evaluation of cost-effectiveness. This will not be easy to accomplish, however, for reasons including ethical restrictions on the use of human subjects in health experiments, the requirements for longitudinal studies to establish the permanency of results, the absence of adequate data systems, and the controversy among policy makers over the importance of monetary and health benefits associated with spending for various programs (see Green, 1977).

Efficiency of Health Education

It augurs poorly that health education is a field which does not inspire confidence. Unflattering stereotypes abound (e.g., dispensers of hackneyed advice, well-intentioned but poorly equipped do-gooders), and they have made it difficult for health education to attract its fair share of talented young men and women. The situation may be improving with the redirection of public policy from illness treatment to disease prevention and health maintenance. Membership in the health education section, one of the many occupation sections composing the American Public Health Association, is currently said to be one of the most rapidly growing (American Public Health Association, 1977b). On the other hand, health education positions continue to be among the first eliminated in elementary and secondary school cutbacks, apparently on the assumption that they accomplish little good. The impoverished state of health education models and the paucity of evidence demonstrating the cost-effectiveness of attempts to inculcate good health practices and eliminate harmful life styles lends justification to the criticism.

The most highly visible work in the construction of health education models remains pegged to getting individuals to seek early disease detection and treatment, despite mounting medical skepticism about the benefits of such an approach for dealing with the disease priorities of a highly developed society, which are largely chronic and multifactorial in nature. Another frequently overlooked problem is that the models have not moved much beyond the theoretically interesting stage. For example, the health belief model is often singled out by behavioral scientists working in the health education area as having the greatest potential for influencing and predicting disease prevention behavior when, in fact, it is associated only modestly with how individuals actually behave. The range of successful predictions is from 10 to 20 percent (Kasl, 1974, pp. 106-27; see also Battistella, 1968).

Attempts to improve compliance with medical orders following the onset of treatment for serious illnesses like heart disease, hypertension, and diabetes are also in the rudimentary stage (see, for example, Dollery et al., 1976, pp. 37-47). Data thus far indicate that compliance remains a problem which intensifies with the length and complexity of treatment. Compliance with medical orders ostensibly is a serious problem even when relatively simple behaviors are involved, such as the taking of medication according to prescription (Kasl, 1974, pp. 113-14). Noncompliance is complicated whenever unpleasant side effects are common. In the case of the clinical management of hypertension, they may include drowsiness and dizziness. These side effects, in turn, are known to contribute to serious automobile accidents and other mishaps. The risk of impotence encountered by adult males can be an especially discouraging obstacle to compliance. (For a description of the side effects of treatment, see, for example, Peart, 1978, pp. 981-82; American Medical Association, 1977, pp. 52-75; Laragh, 1973, pp. 901-09.) While mortality due to hypertension has dropped significantly in recent years, it remains to be proven whether this is due to improvements in detection and treatment or some other factor, such as lowered salt intake in daily diets (see Freymann, 1974, pp. 72-73). The efficacy of the clinical treatment of hypertension has been challenged by Cochrane (1976, p. 261) on the grounds that the evidence is unreliable.

Getting individuals to change enjoyable but harmful behavior is even more difficult when physical or psychological addictions are involved. In the case of cigarette smoking, for example, three-fifths of all smokers report that they have tried to stop one or more times and almost one-third say that a doctor has told them to give up the habit (U.S. Department of Health, Education, and Welfare, 1976a, p. 14).

Despite the many problems involved, interest in voluntary behavior change remains strong. This may reflect the unattractiveness of other solutions. Knowledge of the unsuccessful attempts to legislate behavior (e.g., alcohol and drug abuse, sexual promiscuity and venereal disease) inveighs against the use of legal prohibitions; and the use of involuntary techniques and procedures (such as psychosurgery, electroconvulsive therapy, and chemotherapy) continue to be morally condemned as evils greater than the disease.

Behavior Modification

The meager capabilities for changing life styles are obfuscated by the promotion of behavior modification techniques. They possess a higher status than other health education methods—presumably because they derive from the field of experimental psychology, which has a more powerful scientific image than the sociological and media-oriented methods of health education falling outside the stereotype of carefully controlled laboratory studies. The enthusiasm is in no small part a derivative of the utopian visions sparked by research in operant conditioning led by B. F. Skinner. (On the origins of behavior modification and influence of Skinnerian theory, see Simonds, 1976, pp. 105-08; Bass, 1976, pp. 127-31.)

Behavior modification encompasses a cluster of techniques, including (1) positive reinforcement through use of token economies and modeling; (2) aversion controls incorporating electric shock, social isolation, drugs inducing vertigo and nausea; (3) overcorrection, a method combining positive reinforcement and aversion controls; (4) systematic desensitization, a procedure of gradual progressive exposure to feared situations and assertiveness training designed to overcome diffidence through combinations of the above techniques (U.S. Department of Health, Education, and Welfare, 1975, pp. 1-9).

The simplistic notion inherent in behavior modification inhibits an adequate appreciation of the complexity of behavior and the role of genetics, free will, emulation, and other factors. The magnitude of what is unknown about behavior, and the practical and ethical constraints in research involving human subjects, contribute to the anarchy evident in the array of diagnostic and treatment practices followed in programs seeking to alter behavior, whether for purposes of improved interpersonal relations in which participation is voluntary, or the forced rehabilitation of the mentally ill and legal offenders. The diversity can range from the bizarre (e.g., sensitivity and assertiveness therapies in which individuals may be clothed or unclothed, touch or shout at one another in a variety of unconventional settings, including verdant fields, unlit rooms, and swimming pools) to conventional applications of group dyanmics theory involving peer pressures and chemotherapy. (For further information on limitations in the diagnosis and treatment of behavioral problems, see Torrey, 1974; Rosenham, 1974, pp. 267-86.) Generally speaking, success rates are low, even for aggressively interventionists programs involving aversion chemotherapies like methadone and antabuse for heroin and alcohol abuse respectively, and for highly structured therapeutic communities for the treatment of drug abuse and juvenile delinquency. (For a critical evaluation of the shortcomings of aggressive chemotherapy methods, see Etzioni and Remp, 1973.)

When all is said and done, understanding of human motivation is limited and it remains a mystery for the most part (see Coffer and Appley, 1967, pp. 808-38). Since most self-induced illnesses commonly mentioned in discussions of the potential of behavior modification involve risky life styles which bring pleasure to individuals, it is unlikely that much will be done about problems associated with obesity, alcohol and drug abuse, unsafe motor vehicle driving practices, etc. Behaviors of this sort are more easily turned on than off. Even in cases where motivation can be presumed to be highly favorable, such as in the use of preventive health services either prior to or following the onset of symptoms, participation rates are meager. Among high-risk groups the voluntary use of preventive health services is disappointingly low in immunization programs (polio, rubella, diphtheria, typhoid, and pertussis) and in programs for the early detection of serious conditions like glaucoma, cancer, and cardiovascular disorders (U.S. Department of Health, Education, and Welfare, 1976c, pp. 272-85).

While improvement in the identification of populations at risk on a disease-specific basis and the targeting of treatment among individuals who are properly motivated can generate efficiency in efforts to change behavior, the efficacy of alternate forms of treatment need to be better demonstrated in cost-efficiency terms. Equally important, calculations of cost must be extended whenever the probability of recidivism is high following successful initial treatment, such as with smoking, alcohol and drug abuse, and obesity, where the physiological and psychological factors involved can be very complex. The costs of follow-up may prove prohibitive. Depending on the mix of professional and nonprofessional staff, choice of accounting method for the assignment of overheads, the number, length, and intensity of patient visits necessary, transportation costs, etc., the amount required could run anywhere from several hundred to a thousand dollars or more. On balance, however, the state-of-the-art of behavior-change techniques is so low that proponents of responsible spending may regard it as a good thing that government spending for health education and behavior modification remains minuscule.

The limited capabilities of health education and behavior modification are underscored by the propensity of those who wish to influence life styles to look to commercial marketing and advertising for leadership. The assumption is that the same skills so successful in the inculcation of harmful life styles can, with the proper incentives, be turned around to proselytize good health behavior. Whether inspired by doctrinaire belief in the superior efficiency of business, disingenuousness, or wishful thinking, clarion calls cannot substitute for the gaps in fundamental knowledge about motivation. The problem centers on how to get people to stop doing many of the things they enjoy doing which are bad for their health. Except for the occasional zealot, health more often than not is valued less as an end than as an instrumentality for the pursuit of other life goals, including pleasurable, but potentially harmful, activities. Advertising campaigns which seem successful on the surface, such as the no-cholesterol ads, have yet to be proven in cause-and-effect terms. On the amount of research done to determine advertising effectiveness it has been said: "I doubt that there is any function in industry where management bases so much expenditure on such scanty knowledge . . . probably no more than one-fifth of 1 percent of total advertising expenditure is used to achieve an enduring understanding of how to spend the other 99.8 percent" (Forrester, 1959). And for every example of positive advertising, there remains the question of what to do about the countless ads which encourage and condone harmful life styles. Ranked among the highest absolute spenders for advertising are firms pushing drugs, automobiles, food, and tobacco. Drugs and cosmetics, gum and candy, together with soaps, are the highest spenders relative to percentage of sales (as reported in Kotler, 1976, p. 347).

The report of the National Institutes of Health and the American College of Preventive Medicine (1976, pp. 38-44, 119-27) displayed ambivalence about the role of commercial advertising and television, ranging from moral condemnation of the social irresponsibility and duplicity practiced by the industry to abject awe of its enormous power for benevolent indoctrination. Unlike the situation in health education, there is no professional service ethic among commercial advertisers to restrain them from manipulating and exploiting human wants and values. Too often *caveat emptor* is the overarching principle and profit maximization is the overriding goal.

The enormity of the task of combatting harmful behaviors promoted by commercial advertisers is disclosed partially in the results to date of government-sponsored warnings against smoking and drinking. While there has been, over the past decade, a 25 percent decline in cigarette smokers among adult males, almost two-fifths continue to smoke and the proportion of smokers among adult women has remained unaffected for the most part. What is far more discouraging is that cigarette smoking among teenagers generally has not declined. In fact, smoking among young women is on the increase. The situation with respect to alcohol is also disappointing. Approximately two-fifths of adult males and about one-half as many adult females are classified as moderate to heavy drinkers, and consumption levels for the population as a whole are rising steadily (U.S. Department of Health, Education, and Welfare, 1976a, p. 14).

Political and Moral Ramifications

Future improvements in health behavior will be slow going; they require massive changes in the range, intensity, and consistency of social controls, whether the goal is to keep individuals from falling into bad habits or to discard established harmful life styles. The feedback and reinforcement received from family, friends, and doctors must be made more consistent for individuals struggling with decisions to seek preventive care or to comply with medical advice (Kasl, 1974, pp. 120-21). The widely varying perceptions and attitudes toward health and illness behavior rooted in sociocultural differences complicates matters additionally. The profound difficulty in all this appears more clearly when one ponders the political ramifications of any attempts by government to curb detrimental private sector advertising which promotes—behind the escutcheon of free enterprise—harmful foods, medications, and behaviors. One can expect that such efforts will be strongly resisted by business as overly repressive and totalitarian.

Fear of controls includes the possible misuse of behavior modification methods among involuntary subjects. Indeed, behavior modification has been employed widely among institutionalized populations and the scale of civil rights abuse has been recorded in hearings conducted by the United States Senate (U.S. Senate, 1974).

The testimony of proponents that behavior modification practitioners would work mainly with clients in planning therapeutic goals and procedures is not very reassuring. The language is deceptively soothing. If clients possess, in principle, more autonomy than conventional patients who have, by definition, relinquished sovereignty to professionals, the significance of the distinction may still be academic—especially during times when thresholds for deviancy and idiosyncracy may diminish because of the pressures of modern living and public reaction against the high cost of treating self-induced illnesses. Rather than face prison, incarceration in a mental hospital, or the loss of economic and service entilements, drug addicts, drunken drivers, child molesters and spouse beaters may opt for behavior modification therapy, when given a choice. For institutionalized populations like the mentally ill and the mentally retarded, free will and consumer sovereignty seem even more farfetched.

Any attempt to limit behavior in the area of harmful life styles, no matter how carefully justified as a means to minimize treatment cost and lost economic productivity, probably will clash with traditional ideological teachings of individual liberty, in which a person is believed to have a right to do anything, including the risking of life, providing that in so doing the rights of others are not infringed. In this arena, the thrust of health education today represents a politically radical break with orthodox public health teachings, which advocated that intervention be carefully circumscribed to the control of dangerous forms of contagion. Interest among policy makers in lowering expenditures for avoidable illness is understandable, given the growth of the government's responsibility for health financing, but whether public opinion is ready to support a liberalization of the justification for intervention is uncertain. Some measure of the controversy which can spring from the pursuit of disease prevention and health education strategies which fail to take into account the depth of ideological feelings involved is apparent in the pervasive acrimony accompanying proposals to: (1) use public funds for abortions or the sterilization of the mentally retarded and welfare recipients, (2) legalize marijuana and heroin, (3) make the fluoridation of drinking water compulsory, and (4) restrict the rights of smokers in public places.

Moral concerns also encompass the implications of behavior modification for human dignity. Many of the techniques of behavior modification are characterized by a manipulative orientation to interpersonal relations, whereas others feature a simplistic materialistic understanding of behavior debasing to the human spirit.

Finally, the quest for short-term payoffs, when successful, will contribute to and compound undesirable long-term side effects. Any additions to life expectancy during a period of declining or stable birth rates ironically adds to the burden of future generations of workers because of negative contributions to the dependency ratio and strains on retirement systems. Successful disease prevention results in greater spending for health services in the long run, for the reason that more people reach advanced ages where the need for costly health and social support services is greatest. The cost crisis in Medicare, for example, is to a large extent a consequence of turn-of-the-century public health triumphs over smallpox, typhoid, diarrhea, and other childhood diseases, which have made it possible for more persons to reach old age. Thus, while persons sixty-five and over constitute only about one-tenth of the population, they use nearly one-third of all the money spent annually for personal health services. Of the total spent for the aged, hospital care accounts for nearly one-half and nursing home care roughly one-fourth. Almost four-fifths of all public expenditures for the health care of the aged (i.e., Medicare and Medicaid) are for hospital and nursing home care (figures compiled from Social Security Administration, 1977).

SUMMARY AND CONCLUSIONS

While institutional reform is a far more effective strategy for disease prevention, the indications are that it will be subordinated in the foreseeable future to strategies aimed at changing individual behavior. This forecast is based less on the venality and ineptitude of policy makers than on the recognition of the difficulty of the tradeoffs involved. Upon balancing uncertain long-term health benefits with certain short-term economic dislocations, both individuals living at the margin, and government officials concerned about how to raise revenues to support rising demands for publicly financed services, can be expected to want to put off changes interfering with employment and economic growth. Improvements in such key areas as environmental health, occupational health, and food and drugs will depend heavily on the state of the economy. Unless conditions improve unexpectedly, the prospects are that change in these areas will be slow and uneven. Stepping backward often may be a precondition for moving ahead.

Along with being more acceptable politically than measures compelling large-scale social change, efforts to influence behavior possess great expediency for diffusing blame for the alarmingly high rates of increase in health care expenditures from government, hospitals, and doctors. Insofar as illness is self-induced and health status can be affected by life style choices, individuals also are partly to blame.

The panic in government over the cost of illness treatment services inclines decision makers to magnify the potential savings from disease prevention and health education. Health education provides an expedient opportunity to arrest dependence on public financing by getting individuals and families to assume a larger share of responsibility for disease prevention, health maintenance, and the treatment of routine, uncomplicated illness.

There is an assumption at the core of the health education strategy that individuals can be taught almost anything at little cost or effort. Knowledge available in the behavioral sciences suggests, however, that this is wishful thinking, since understanding of human motivation remains slight. No amount of effort to invoke the vaunted powers of commercial advertising or the scientific trappings of behavior modification can substitute for this gap in knowledge. Nor is it a problem which can be overcome simply through the spending of more money in the training of more professionals in health education.

Until individuals themselves admit to having a problem and seek actively to correct it, the prospects are poor that much progress can be made in the elimination of harmful life styles which are a source of pleasure to individuals. The prospects are bleaker still when mental and physical forms of dependence are involved. Given the nature of illness today and its relationship to old age, it is unlikely that research and new technologies for illness treatment can provide a solution. This is not to claim that behavior is immutable. Individuals can and do change for reasons which may include life cycle variations in biology and social role demands, personal interests, or peer pressures, as well as the influence of fashions and other cultural phenomena. The point is that techniques for programming behavior are primitive and the possibilities for control and fine tuning remain visionary. Along with the issues of effectiveness, available techniques have not been properly evaluated in cost-efficiency terms and they raise, moreover, some very troublesome ethical concerns.

The social control aspects of behavior modification and other measures for disease prevention conflict sharply with traditional values of individual choice in a free society and pose grave ethical questions regarding the use of techniques debasing to humanistic concepts of man. To the extent that gradual changes in social institutions occur which do improve life expectancy, the effect ironically may be to exacerbate moral issues involving the sustaining of life through the use of costly medical technologies and social supports for population groups which do not contribute to the economy.

If there is a useful role for health education in all this, it centers on the challenge and opportunity to inform policy makers about the limitations of life style solutions to health care costs and disease prevention, and to alert the public to the way in which social institutions contribute to unnecessary illness, disability, and premature death. Such information is a vital underpinning to the intelligent calculation and choice of tradeoffs. Consistent with these purposes, the dissemination of information to individuals about the risks associated with life style choices within their personal control will remain an important function.

If the dilemmas of health policy can be expected in the years ahead to strain the integrity of government, the demands will also be heavy on public health to provide prudent leadership which balances the self-interest of the profession with the interests of individual citizens and families. For both government and public health, the litmus test of their commitment to health promotion will be found in the persistence and depth of political courage displayed at the nexus of political-economic expediency and democratic-humanitarian values.

REFERENCES

American Medical Association. *AMA Drug Evaluations* (3rd ed.). Littleton, Mass.: Publishing Sciences Group, 1977.

American Public Health Association. *Abstracts of the 105th Annual Meeting.* Washington, D.C.: The Association, 1977a.

American Public Health Association. "Membership Soars." *Nation's Health* (October 1977b): 1.

Bass, F. "Behavior Modification: A Review of Basic Concepts and Recent Research." *Promoting Health,* edited by A. R. Somers. Germantown, Md.: Aspen Systems, 1976.

Battistella, R. M. "Limitations in Use of the Concept of Psychological Readiness to Initiate Health Care." *Medical Care* 6 (July/August 1968): 308-19.

Belloc, N. B., and Breslow, L. "The Relation of Physical Health Status and Health Practices." *Preventive Medicine* 1 (August 1972): 409-21.

Bergman, A. B. "The Menace of Health Screening." *American Journal of Public Health* 67 (July 1977): 601.

Burnham, D. "One in Four Americans Exposed to Hazards on Job." *New York Times* (September 28, 1977a): 1.

Burnham, D. "Califano Urged Overhaul of Law on Drug Safety." *New York Times* (October 6, 1977b): 1.

Carlson, R. J. *The End of Medicine.* New York: John Wiley & Sons, 1975.

Cochrane, A. "Some Reflections." *A Question of Quality?,* edited by G. McLachlan. London: Nuffield Provincial Hospitals Trust, 1976.

Coffer, C. N., and Appley, M. H. *Motivation: Theory and Research.* New York: John Wiley & Sons, 1967.

Council on Wage and Price Stability. *The Problem of Rising Health Care Costs.* Washington, D.C.: Executive Office of the President, 1976a.

Council on Wage and Price Stability. *The Complex Puzzle of Rising Health Care Costs: Can the Private Sector Fit It Together?* Washington, D.C.: Executive Office of the President, 1976b.

Dollery, C., et al. "The Care of Patients with Malignant Hypertension in London in 1974-5." *A Question of Quality?,* edited by G. McLachlan. London: Nuffield Provincial Hospitals Trust, 1976.

Etzioni, A., and Remp, R. *Technological Shortcuts to Change.* New York: Russell Sage Foundation, 1973.

European Public Health Committee. *Screening as a Tool of Preventive Medicine.* Strasbourg: Council of Europe, 1974.

Executive Office of the President, Office of Management and Budget. *Special Analyses: Budget of the United States Government, FY 1978.* Washington, D.C.: Government Printing Office, 1977.

Foltz, A. "The Development of Ambiguous Federal Policy: Early and Periodic Screening Diagnosis and Treatment (EPSDT)." *Milbank Memorial Fund Quarterly, Health and Society* 53 (Winter 1973): 35-61.

Forrester, J. W. "Advertising: A Problem in Industrial Dynamics." *Harvard Business Review* 37 (March/April 1959): 102.

Fox, R. C. "The Medicalization and Demedicalization of American Society." *Daedalus* (Winter 1977): 9-22.

Freymann, J. G. *The American Health Care System: Its Genesis and Trajectory.* Baltimore: Williams & Wilkins, 1974.

Fuchs, V. R. *Who Shall Live?* New York: Basic Books, 1974.

Green, L. H. "Evaluation and Measurement: Some Dilemmas for Health Education." *American Journal of Public Health* 67 (February 1977): 155-61.

Greenberg, D., and Randal, J. E. "The Questionable Breast X-Ray Program." *Washington Post* (May 1, 1977): 5-C.

Gruenberg, E. M. "The Failure of Success." *Milbank Memorial Fund Quarterly, Health and Society* 55 (Winter 1977): 3-24.

Holland, W. W. "Prevention: The Only Cure." *Preventive Medicine* 4 (December 1975): 387-88.

Holsendolph, E. "Congress Nears a Final Decision on Auto Safety." *New York Times* (September 29, 1977): A-21.

Holtzman, N. A. "The Goal of Preventing Early Death." *Papers on the National Health Guidelines: Conditions for Change in the Health Care System* (Publication no. 78-642). Washington, D.C.: HEW, 1977.

Illich, I. *Medical Nemesis.* New York: Pantheon, 1976.

Kasl, S. "The Health Belief Model and Behavior Related to Chronic Illness." *The Health Belief Model and Personal Health Behavior,* edited by M. H. Becker. Thorofare, N.J.: Charles B. Slack, 1974.

Kinzer, D. M. *Health Controls Out of Control.* Chicago: Teach 'Em, 1977.

Knowles, J. H. "The Responsibility of the Individual." *Daedalus* (Winter 1977): 57-80.

Kotler, P. *Marketing Management* (3rd ed.) Englewood Cliffs, N.J.: Prentice-Hall, 1976.

Kristen, M. M.; Arnold, C. B.; and Wynder, E. L. "Health Economics and Preventive Care." *Science* 195 (February 4, 1977): 457-60.

Laragh, J. H. (ed.). *Hypertension Manual.* New York: Yorke Medical Books, 1973.

Lazarus, W.; Schorr, L.; and Weitz, J. H. "Reaching Needy Children with Health Care." *Papers on the National Health Guidelines: Conditions for Change in the Health Care System* (Publications no. HRA 78-642). Washington, D.C.: HEW, 1977.

McKeown, T. *The Role of Medicine: Dream, Mirage or Nemesis?* London: Nuffield Provincial Hospitals Trust, 1976.

National Institutes of Health and the American College of Preventive Medicine. *Health Promotion and Consumer Health Education.* New York: Prodist, 1976.

National Leadership Conference. *Controlling Health Care Costs.* Washington, D.C.: National Journal, 1977.

Office of Health Economics. *The Work of Primary Care.* London: The Office, 1974.

Peart, W. S. "Arterial Hypertension." *Textbook of Medicine* (14th ed., vol. 2), edited by P. B. Beeson and W. McDermott. Philadelphia: W. B. Saunders, 1978.

Powles, J. "On the Limitations of Modern Medicine." *Science, Medicine and Man* 1 (April 1973): 1-28.

Rosenham, D. L. "On Being Sane in Insane Places." *Health and the Social Environment,* edited by P. M. Insel and R. H. Moos. Lexington, Mass.: Lexington Books, 1974.

Rushmer, R. F. *Humanizing Health Care.* Cambridge, Mass.: MIT Press, 1975.

Schultze, C. L. "Federal Spending: Past, Present, and Future." *Setting National Priorities,* edited by H. Owen and C. L. Schultze. Washington, D.C.: Brookings Institution, 1976.

Simonds, S. K. "Health Education in the Mid-70's—State of the Art." *Promoting Health,* edited by A. R. Somers. Germantown, Md.: Aspen Systems, 1976.

Social Security Administration, Office of Research and Statistics. "Age Differences in Health Care Spending, Fiscal Year 1976." *Research and Statistics Note* (no. 12). Washington, D.C.: Government Printing Office, 1977.

Somers, A. R., and Somers, H. M. "A New Framework for Health and Health Care Policies." *Papers on the National Health Guidelines: Conditions for Change in the Health Care System* (Publication no. 78-642). Washington, D.C.: HEW, 1977.

Torrey, F. E. *The Death of Psychiatry.* Radnor, Penn.: Chilton, 1974.

U.S. Congressional Budget Office. *Expenditures for Health Care: Federal Programs and Their Effects.* Washington, D.C.: Government Printing Office, 1977.

U.S. Department of Health, Education, and Welfare. *Report of the President's Committee on Health Education.* Washington, D.C.: HEW, 1973.

U.S. Department of Health, Education, and Welfare. National Institute of Mental Health. *Behavior Modification: Perspective on a Current Issue* (Publication no. ADM 75-202). Washington, D.C.: HEW, 1975.

U.S. Department of Health, Education, and Welfare. *Forward Plan for Health, FY 1978-82* (Publication no. OS 76-50046). Washington, D.C.: HEW, 1976a.

U.S. Department of Health, Education, and Welfare. *Trends Affecting U.S. Health Care System* (Publication no. HRA 76-14503). Washington, D.C.: HEW, 1976b.

U.S. Department of Health, Education, and Welfare. *Health: United States, 1975* (Publication no. HRA 76-1232). Washington, D.C.: HEW, 1976c.

U.S. Department of Health, Education, and Welfare. *Papers on the National Health Guidelines, Baselines for Setting Health Goals and Standards* (Publication no. HRA 77-640). Washington, D.C.: HEW, 1977.

U.S. Senate, Committee on the Judiciary. *Individual Rights and the Federal Role in Behavior Modification* (93rd Congress, 2nd session, 1974).

Washington Business Group on Health. *A Private Sector Perspective on the Problems of Health Care Costs.* Working Paper submitted to the Secretary of Health, Education, and Welfare, 1977.

Winikoff, B. "Nutrition and Food Policy: The Approaches of Norway and the United States." *American Journal of Public Health* 67 (June 1977): 552-57.

11

The Future of Primary Health Services

Selection by Roger M. Battistella and Thomas G. Rundall

The emergence of primary care as a topic of national health policy in the United States in the 1970s may not appear particularly significant when taken in isolation. Subject to numerous definitions, primary care generally refers to those fundamentals of medical education and practice long associated with general practice and lower-level medical specialties dealing with the routine complaints and illnesses which cause individuals to seek medical care most of the time (see, for example, Gross, 1974; Parker, 1974; Fink and Owen, 1976; U.S. Department of Health, Education, and Welfare, 1970).

Because of the preoccupation throughout most of this century of medical education with scientific-technological progress and the superior status now accorded to upper-level medical specialties for the treatment of rarely occurring illnesses, the stereotype which primary care summons to mind is that of a hectic, but essentially humdrum, activity removed from the mainstream of professional achievement and innovation (see, for example, Freymann, 1974, pp. 60-76). This characterization of primary care may be too simplistic and a hindrance to an appreciation of its potentially vast implications for the restructuring of health services. The image does not invite an examination of the assumptions underlying health policy or recognition of the values and goals of vested-interest groups which may restrain the development of primary care along preferred lines.

The purpose of this paper is to describe some of the more significant factors associated with the rising importance of primary care, and to answer some of the questions about its role and organization by revealing some hidden as-

This selection, "The Future of Primary Health Services in the U.S.: Issues and Options," was prepared especially for this volume.

sumptions and issues. Leading alternatives are assessed in terms of short- and long-term consequences. Appropriate economic, political, and medical effects are considered from a predominantly sociological vantage point in which the accessibility of health services and responsiveness of professionals to the day-to-day health needs of the population are regarded as a major feature of contemporary quality-of-life expectations.

COST AND AVAILABILITY OF HEALTH SERVICES

The growth of interest in primary care is correlated closely with deepening fears among policy makers that uncontrolled growth of medical science and technology is largely responsible for the unacceptably high rates of inflation in health spending and for the unavailability of services for the care of commonplace health care needs. Medical science and technology are at the heart of the dilemma in government arising from (1) the alarm over the size and rate of increase in annual spending, which has stiffened resolve to impose cost discipline within the health sector; and (2) the pressures to increase the availability of services for neglected disease priorities and for underserviced populations (see Council on Wage and Price Stability, 1976, p. 29; U.S. Department of Health, Education, and Welfare, 1977, pp. 57-58). The apparent incompatibility of these two concerns frustrates decision makers. Resolution of the conflict is essential to breaking the deadlock and preparing a clear and consistent policy for guiding the future development of the health sector.

Cost of Health Care

The cost problem is preeminent among the concerns of health policy makers. Without doubt it has been the chief obstacle to the enactment of national health insurance following the dissipation of previously strong opposition to the concept in the late 1960s.

Since 1965 aggregate health spending has more than tripled. About half of the increase is due to inflation and about two-fifths to greater per capita use of health services and to increased technology and complexity of care (U.S. Department of Health, Education, and Welfare, 1977, pp. 63-64).

A vast program of investment undertaken by the federal government in the postwar era increased the number of nonfederal hospital general and surgical beds from 3.4 per 1,000 population in 1948 to 4.3 in 1975 (U.S. Department of Health, Education, and Welfare, 1975a, p. 7), and accelerated the innovation and diffusion of expensive technologies. In the period from 1963 to 1973, the proportion of all hospitals reporting electro-encepholography services doubled from 20 percent to 40 percent; those reporting intensive-care units rose from 19 percent to 55 percent; those with radioisotope facilities rose from 22 percent to 61 percent; and those with radium therapy went up from 14 percent to 22 percent (compiled from U.S. Department of Health, Education, and Welfare, 1976a, p. 138). The effect of this spread of new technologies on the cost of treatment has been enormous. For example, the cost for treatment of heart attacks rose from $1,449 to $3,280—an increase of 126 percent; treatment for breast cancer conditions went up from $1,559 to $2,557—an increase of 64 percent; the cost for maternity care rose from $523 to $807—a 53 percent increase; and the cost of treatment for appendicitis jumped from $592 to $1,063—an 80 percent increase (Council on Wage and Price Stability, 1976, p. 5).

As the main locus for new therapies made possible by advances in specialization and technology, the hospital has become the most important component of the health economy—accounting for two-fifths of all spending and over one-half of the labor force. Admission rates have risen to the point where one in nine Americans is now hospitalized annually (U.S. Department of Health, Education, and Welfare, 1976a, p. 307). There is disturbing evidence, however, that a considerable amount of hospitalization is unnecessary or harmful.

Roughly 15 percent or more of all hospital admissions are believed unnecessary, and it is said that one-fifth of the bed supply could be eliminated without endangering the health status of the population (McClure, 1976). It is claimed that as much as 20 percent of all the surgery performed is either medically questionable or unnecessary (Williams, 1971, p. 13), and that more than 7 percent of all hospitalized patients incur compensable injuries in the course of treatment (Pocinki, Dogger, and Schwartz, 1973, p. 50).

Cost increases generally have not been accompanied by a corresponding increase in benefits. Measured in terms of life expectancy and quality of survival, it is costing more and more to accomplish less and less—primarily because of the aging of the population and the growth in importance of chronic-degenerative illnesses and disabilities for which modern medicine can do little (see, for example, Thomas, 1977). Nevertheless, public faith in the value of medicine, especially hospital-oriented, acute-episodic treatment services, remains high and there are powerful political pressures on government to go beyond present programs (e.g., Medicare and Medicaid) for the financing of illness treatment services, and to make high-technology services more widely available through catastrophic health insurance.

As well as exacerbating problems involving the cost and quality of health care, the heavy concentration on highly specialized services for the treatment of acute-episodic illness steers medical manpower away from disease prevention and the care of the chronically ill. The medical neglect of patients in nursing homes and mental hospitals, together with the low performance of the U.S. in world standings comparing immunization levels among children and other measures of disease prevention, are painful reminders of the consequences of this imbalance (U.S. Department of Health, Education, and Welfare, 1976a, pp. 158-71).

Decline of General Practice

The growth and prestige of science and technology has transformed medical practice from a generalist to a specialist activity. The proportion of active general practitioners has declined from 80 percent in 1931 to 28 percent in 1963 and to less than 15 percent today. At least two-thirds of all medical graduates in the postwar period have become formally certified in a specialty. Among those uncertified, an unknown but large number have become self-designated specialists (compiled from Parker, 1974, p. 35; Macy Commission, 1976, p. 70). The training and practice of medicine has evolved from a simple generalist base to an elaborately complex structure of forty-five recognized specialty and subspecialty areas, and an equally complex proliferation of specialization and subspecialization among nonmedical health professionals (Stevens, 1971, pp. 3, 342). The fragmentation of services accompanying this development has produced pressures for coordination through organizational reforms and the revival of the medical generalist.

The decline of general practice has constricted the availability of medical services. In relation to specialists, general practitioners typically not only work longer hours and see more patients, but are more likely to make home visits and to practice in rural areas and within low-income urban areas. As reported in a recent government survey of use of ambulatory care services (U.S. Department of Health, Education, and Welfare, 1976b, p. 9), nearly 42 percent of all visits to office-based practitioners are to general and family practitioners in contrast to 25 percent to medical specialists and 28 percent to surgical specialists. In contrast to the situation at the turn of the century when there was roughly one doctor for every 500 persons, of whom 90 percent were generalists in office practice, the ratio of doctors readily available to care for everyday illness complaints declined to about 1:3,000 in the 1970s, counting only active generalists in private practice (Silver, 1976, p. 47).

The larger populations necessary to provide sufficient clinical material to assure the full employment of specialists promotes centralization and compounds problems of access and convenience of services. Over two-thirds of all outpatient doctor contacts now occur in doctors' offices. Home visits are a phenomenon of the past, accounting for only 1 percent of visits in 1973, and 5 percent a decade previously. Nearly 11 percent of all ambulatory visits occur in hospitals, either in outpatient clinics (6.8 percent) or emergency rooms (3.9 percent) (U.S. Department of Health, Education, and Welfare, 1976a, p. 293).

IMPLICATIONS OF PRIMARY CARE FOR THE RESTRUCTURING OF HEALTH SERVICES

That much of what has been written about primary care has been depicted as "vacuous and contradictory" (Lewis, Fein, and Mechanic, 1976, p. vii) belies some profound implications for the restructuring of health services. The indictment may reflect the displeasure stirred by a concept which appears somewhat backward by the values of scientific medicine. On the other hand, it may be an oblique reflection of the anxieties within high-technology medicine, fearful of a loss of independence and financial support should primary care achieve competitive status. The term *high-technology medicine* refers here to complex and costly treatments (mainly hospital-based), the safety and/or efficacy of which often have not been proven conclusively (e.g., cardiac care units, anticoagulant therapy, cardiac bypass surgery, and radical mastectomies), and to procedures of demonstrated value which are used inappropriately (e.g., radiation, laboratory tests, respiratory therapy, and heroic interventions in medically hopeless cases).

Primary care is a concept foreign to health services organized along laissez-faire, free-enterprise lines. It derives from the theory of planning, in which health services are conceived within a hierarchically organized division of labor based on technocratically determined economies of scale and quality control desiderata (see Pearson, 1976; Parker, 1974). Primary care implies, therefore, a planned organization and integration of elementary first-contact medical and related services. The consequences depart radically from solo fee-for-service practice, in which doctors, once licensed, are free to take on any medical procedure, regardless of the complexity of treatment and without a periodic demonstration of competence through continuing education and reexamination.

The principles of division of labor and economies of scale intrinsic to planning are used in practice to justify the differentiation of services—typically into three levels of specialization and intensity of care, ranging in descending order from the full array of hospital-based medical specialty services and large-scale teaching and research capabilities (tertiary care) to the most commonly employed hospital-based specialty services (secondary care), and the most basic level of specialty and generalist services organized outside hospitals (primary care). In such a system the welfare of specialty and superspecialty medicine invariably becomes more, rather than less, dependent on patient referrals under the control of primary care practitioners. In the gatekeeper role, the doctor-of-first-contact holds the key to effective use of costly hospital and specialty services. Ideally, he is also freed to spend more time in disease prevention and health promotion activities which can reduce serious illness and the need for costly treatment. Indeed, these goals are the justification for primary care in such highly planned health care systems as England and the Soviet Union (see Fry, 1969, pp. 58-101).

In addition to revising traditional power relationships, the smooth functioning of a formalized system of division of labor requires a predictable and stable supply of practitioners by specialty obtainable only through manpower planning. Primary care also entails, therefore, some controversial changes for the way medical education is structured in the U.S., which historically has been attuned to the values of individual freedom in choice of career specialty and of governmental noninterference in medical school curricula.

Related Policy Developments

Amidst all the confusion about the purpose and objectives of primary care, several strands of consensus are identifiable. First, in coupling ambulatory treatment with primary care in the new medical manpower legislation (Health Professions Educational Assistance Act of 1976), the federal government has made explicit the importance it attaches to the need for services less dependent on the use of costly hospital beds. A reaction against excessive hospital-oriented medical specialization is at the core of this shift in policy. The legislation mandates for the first time a system of manpower planning, which sets quotas on the numbers of medical students entering specialty training (U.S. Congress, 1976). The significance of this development looms larger when juxtaposed with two other initiatives undertaken by the federal government to restructure health services: mandatory peer review of medical decisions and national health planning and resources development.

The Professional Standards Review Organization (PSRO) program is designed to reduce admissions to and length of stays in acute hospitals and skilled nursing homes, and to subject clinical decision making to systematic monitoring and evaluation. The aims are to contain costs and safeguard quality (U.S. Department of Health, Education, and Welfare, 1975a, pp. 142-57). The National Health Planning and Resources Development Act of 1975 strengthens and expands preexisting planning and regulatory machinery (Sieverts, 1977). The aim is to improve access to quality services at reasonable cost by reducing the supply of unnecessary hospital beds, by controlling the diffusion of expensive new technologies, by promoting the growth of primary care capabilities, and by imposing a division of labor within the framework of hierarchically structured regional systems.

Further progress in planning for regionalization and health manpower will depend on the acceptance by the public of two crucial assumptions which run counter to traditional thinking. First, the uncontrolled training of medical practitioners is dysfunctional because the momentum of modern medicine causes an overproduction of specialists, particularly surgeons, at the expense of primary care, the care of the chronically ill, and the needs of populations in rural and economically depressed areas. Second, the uncontrolled development and proliferation of new technologies is dysfunctional because of the momentum in medicine which causes small and medium hospitals to emulate the mix of services provided by large teaching hospitals symbolizing the apex of clinical excellence. Illustrative of this point are the public investments in specialization and technology which have occurred without much attention to the implications for duplication, fragmentation, and quality of care. Consequently, there is little difference in the technology and staffing mix of services provided by acute hospitals, regardless of difference in size. Except for hospitals under 100 beds, the profile of U.S. hospitals is more flat than pyramidal (Freymann, 1974, pp. 355-63).

Beyond the conflict generated over implicit and explicit goals, discussion about the future of primary care was fraught with the conflict inherent in any attempt to carry out large-scale social change. While it may be intended that primary care should relate closely to the patients' commonplace needs and wants and feature a nonhospital orientation, it cannot be assumed that this will occur. The political realities of conflicting and competing pressures from diverse interest groups in the health sector seeking to preserve or increase their control of limited resources (often in the name of reform and greater responsiveness to consumer wants) could seriously compromise and cripple intended objectives.

UNRESOLVED ISSUES IN THE ORGANIZATION
OF PRIMARY CARE SERVICES

Hesitancy about the future of primary care is advisable, given the degree to which faith in high-technology values dominates in medicine and the tensions which can be expected from any attempt to alter customary practices in medical education and practice. The unresolved issues which will focus the struggle are numerous. Who will deliver primary care services? What services are to be provided? Where shall primary care be provided? And, as is increasingly the issue in health services, will primary care contribute to the already spiraling economic inflation observed in the health sector? The sharply different ways in which other advanced industrial nations have structured primary care suggests that there are no pat answers.

Designation of Responsibility

The assignment of responsibility is fundamental to the establishment of a smoothly functioning division of labor and clear lines of accountability. Disagreement over which of the different types of doctors trained in the U.S. should have the responsibility for primary care is not surprising, given the laissez-faire tradition in the health sector.

Rather than debating the merits of the generalist in an age of specialization, pragmatism has prevailed for the most part. Primary practice has been defined flexibly in the past to consist of a mix of generalist and front-line specialists (i.e., general practice, internal medicine, pediatrics, and obstetrics and gynecology) in accord with statistical studies of first-contact utilization (see, for example, U.S. Department of Health, Education, and Welfare, 1976a, pp. 105-06). The problem with this approach, however, is that it begs the issue of how services ought to be provided and condones, in the name of free enterprise and pluralism, shortcomings in the organization and delivery of services. The confusion and contradictions which can result are apparent in some recent changes in medical education.

Generalist vs. specialty practice

The American Medical Association's designation of family medicine in 1969 as a recognized specialty culminated an organized campaign begun by general practice in 1956 to preserve and renew the generalist's role in health care delivery in the wake of diminishing influence and prestige from competition with specialty medicine. Spurred largely by financial incentives from government and philanthropy, family practice rapidly is becoming established as the answer to the primary care dilemma. Many state governments, in reacting to the declining availability of doctors for routine medical needs, have required medical schools to establish separate departments of family practice as a condition for receiving state aid. By 1974 over half of the nation's medical schools sponsored training in family practice, either as part of the undergraduate curriculum, mostly on an elective basis, or the residency structure of the graduate program, or both. Family practice has a specialty board which, unlike other boards, requires that diplomates be reexamined every six years (Lewis, Fein, and Mechanic, 1976, pp. 76-91).

Family medicine can be summarized as an attempt to upgrade the credibility and standing of general practice through the amalgamation of internal medicine, pediatrics, and obstetrics and gynecology. Because training cuts across these three older and better established specialties and, moreover, overlaps in actuality with general surgery, family practice understandably is a nebulous and controversial innovation.

Resistance from threatened specialty interests, together with doubt over the value of the generalist in an age of specialization, places the future of family practice in doubt. Further uncertainty will ensue if current attempts to limit surgery to board-certified practitioners are followed by a comparable restriction of access to medical beds. Papering over the issue by the granting of specialty status to family practice has not helped to resolve conflicts and uncertainty, only to conceal them from the uninformed.

Restricting the supply of specialists is an acknowledged means for controlling costs. As put by a former high-ranking HEW official, "That European medicine tends to train fewer specialists serves to keep the cost of medical care somewhat below that of the United States; specialists not only demand higher fees than general practitioners, but they have to be served by an army of technicians and professionals as well as by a vast amount of expensive instruments and equipment" (Silver, 1976, p. 236).

The increase in family medicine residencies since the birth of family practice as a specialty has been proclaimed spectacular, but the percentage growth figures look good simply because they start from a base of zero. There also is evidence that the data are inflated. They are based on the number of students entering the first year of the required three-year residency training and fail to disclose the number of residents subsequently entering subspecialties (particularly those in internal medicine) in later years of their training (U.S. Congress, 1977, p. 11).

Annual production of family practitioners is now only slightly more than that of new neurologists—about 1,600. At present rates of output, most of the next generation of physicians capable of giving primary care will continue to be in internal medicine, pediatrics, and obstetrics. Calling these specialists primary care practitioners will not necessarily transform them to fulfill the functions important in first-contact care (Freymann, 1976, p. 25).

Role of medical surrogates and substitutes

Together with family practice there has emerged a bewildering array of new programs for the training of lower-grade functionaries for the purpose of plugging gaps in the supply and distribution of first-contact medical practitioners. Justified at their onset in the mid-1960s as a way to improve access and convenience by boosting the productivity of doctors through providing them with assistants specially trained to perform under medical supervision uncomplicated procedures (e.g., medical histories, physical examinations), the philosophy has since changed so that they are seen also as substitutes capable of working independently of medical supervision in underserviced areas. (Indeed, the Rural Health Clinics Services Act, PL 95-210, enacted in December 1977, permits Medicare and Medicaid to reimburse services of physician assistants and nurse practitioners rendering care in rural outpatient clinics.) The thinking on substitute personnel is patterned after the example of the feldshar and the barefoot doctor in rural parts of the Soviet Union and China, respectively. The assumption is that persons less highly trained in preventive, diagnostic, and treatment methods will be more willing to work in areas unattractive to doctors, especially if they are recruited from the ranks of poor and rural populations indigenous to underserviced areas.

The two most important types of training programs to emerge are those for physicians' assistants and nurse practitioners. They overshadow the many other programs which train team workers for special health settings such as child health and mental health (see, for example, Mahoney, 1973, pp. 124-41).

Since they are sponsored and accredited by several medical specialties (pediatrics, internal medicine, and family practice), the training programs for physicians' assistants do not vary much. There were a total of forty-three accredited programs in 1974 and their chief objective was to train assistants to help increase the productivity of primary care practitioners. The nurse practitioner programs are, on the other hand, extremely heterogeneous in curriculum and mission. Training programs vary in length from six weeks to two years, and range in focus from child health to obstetrics-gynecology, family medicine, geriatrics, and mental health. The estimates for 1976 are that there may be as many as fifty physicians' assistant and 200 nurse practitioner programs, with the number of graduates to date totalling 3,000 and 6,500 respectively. Due to the breadth of sponsorship and diffuseness of support from government and foundation funds, these programs have not been evaluated closely (Lewis, Fein, and Mechanic, 1976, pp. 111-26).

It is hard to say whether these new functionaries have improved access to first-contact care. Since the physicians' assistants are compelled to work under the supervision of a licensed doctor, it is unlikely that they can have done much about the geographic maldistribution of services. While nurse practitioners often have more independence, there is no reason to believe that they are any more willing than doctors to withstand status deprivation and cultural isolation. Nor are there any data to show that these new functionaries have helped to lower psychological and social barriers to first-contact care because they are more down to earth, have more in common with patients, or get on better with people than do doctors. Even if medical surrogates were free to practice independently, there is no reason to assume they would be accepted by underserviced populations. Given the consciousness-raising effect of higher education and mass communications, and the important role of relative deprivation in the interest group politics characteristic of advanced industrial societies (phenomena described by Janowitz, 1976, pp. 100-10), it is far more likely that underserviced populations will want to receive treatment by the same type of practitioners common to the rest of the population. Indeed, the Soviet Union reportedly is, for this reason, intent on replacing feldshars with doctors of medicine.

The assumption that medical substitutes, as distinct from assistants, are necessary to overcome problems of recruitment is specious, considering the number of qualified students denied admission to medical schools. The national average application-admission ratio of roughly 3:1 does not indicate a shortage of potential medical talent (Macy Commission, 1976, p. 73). What may be indicated, instead, is that the values of modern medicine cause medical schools to eschew low-technology training and behavioral science instruction, vital to the doctor-patient relationship in primary care, as unscientific, and to spin off responsibility for these functions (Pellegrino, 1973, pp. 57-72). Indeed, in summing up the history of attempts stretching back to the 1950s to establish primary care teaching and research capabilities in the U.S. medical schools, Reader and Soave (1976) concluded that the record is one of failure, mainly because of opposition from faculty power structures committed to high-technology medicine.

Definition of primary practice in federal manpower legislation

The new manpower legislation (U.S. Congress, 1976) does nothing to lessen the confusion over the definition of primary care practice, or the turmoil over whether first-contact care is best provided by generalists, specialists, or less highly trained nonmedical substitutes. Instead, it sanctions multiple approaches in the name of experimentation and pluralism. Except for the exclusion of obstetrics and gynecology and the inclusion of family practice, the definition of primary care remains unchanged, and support for the training of family practitioners and medical assistants and surrogates has been expanded. In interpreting future statistics on the supply of primary care personnel, the lumping of apples with oranges will continue to be a problem.

The question of what proportion of the practitioners actively caring for patients should be generalists is debatable. The experience of other highly developed free-market countries, noted for having preserved a strong foundation of general practitioner services, may provide a rough guide. The proportion of doctors in general practice ranges from 40 to 55 percent in Australia, Canada, West Germany, France, the Netherlands, and the United Kingdom (U.S. Department of Health, Education, and Welfare, 1975b). Although the issue is clouded due to differences in the definition of the generalist, the United States appears headed in this direction. Controls introduced by the federal government on the training of specialists have designated a target of 50 percent of medical school output for primary care by 1980.

Control of Hospital Beds

The right of first-contact medical practitioners to admit and care for patients in hospitals is a distinctive feature of American medicine. It runs counter to the pattern followed in most industrial countries in which first-contact medicine is centered almost exclusively on ambulatory services. The principle of non-differentiation is acclaimed generally in the U.S. as an expression of egalitarianism within the medical profession and as essential to good patient care, on the assumption that quality medicine cannot be practiced outside the hospital (Freymann, 1976, p. 23). The justification for restricting hospital privileges in other countries is that rapid advances in medical knowledge require confining complex procedures to highly qualified practitioners undergoing prolonged training, and that the realities of ambulatory care and hospital services differ markedly.

Medical experts in the U.S. and England disagree somewhat, but it does not appear that the vast majority of the work in primary care requires lengthy technical training. Anywhere from 75 to 90 percent of patient visits consist of complaints and illnesses which either are self-correcting or responsive to simple therapies (see, for example, Fry, 1966, pp. 8-11; Stead, 1973, p. 146; Marsland, Wood, and Mayo, 1976, pp. 38-74; U.S. Department of Health, Education, and Welfare, 1976b, pp. 20-21).

The trend in the U.S., foreshadowed by the growth in voluntary quality controls and the prospects inherent in the PSRO initiative, is to limit the performance of complex procedures to formally certified practitioners. The effect of voluntary controls in hospitals is illustrated in New York City, where approximately one-fifth of active practitioners do not have hospital privileges (Freymann, 1976, p. 23). This is no doubt due to the large number of medical school-affiliated teaching hospitals which are more demanding in the awarding of medical staff privileges than are community general hospitals. The growing worry among surgeons about an oversupply of manpower and underemployment of skills can be expected to accelerate the movement towards a division of labor in medicine, based on formal certification (American College of Surgeons, 1975, pp. 77).

Whether primary care practitioners ought to have hospital privileges and over what type of beds is hotly contested. Among primary care practitioners trained and socialized in conventional medical schools, there is a natural desire to have access to hospital beds. In responding to the cross-pressures of cost and quality controls and the expectations of conventionally trained doctors, policy makers may find attractive the option of granting primary care practitioners the responsibility for the care of the chronically ill in long-term beds. The Finnish government did this as part of a broad-sweeping reform of health services enacted in 1972 which also included access to a limited number of acute beds for uncomplicated deliveries and the nonseriously ill (Hakkarainen, 1975).

While primary care practitioners on the surface may be better disposed in outlook and training to care for the long-term ill, who require a greater emphasis on care than cure, there is the risk that attitudes formed in medical schools, combined with feelings of status deprivation in relation to more prestigious specialties, will make it difficult for the government to withstand pressures for more elaborate staffing and equipment than is needed. Long-term care facilities which attempt to duplicate the resources of acute hospitals represent a disastrous waste of resources.

Health Centers

Broader in scope and more highly organized than group practice, the health center is the apotheosis of currently popular principles of management, efficiency, and quality of care. Previously the exclusive and controversial hallmark of U.S.S.R.-style health services planning, the problems associated with increased public financing of health services have led governments in the West to introduce and expand material incentives designed to get doctors to give up solo practice in favor of group practice and practice in health centers (see, for example, Maxwell, 1975, p. 25; Abel-Smith, 1974, pp. 23-24).

The weight of opinion among medical educators in England, for example, favors more governmental incentives for moving general practitioners from solo and partnership practice into specially equipped health centers staffed by up to twelve practitioners, with ample clerical-secretarial support and nursing and social work backup, including home visitors and domestic helpers (Royal Commission on Medical Education, 1968). A concern for critical mass sufficient to justify the cost and to assure everyday interaction with a broad range of relevant allied health and social service personnel underlies this outlook (Forsyth, 1973, pp. 209-10).

The multiprofessional health center practice is considered by proponents in all countries to be the best way to reduce dependence on costly hospital services by providing as much care in the community as possible, and to obtain optimal use of hospital services by a system of referral for putting the right patient in the right bed at the right time (see, for example, Silver, 1976, pp. 132-38; Fry, 1969, pp. 194-209; Macy Foundation, 1973).

Staffing and technology mix

Two of the more important questions on the organization of health centers involve staffing and technology. In matters of staffing, the choices, as represented in the experience of highly developed countries, involve a purely medical model or the bringing together of medical and social services personnel.

The basic issue with regard to medical staffing centers on single versus multispecialty practice. In the Soviet Union, the country with the longest and most extensive experience with health centers, the preference is for the medical model exclusively, consisting of multispecialty medical staffing supplemented by allied health workers, including physical therapists. In England and Scandinavia, the practice is to staff health centers on a single-specialty basis, in which general practitioners are assisted by allied health workers. The mixing together of medical and social models varies in the West. In England and Sweden, for example, the preference is to include social workers and related social services personnel, whereas in Finland the Soviet example of excluding social workers is followed (Battistella, 1977).

The multispecialty composition of primary care in the U.S. provides a built-in predilection to follow the Soviet approach to medical staffing. The variable experience with such possible precursors as neighborhood health centers and health maintenance organizations, which has been summarized by Lewis, Fein, and Mechanic (1976, pp. 188-206, 220-40), suggests that, unlike the countries mentioned, the role of social work remains an open question.

The issue of what and how much technology primary practitioners should have in their offices will have far-reaching consequences for providers, consumers, and government. Independently of economic incentives and the threat of malpractice, ease of access to sophisticated diagnostic technology is an inducement to the ordering of costly tests. Thus, for example, the rate of use of clinical laboratory services among doctors in office-based practice is lower in England than in the U.S., where these services are more readily available to doctors. Outside of the new health centers, general practitioner offices in England contain little of the diagnostic technology taken for granted in the U.S. (Mechanic, 1972, pp. 152-53).

The probability for error will grow with increased use of complex diagnostic equipment. Conceivably, false test results could lead to forms of treatment which are hazardous to patients (see, for example, U.S. Department of Health, Education, and Welfare, 1975a, pp. 147-48). Decision making in technologically intensive environments is likely to be structured against less costly, low-technology, and natural methods which may be just as effective and possibly safer. Whenever given a choice, the knee-jerk reaction of a high-technology environment is to opt for complexity rather than simplicity.

The experience with neighborhood health centers and services provided in hospital outpatient departments reveals that the economic effect of organizing primary services in technology-intensive and organizationally complex interprofessional team settings is to raise the cost of each patient visit by a factor of from two to three times over the cost of what doctors in conventional practice charge for an office visit (see, for example, Sparer and Anderson, 1972). Whether the added cost can be justified in better treatment outcomes and patient satisfaction has not been demonstrated.

Duplication of hospital services

Proposals to upgrade the scientific credibility of primary care by moving practitioners into highly equipped health centers will encounter little resistance within segments of the medical community placing great value on specialization and technology. Primary care practitioners anxious to improve their status both among the public and within the medical community also will be receptive. This psychology is evident in the location of CAT scanners (costing from $300,000 to $700,000 each, and from $300,000 to $400,000 to operate per year) and similar diagnostic equipment in ambulatory settings, when their accessibility in hospitals is restricted by planning agencies. The lack of authority to prevent this is a major limitation of the new health planning machinery now being implemented in the United States. About 15 percent of all scanners are owned by doctors and located outside the scope of hospital controls (Office of Technology Assessment).

A blurring of the differences between primary care and hospital-based services also will appeal to persons who worry about problems of recruitment and high rates of turnover in primary care, because of the greater prestige and material rewards of technology-intensive medicine. In addition, hospital-based interest groups may welcome a lessening of distinctions, as security against the possibility of primary care being used by government to restrict access to high-technology beds and to shift public financing to less costly ambulatory and home care services.

Any move to increase the role of technology and specialization in primary care predictably will introduce economic pressures for economies of scale and the centralization of services in health centers, which could further restrict access. Increased travel time as well as the aggravation of traffic might discourage the gainfully employed from initiating care. And the decrepit state of public transportation would pose serious problems for aged and poor individuals who are either without automobiles or unable to drive themselves. Short of reversing the trend among doctors against making home calls, the only alternative is to develop publicly financed ambulance systems for which the costs may be prohibitive. Without such transportation, the effect of present strategies to deinstitutionalize the treatment of illness (both in the acute and long-term areas) may do more to lower than raise standards of patient care.

Need for professional management

The risks of overmanagement generally are not well recognized. The running of large, complex health centers creates demands for professionally trained managers whose value systems and career needs may equate size and growth with power and progress (see, for example, Gordon, 1945, pp. 305-07; Burns, 1974). The impulse for growth is possibly as strong a motivating element among professionally trained managers as the technological imperatives which drive doctors to emulate the conditions of practice characteristic of teaching hospitals, and which cause surgeons to want to operate when the diagnosis and course of treatment are unclear.

Appeals to better management and more rational organization for getting on top of the cost problem may be self-defeating—any gains in lower unit cost may be miniscule in relation to changes in greater aggregate expenditures. The inclination of boards of trustees and managers themselves to evaluate managerial performance using narrow short-run criteria of efficiency precludes proper consideration of second- and third-order consequences so that (as advanced by Bower, 1974) decision making is slanted in a socially dysfunctional direction.

Justification for economies of scale

Pressures for centralization also could, as argued by Halberstam (1971), carry bureaucracy to the point of diseconomies in terms of patient dissatisfaction and the paralysis of professionals by too much coordination and red tape. The amount of effort spent on conflict resolution, coordination, and accountability certainly will rise with increases in the numbers of different medical specialists and in allied health and social service workers. An evaluation in Australia of recently introduced multiprofessional health centers disclosed that close to two-fifths of staff working time is absorbed by administrative activities (Moran and McCarthy, 1976).

The problems inherent in the bureaucratization of primary care suggest the need for research on the psychology of growth and diseconomies of scale. When looked at comprehensively, simple nonbureaucratic solutions may be preferable to organizationally complex solutions. It has been noted (Galbraith, 1973, p. 57) that in cases where no (or simple, inexpensive) technologies are involved, the advantages of organization for economy are marginal, at best. The inability of economists to demonstrate conclusively that economies of scale have been attained in primary care is a further cause for skepticism (Weisbrod, 1975, pp. 645-46). The prevailing assumption in health planning is that general managerial economic principles applicable to tertiary and secondary services ought to hold for primary care. However, the differences in purpose, and in types of patients, suggest, instead, that the approach taken might better vary by level of technological intensity.

The solution to keeping the scale of organization within human dimensions, while creating a structure which is both supportive of patients' total needs and a check against the unnecessary use of costly service, centers on what services practitioners in primary care ought to be allowed to perform and with what technologies. Under carefully circumscribed conditions, practices of limited scale consisting of several practitioners with nursing and related help could be vastly preferable to large health centers for reasons encompassing economy, access, continuity, and relevance of care. The limiting of services to simple and intermediate technologies would both lower the cost of the treatment and make it possible to locate services closer to where patients live.

The association of individual patients with fewer practitioners in small-scale practices would facilitate doctor-patient relationships better suited to continuity of care. Furthermore, the highly personalized doctor-patient relationship characteristic of nonbureaucratic practice provides a better environment for patient education in disease prevention and for affecting changes in behavior that help control the progression of pain and disability associated with chronic-degenerative illness. The growing importance of psychosocial illness and self-induced illness, and the increased recognition of the therapeutic potential of the doctor-patient relationship itself, caution against the uncritical acceptance of bureaucratic solutions (see, for example, Parsons, 1975; Balint, 1957; Ornstein, 1977).

Efficiency and Productivity

There is limited information on how to improve the efficiency of primary care practice. While the governments of advanced industrial nations have become more involved in the financing of health care, they have not been deeply involved with organizational matters—especially in the West, where they have opted to supplement purchasing power while interfering as little as possible with the status quo (Battistella, 1972). Even in England and the Soviet Union, where primary care services are highly structured, progress in studies of efficiency and productivity has been slow because of difficulties in establishing reliable information systems for measuring the volume of symptomatic and asymptomatic morbidity present in populations, and in operationalizing multidimensional outcome measures. In other countries, diversity in the organization of first-contact services encompassing solo, group, and health center practices, with large differences in the number and type of supportive personnel and equipment, present additional problems.

The *Journal of the Royal College of Physicians* (1972) has reported data which indicates that the average number of patients cared for by primary care practitioners varies from 2,500 in England to 5,000 or more in Scandinavia. (In the largely unstructured free enterprise climate of U.S. medical practice, it is rare for doctors in first-contact medicine to know the exact number of patients whom they care for.) Fry (1969, p. 92) has presented data which show that the average time spent for each patient varies considerably among countries. The time spent per patient for office calls is six to seven minutes in England, contrasted with twelve minutes in the U.S.S.R. and twenty-five minutes in the U.S. In the case of home visits, the time spent per patient ranges from less than twenty minutes in England to thirty minutes in the U.S.S.R. and the U.S. Doctors of first contact in the U.S.S.R. are required to spend half of each working day making home calls, whereas home visits in England have been declining and have all but disappeared in the U.S. In the Soviet Union doctors are also required to spend the equivalent of one-half day per week on preventive services.

Upon reviewing carefully kept records of the changes in his general practice in England which occurred over twenty-one years, Fry (1972) reported that it is possible for two general practitioners to provide sound care for as many as 9,000 people in stable populations not disrupted by high rates of migration. Advances in antibiotics for infections, better diuretics for congestive heart failure, and improvements in drugs for the management of asthma, arthritis, depression, anxiety, and skin conditions have made it possible to reduce the number of times patients have to be seen which, together with encouraging patients to seek care in the doctors' offices rather than at home, has resulted in an overall reduction of work during the past several decades. The addition to the practice of another practitioner, a nurse clinician, a home visitor, and a secretary/receptionist, together with the introduction of a full appointment system, also were important factors. During the two decades, Fry reduced his workload by one-third and shortened his workweek by sixteen hours.

The implications of Fry's observations for the future of health services in the U.S. are mindboggling. It is estimated that the ratio of primary care practitioners to the population is likely to grow from one per 1,500 persons in 1970 to one per 1,100 in 1990 (U.S. Department of Health, Education, and Welfare, 1977, p. 106). This suggests that the real problem of primary care in this country is organizational, rather than a manpower shortage.

The overmedication and questionable treatment which could result from a surplus supply of primary care practitioners is a disturbing prospect, particularly under conditions of fee-for-service reimbursement. A surplus might also invite further medicalization of social and behavioral problems which could be treated equally well or better, and for less money, outside the health sector (e.g., crime, mental stress, alcohol and drug abuse, obesity, and smoking); it is also sure to result in demands for a shortening of the workweek without a reduction in income, and a compounding of controversies over the tradeoffs between productivity and quality.

Reimbursement incentives

The effects of reimbursement as an incentive for referring too many or too few patients and for overservicing and underservicing are not well understood (Glaser, 1976). Fee-for-service is believed, in principle, to discourage referrals and to give doctors an incentive to provide questionable and unnecessary services, whereas capitation and salary are thought to provide a greater interest in prevention. On the negative side, they are criticized for encouraging too many referrals or the withholding of services. Fee-for-service may be superior to other alternatives for increasing provider receptivity to patients and for maximizing both consumer and provider satisfaction where purchasing power is sufficient.

The effect of reimbursement on provider satisfaction appears to depend on a blend of ideological preference and the adequacy of income relative to preferences for leisure (Anderson, 1972, pp. 191-201).

In the U.S., the desire of the federal government to test how alternative forms of remuneration can reduce hospitalization and contain costs led to the introduction in 1973 of legislation and subsidies fostering the spread nationally of prepaid group practice (HMOs), in which doctors are paid in advance for caring for a defined population, and the medical group is placed at risk for any end-of-year deficits. Though plagued by controversy over amendments and inadequate funds, sufficient experience has been obtained (Gaus, Cooper, and Hirschman, 1976) to show that doctors on salaries in organized group practices utilize two-and-a-half times less hospital beds and operate at half the rate of doctors paid by fee-for-service.

The priorities for cost containment and predictability in budgeting, which were so instrumental in winning governmental support for the HMO program, suggest there will be strong pressures in any system of national health insurance either to place doctors on salary, or to organize them into groups which have a financial interest in controlling utilization. The HMO initiative can be interpreted as a clever strategy for speeding up the transition from solo to health center types of practice and for curbing the access of consumers and providers to hospital services through the manipulation of free enterprise values in American medicine.

Where and How Should Primary Care Practitioners be Trained?

As suggested previously, the work of primary care includes more than the purely technical functions of disease prevention, diagnosis, and treatment. At least three other roles are identifiable: (1) the sorting out and referral of patients to the right specialist; (2) the pastoral role of providing sympathy, understanding, and advice to the worried well and to the sick for whom modern medicine can do little; and (3) the social work role of assuring that rehabilitation of the seriously ill and disabled is not impeded because of the failure to assure proper coordination of medical services with such social services as income maintenance, housing, job retraining, and physical and occupational therapy. The neglect of the aged in nursing homes and of the institutionalized mentally ill and mentally handicapped suggests a fourth role—the humane care and medical supervision of the institutionalized incurably ill and dying. Balanced instruction and training for primary care requires (as described by Freymann, 1974, pp. 163-202) competence in the behavioral sciences, health education, and disease prevention, as well as the biomedical sciences.

This is apparent in the growing importance of sociomedical problems, the intertwining of psychological and somatic factors among the sick aged, and the tendency to medicalize disorders previously the responsibility of the individual, the courts, or the church—such as obesity, alcoholism, depression, sexual deviations, and strained family relationships.

But behavioral and social subjects at best are marginally represented in medical school curricula. Rather, the focus is on narrowly defined technical functions of an engineering nature, tilted toward acute intervention for rarely occurring illnesses. The predisposition of scientific medicine is to dismiss the nontechnical aspects of patient care as prescientific primitivism (see, for example, Freymann, 1974, pp. 290-300; Ehrlich, 1973, p. 71). The bias in modern medicine for the technical role is the result of a pervasive system of reinforcing interests encompassing national biomedical research policy geared to innovation and diffusion of high-technology therapies, the measures used in the selection of medical students which are weighted against individuals wanting to work directly with people, the biomedical and research thrust of the medical school curriculum, and the control of medical school faculty and teaching hospital power structures by specialists (see Freymann, 1974, pp. 147-202).

The superior status and prestige assigned specialists in medical schools and teaching hospitals places them in the leadership of standard-setting activities. Their values lead them to evaluate colleagues in primary care almost exclusively by their ability to diagnose and treat accurately rarely occurring physical ailments. Their evaluative criteria seldom allow for how well a primary practitioner does in sustaining the ability of patients to carry on in the face of emotional stress and chronic impairments. It is understandable that primary practitioners socialized in a milieu dominated by specialists should come to evaluate themselves in a similar way. The values and reward systems of medicine today inevitably tip decisions in the direction of making too many physical diagnoses, rather than too few—a natural disposition which is strengthened by the growth in medical malpractice (see, for example, Mechanic, 1972, pp. 9-23).

The near total restriction of all clinical instruction (undergraduate, graduate, and continuing education) to the confines of the teaching hospital is an equally important barrier to the future development of balanced instruction for socially responsive primary care. The interdependence between the teaching hospital and medical faculty produces an environment with an outmoded emphasis on inpatient care and acute intervention (Freymann, 1974, pp. 196-202). The esoteric and statistically rare nature of the clinical material found in teaching hospitals further distorts the reality of day-to-day practice in primary care. White (1961) has estimated that within a hypothetical population of 1,000 adults as risk, 75 percent have some identifiable medical problems, 25 percent obtain some medical care, 10 percent are admitted to a community general hospital and only 1 percent are admitted to a university teaching hospital where medical students receive their training.

The temptation to dismiss outright established educational and training capabilities in favor of environments more supportive of primary care treatment must be moderated somewhat. England's National Health Service indicates that primary care practitioners can be trained side-by-side with specialists going into hospital practice, provided that the stresses from competition for status and income can be accommodated successfully. The stresses can be quite severe, however, and the potential for cooptation is high. The likelihood of undesirable cooptation will not be lessened soon, considering that the power structure of medical education is controlled by individuals who may be several decades away from retirement. Progress in replacing them with individuals more supportive of primary care will be slow.

Perhaps the time has come to consider the option of establishing a new generation of medical schools in which all of the organizational incentives are skewed towards educational concepts and research more in line with public policy priorities for less costly technologies and noninstitutional care. In this regard, the combining of relevant components of public health and social work with primary care opens some attractive possibilities. A separate and independent learning environment encompassing a strong coalition of community-oriented interests would be less susceptible to cooptation by high technology and ostensibly better suited to the development of progressive theories of noninstitutional care. It also would be more open to cost-efficiency studies of alternative medical and social services treatment models, especially for geriatric patients and the mentally ill, where the benefits of physical and occupational therapy and social work may surpass the benefits of orthodox medical treatment. At the very least, the period of training following graduation should be shifted from teaching hospitals to places where medical residents could obtain a more authentic exposure to the world of primary care, notably, health centers and physicians' offices.

Ironically, the need for more highly personalized and commonsense approaches to primary care, combining the technical role with pastoral and social work aspects, is increasing at a time when medical schools are moving to strengthen the curative aspects of medicine. Toward the end of unifying previously fragmented responsibility for undergraduate training, residency training, and continuing education provided in teaching hospitals, there is a trend toward bringing teaching hospitals more closely under the control of the medical schools. The number of teaching hospitals affiliated with medical schools has grown substantially since 1968, so that the ratio of residency programs in affiliated hospitals to those in nonaffiliated hospitals has shot up from 2:1 to 3:1 (Anlyan and Bucci, 1973, p. 119).

Consumer Participation

The controversy and confusion generated by the question of consumer participation in health planning and the administration of health centers (i.e., neighborhood health centers, health maintenance organizations, and community mental health centers) has been extensive and unrelenting, since it first became a major issue in the health politics of the mid-sixties. This may be attributed to the way it has been used freely by different interest groups for widely different purposes, ranging in extreme from utopian visions of anarchistic decision making in which crass professionals are stripped of authority by the enlightened underprivileged, to the cynical manipulation of consumers for the entertainment and aggrandizement of professionals.

Introduced initially as a means for educating professionals to the real, rather than assumed, needs of medically underserviced, low-income populations, and for equipping poor minorities to achieve a standard of utilization commensurate with that of the middle class, consumer participation from the start had overtones of Marxist class conflict. Most recently the intent behind the consumer majorities required in the National Health Planning and Resources Development Act of 1974 is to check the expansion of high-technology services and to subject professionals to cost discipline (Vladeck, 1977).

Many health professionals initially perceived the consumer participation movement as a threat to their monopoly powers in diagnosis and treatment, and as a rebuff to their willingness to abide by principles of trust and restraint of self-interest contained in the service ethic, which justifies their perquisites of status and freedom in clinical decision making. In the wake of experience which has left their authority intact, professionals have grown more relaxed and are coming to recognize the positive aspects of a closer association with consumers. These positive aspects can include the provision of advice and information for more responsive health services planning and delivery, the legitimization of previously suspect allocation decisions, and the broadening of demand for services which can offset pressures for steady-state budgets and retrenchment.

In retrospect, much of the rhetoric predicting that consumer participation would culminate in a radical transformation of power in which the masses would bring errant professionals to bay was naive. As noted by Rossi (1965), professionals can spend more time dealing with health problems specifically (professionals are employed full time whereas consumers must divide their time among competing demands), have more skill in the marshalling and organization of human effort, and have more control over the collection and interpretation of esoteric knowledge and technical information.

Consumers also have a tendency to defer to medical authority for reasons of trust and respect. Opinion polls consistently show greater public confidence in medicine than in business, government, education, and the scientific community. Moreover, consumers believe even more intently than doctors in the benefits of health service, not simply because of conditioning by medical propaganda, but because they are predisposed to do so. Since many of the things people enjoy most are harmful to their health, it is understandable that they should hope for and believe in the availability of a technological fix, whether in the form of drugs or surgery, rather than agree to unpleasant and unwanted changes in life styles. The emotional significance of illness and death is a fundamental reason for public faith in the benefits of medical intervention. And the unique vulnerability of the sick to exploitation of all sorts causes them to want to believe in the integrity of their personal doctor and to expect more socially responsible behavior from the medical profession than from other professions and occupations.

As the sophistication of professionals deepens to the point where the contributions of consumer participation to the political support of programs in a period of economic retrenchment are better recognized, government officials may find themselves mired in the contradiction of withdrawing support for consumer participation previously mandated either on egalitarian grounds or as a check against professional imperialism. Given the public's faith in the benefits of modern medical treatment and the confidence it places in the medical profession, any strategy for cost containment which seeks to pit consumers against doctors would be myopic. More important than the risks of failure are the longer-run implications for increased social alienation and unrest which could result from a weakening of public confidence and trust in medicine. As pointed out by Janowitz (1976, pp. 1-16), health and related social services play a key role in maintaining the social and political stability essential to the well-being of advanced industrial nations. A wiser and more successful course of action might involve a systematic program for informing the public of the limitations of modern medicine, side by side with the training of a new generation of doctors motivated and trained for practice in primary care who are themselves more understanding of the limitations of medical science and technology.

SUMMARY AND CONCLUSIONS

The severity of the economic and social problems experienced within the health sector in an era of advanced medical specialization and technology warrants a reexamination of the role of primary care services. If attuned appropriately to contemporary exigencies, primary care could contribute substantially to the harmonization of conflicting policy aspirations for cost containment and the expansion of health services. This may require, however, a willingness and ability among policy makers to challenge conventional medical alternatives about how best to train and organize primary care practitioners.

Piecemeal strategies overly concentrated on reducing dependence on costly hospital service will probably fail and possibly be counterproductive. A coordinated division of labor, with separate but complementary arrangements for services designed to meet the different realities of front-line medical practice and secondary and tertiary lines of medical care, is consistent with the trend in medicine toward manpower planning and the differentiation of services by levels of medical intensity and complexity.

A strong foundation of simple and inexpensive services, for the treatment of routine illness and the care of illnesses for which medicine can do little apart from the relief of suffering, is essential if growing demands for more health services, due to changes in population structure and disease patterns, are to remain within the bounds of available resources. The experience of other highly developed countries suggests that the granting of controls over referrals to first-contact practitioners is the fulcrum for making more economic use of costly hospital services while maintaining the convenient availability of services responsive to the everyday medical needs of individuals and families.

The importance of personalized relationships for the treatment of illnesses in which psychological and physical factors are heavily interconnected, the necessity to influence life styles in the management of chronic illness, and the compelling obligations for the humane care of the incurably long-term ill and dying indicates that the traditional doctor-patient relationship displaced by progress in scientific medicine ought to be restored to primary care training and practice. The obsession of medicine with acute treatment departs from the real needs of the population in a highly developed society: the mentally handicapped, the physically disabled, the mentally ill, and the aged. The degree to which this population group is presently improperly cared for reflects the narrowness of values in conventional medical education.

Both the human aspects of good patient care and the priorities for economy and efficiency caution against the emulation of economy-of-scale principles appropriate for technology-intensive services provided within hospitals. Smaller scale and limited bureaucratic arrangements in primary care provide greater opportunities for personalized treatment. They also place fewer demands on capital and tend to constrain professional and organizational incentives to view growth as a surrogate for success.

The domination of medical education and practice by proponents of high-technology medicine is a formidable barrier to the deployment of primary care against deficiencies in the accessibility and cost-effectiveness of medical services. Convincing high-technology interests of the value of more modest therapies and the legitimacy of having medical practitioners assume responsibility for the care of routine illness is critical to how primary care will develop and what it can contribute to improving the organizational efficiency and responsiveness of health services.

REFERENCES

Abel-Smith, B. "Value for Money in Health Services." *Social Security Bulletin* 37 (July 1974): 17-28.

American College of Surgeons and Surgical Association. *Surgery in the United States.* Chicago: American College of Surgeons, 1975.

Anderson, O. W. *Health Care: Can There Be Equity?* New York: John Wiley & Sons, 1972.

Anlyan, W. G., and Bucci, B. E. "Current Curricular Changes in Medical Education." *National Health Services,* edited by J. Z. Bowers and E. Purcell. New York: Josiah Macy, Jr., Foundation, 1973.

Balint, M. *The Doctor, His Patient, and the Illness.* New York: International Universities Press, 1957.

Battistella, R. M. "Postindustrial Europe and Its Health Care." *International Journal of Health Services* 2 (1972): 465-77.

Battistella, R. M. "Study of Macrohealth Planning Developments in Finland, Sweden, Union of Soviet Socialist Republics, England and Northern Ireland." Report submitted to John E. Fogarty International Center for Advanced Studies in the Health Sciences, 1977.

Bower, J. L. "On the Amoral Organization." *The Corporate Society,* edited by R. Marris. New York: John Wiley & Sons, 1974.

Burns, T. "On the Rationale of the Corporate System." *The Corporate Society,* edited by R. Maris. New York: John Wiley & Sons, 1974.

Council on Wage and Price Stability. *The Problem of Rising Health Care Costs.* Washington, D.C.: Executive Office of the President, 1976.

Ehrlich, G. E. "Health Challenges of the Future." *Annals of the American Academy of Political and Social Science* 408 (July 1973): 70-82.

Forsyth, G. *Doctors and State Medicine* (2nd ed.). London: Pitman, 1973.

Fink, P. J., and Owen, D. "The Role of Psychiatry as a Primary Care Specialty." *Archives of General Psychiatry* 33 (August 1976): 998-1003.

Freymann, J. G. *The American Health Care System: Its Genesis and Trajectory.* Baltimore: Williams & Wilkins, 1974.

Freymann, J. G. "Organization of the Health Care System: Logical Fantasy Versus Illogical Reality." Paper presented at the Bicentennial Conference on Health Policy Agendas (University of Pennsylvania, 1976).

Fry, J. *Profiles of Disease.* London: E. & S. Livingstone, 1966.

Fry, J. *Medicine in Three Societies.* New York: Elsevier, 1969.

Fry, J. "Twenty-one Years of General Patterns: Changing Patterns." *Journal of the Royal College of General Practitioners* 22 (1972): 521-28.

Galbraith, J. K. *Economics and the Public Purpose.* Boston: Houghton Mifflin, 1973.

Gaus, C. R.; Cooper, B. S.; and Hirschman, C. G. "Contrasts in HMO and Fee-for-Service." *Social Security Bulletin* 39 (May 1976): 3-14.

Glaser, W. A. "Controlling Costs Through Methods of Paying Doctors: Experiences from Abroad." Paper prepared for the John E. Fogarty International Center for Advanced Studies in the Health Sciences, 1976.

Gordon, R. A. *Business Leadership in the Large Corporation.* Washington, D.C.: Brookings Institution, 1945.

Gross, R. J. "Primary Health Care: A Review of the Literature Through 1972." *Medical Care* 12 (August 1974): 638-47.

Hakkarainen, A. "Introducing Primary Health Services in Nationwide Scale: Centralized Planning-Decentralized Administration." Paris: Organization for Economic Cooperation and Development, 1975.

Halberstam, M. J. "Liberal Thought, Radical Theory and Medical Practice." *New England Journal of Medicine* 284 (May 27, 1971): 1180-85.

Janowitz, M. *Social Control of the Welfare State.* New York: Elsevier, 1976.

Journal of the Royal College of Physicians. "How Many Patients?" *Journal* 22 (1972): 491-93.

Lewis, C. E.; Fein, R.; and Mechanic, D. *A Right to Health Care.* New York: John Wiley & Sons, 1976.

Macy Commission. *Physicians for the Future.* New York: Josiah Macy, Jr., Foundation, 1976.

Macy Foundation and Royal Society of Medicine. *The Greater Medical Profession.* New York: Josiah Macy, Jr., Foundation, 1973.

Mahoney, M. E. "The Future Role of Physician's Assistants and Nurse Practitioners." *National Health Services,* edited by J. Z. Bowers and E. Purcell. New York: Josiah Macy, Jr., Foundation, 1973.

Marsland, D. W.; Wood, M.; and Mayo, F. "Content of Family Practice." *Journal of Family Practice* 3 (1976): 25-74.

Maxwell, R. *Health Care: The Growing Dilemma.* New York: McKinsey, 1975.

McClure, W. *Reducing Excess Hospital Capacity* (HRA 230-76-0086). Washington, D.C.:
    Bureau of Health Planning and Resources Development, 1976.
Mechanic, D. *Public Expectations and Health Care*. New York: John Wiley & Sons, 1972.
Moran, L. J., and McCarthy, N. J. "Community Health Center Evaluation." *Australian Family Physician* 5 (March 1976).
Ornstein, P. H. "The Family Physician as a Therapeutic Instrument." *Journal of Family Practice* 4 (April 1977): 659-62.
Parker, A. W. "The Dimensions of Primary Care: Blueprints for Change." *Primary Care*,
    edited by S. Andreopoulos. New York: John Wiley & Sons, 1974.
Parsons, T. "The Sick Role and the Role of the Physician Reconsidered." *Milbank Memorial Fund Quarterly, Health and Society* (Summer 1975): 257-78.
Pearson, D. A. "The Concept of Regionalized Personal Health Services in the United States." *The Regionalization of Personal Health Services*, edited by E. W. Saward.
    New York: Milbank Memorial Fund, 1976.
Pellegrino, E. D. "Delivery of Medical Care in the United States." *The Greater Medical Profession*. New York: Josiah Macy, Jr., Foundation, 1973.
Pocinki, L. S.; Dogger, S. J.; and Schwartz, B. A. "The Incidence of Iatrogenic Injuries."
    Appendix to Report of the Secretary's Commission on Medical Malpractice (Publication no. OS 73-89). Washington, D.C.: HEW, 1973.
Reader, G. R., and Soave, R. "Comprehensive Care Revisited." *Milbank Memorial Fund Quarterly, Health and Society* 54 (Fall 1976): 391-414.
Rossi, P. H. "What Makes Communities Tick?" *Health and the Community*, edited by A. H.
    Katz and J. S. Felton. New York: Free Press, 1965.
Royal Commission on Medical Education. *Command Paper 3569*. London: Her Majesty's
    Stationery Office, 1968.
Sieverts, S. *Health Planning Issues and Public Law 93-641*. Chicago: American Hospital
    Association, 1977.
Silver, G. A. *A Spy in the House of Medicine*. Germantown, Md.: Aspen, 1976.
Sparer, G., and Anderson, A. "Cost of Services at Neighborhood Health Centers." *New England Journal of Medicine* 286 (June 8, 1972): 1241-45.
Stead, E. A., Jr. "Family Practice: One View." *The Future of Medical Education*, edited by
    W. G. Anlyan et al. Durham, N.C.: Duke University Press, 1973.
Stevens, R. *American Medicine and the Public Interest*. New Haven, Conn.: Yale University
    Press, 1971.
Thomas, L. "On the Science and Technology of Medicine." *Daedalus* 106 (1977): 35-46.
U.S. Congress, House of Representatives. *Conference Report Accompanying the Health Professions Educational Assistance Act of 1976* (Report no. 94-1612, 94th Congress,
    2nd session, 1976).
U.S. Congress, House of Representatives. *Conference Report on the Health Professions Education Amendments of 1977* (Report no. 95-828, 95th Congress, 1st session, 1977).
U.S. Department of Health, Education, and Welfare. *A Conceptual Model of Organized Primary Care and Comprehensive Community Health Services*. Rockville, Md.: Community Health Service, 1970.
U.S. Department of Health, Education, and Welfare. *Forward Plan for Health: FY 1977-81*
    (Publication no. OS 76-50024). Washington, D.C.: HEW, 1975a.
U.S. Department of Health, Education, and Welfare. *National Health Systems in Eight Countries* (Publication no. SSA 75-11924). Washington, D.C.: HEW, 1975b.
U.S. Department of Health, Education, and Welfare. *Health: United States, 1975* (Publication no. HRA 76-1232). Washington, D.C.: HEW, 1976a.
U.S. Department of Health, Education, and Welfare. *The Nation's Use of Health Resources*
    (Publication no. HRA 77-1240). Washington, D.C.: HEW, 1976b.
U.S. Department of Health, Education, and Welfare. *Papers on the National Health Guide-*

lines: Baselines for Setting Health Care Goals and Standards (Publication no. HRA 77-640). Washington, D.C.: HEW, 1977.

Vladeck, B. C. "Interest-Group Representation and the HSAs: Health Planning and Political Theory." *American Journal of Public Health* 67 (January 1977): 23-29.

Weisbrod, B. A. "Research in Health Economics: A Survey." *International Journal of Health Services* 5 (1975): 643-61.

White, K. L. "The Ecology of Medical Care." *New England Journal of Medicine* 265 (November 2, 1961): 885-92.

Williams, L. P. *How to Avoid Unnecessary Surgery.* Los Angeles: Nash, 1971.

12

The Limits of Modern Medicine

Selection by Rick Carlson

Voltaire suggested that "the efficient physician is the man who successfully amuses his patient while nature effects a cure."

Medicine is a conundrum to those who have not had medical training. Three characteristics of medical practice are particularly perplexing to the uninitiated.

First, determinations of the quality of care are made without reference to the actual outcomes of care to the patient. To use a homely example, most of us judge a restaurant on the basis of the taste and quality of the food. Seldom do we inquire as to the chef's lineage or education, or visit the kitchen to inspect the ovens and utensils. The quality of means and the results of health care are matters of different importance and magnitude, but the analogy fits. Unlike the quality of food, the regulatory measures traditionally employed to control the quality of medical care have focused on who renders it and how, more often than on what the results have been.

There is one notable exception, although Florence Nightingale should get similar kudos. In the early 1900s, Dr. E. A. Codman, a surgeon at Massachusetts General Hospital, sought to orient assessment of the quality of medical care from structural or input evaluation—who did it—to process and end-result evaluation—how and why (see Codman, 1914). But first he had to find out what was going on. He started by monitoring 692 hospitals of 100 or more beds. The results revealed shockingly low quality of care; only 89 of the 692 hospitals could

Reprinted by permission from "The Impact of Medicine," *The End of Medicine* (New York: John Wiley & Sons, 1975), pp. 6-29.

meet the standards established for the study. Limited circulation of the results aroused so much controversy that Codman could not at first get his findings published and then could not find sponsors for further research.

Codman's approach was radical and would still be viewed that way today. He argued that patients should be required to pay only for good results, and that people should be aware of the results of their care. This is a slight variation on the practice in Babylon of severing the physician's hand if he failed to cure. Codman practiced his beliefs. He published annual reports that documented the results of his care and his methods of accounting for the results. For example, of the 337 cases he treated between 1911 and 1917, Dr. Codman concluded that 183 (or 54 percent) were managed without undue complications. For the remaining 154 cases that were not satisfactorily managed in his judgment, 204 separate judgments were made to determine why problems arose. In most cases (roughly 76 percent), the problems were found to be due to errors in physician care, including surgical misjudgment, use of faulty equipment, or misdiagnosis.

Second, and more puzzling than the failure of the medical care enterprise to examine its results, is the paucity of research on the impact of care on the health of populations. Controlled clinical trials have been used to measure the impact of medical cures for individual patients. But, historically, with the surrender of medicine to the scientific method, "population" medicine was relegated to the schools of public health, while medicine went to work on the individual. Consequently, we know something about medicine's impact on individual patients but very little about the impact of medical care on populations.

Third, there is even less research on the *relative* impact of personal medical care services and other socioenvironmental factors such as education, housing, air, water, seat belts, and Muzak. In other words, other than some anecdotal and impressionistic evidence, we have virtually no information on the relative weight to assign to the various factors that bear on health, including medical care. In part, this is due to the confusion of medical care with health.

This chapter takes up the impact question. First, evidence about the outcomes of medical care, when it is presumed to be efficacious, is examined. Then the obverse is examined—when the outcomes are adverse as a result of iatrogenesis, or disease "caused" by the medical care system itself. Next, the placebo effect is assessed, followed by a discussion of the importance of caring. The balance of the chapter examines the slender research on the impact of medical care on the health of populations and concludes with a review of the even more sparse work on the relative impact of medical care and other factors on health.

To grapple with this subject, the following definitions developed by the World Health Organization can be used. "Efficacy" is the benefit or utility to the individual of the service, treatment regimen, drug, or preventive or control measures advocated or applied. "Effectiveness" is the effect of the activity and the end results, outcome, or benefits for the population achieved in relation to the stated objectives. "Efficiency" is the efforts or end results achieved in relation to the effort expended in terms of money, resources, and time.

THE IMPACT OF MEDICAL CARE ON PATIENTS

The Outcomes of Medical Care

There is mounting evidence that the quality of medical care is uneven. There is also evidence that it is poor in a surprisingly high number of instances. But we lack a comprehensive body of research. The Center for the Study of Responsive Law incorporated much of the research that has been done in its publication, *One Life–One Physician* (McCleery et al., 1971).

One illustration in the book is the work of Dr. Charles E. Lewis, then of the Harvard Center for Community Health and Medical Care, now at UCLA. Dr. Lewis reviewed the records of the Kansas Blue Cross Association over a one-year period (only two hospitals in the state failed to participate in the review). He tabulated the number of elective operations for removal of tonsils, hemorrhoids, and varicose veins, and the operations for hernia repair, in all the hospitals in each of the state's eleven regions. Variations for the average rate of these four elective surgical procedures ranged from a low of 75 operations per 10,000 persons in one region to a high of 240 operations per 10,000 persons in another. Striking variations were also found between regions within each elective surgical category. The high and low regional incidences (rounded off) per 10,000 persons were: for tonsillectomy, 153 and 432; for hemorrhoidectomy, 11 and 35; for varicose veins, 3 and 7; and for hernia repair, 18 and 43 (Lewis, 1969).

Some of this variation can be explained by differences in patient income, disease incidence, number of physicians, and so forth. There is little doubt, however, that part of the variation is due to the relationship between the medical care provided and the number and type of providers providing it. This relationship can be illustrated by looking at rates of surgery. In the United States, there are twice as many surgeons in proportion to population as in England and Wales. And there is twice as much surgery in the United States as in England and Wales (Bunker, 1970).

Another major study, the National Halothane Study, after adjusting for age, sex, year, diagnosis, physical status, and previous operations, revealed three-fold variations in postoperative mortality among thirty-four distinguished teaching hospitals (Moses and Mosteller, 1956). Despite this variation in mortality—a very real matter—physicians generally refuse to tell patients about to undergo surgery what anesthesia will be used and what the hospital's track record is in patient recovery. If the results of the Halothane study are accurate, many patients are rolling dice with their lives when they seek care.

Other evidence included in *One Life–One Physician* is equally unsavory. In general, the research shows that the quality of medical care varies greatly; many instances of poor care can be found. The data are also remarkable in light of the presuppositions most consumers hold about the quality and reliability of medical care. There is a limitation, however. Most of the studies in the report judge the quality of care by examining the "processes" of care rather than "outcomes" of care. In other words, the "manner" in which care was provided is the focus of most of the studies, rather than the actual "outcomes" of care.

There are few studies on "outcomes." One of the few studies in this emerging area of investigation was conducted by Robert H. Brook et al. (1973). The outcomes for 141 emergency room patients were examined. Initially, only 94 of the 141 patients completed the battery of studies based on diagnostic X-rays; 77 (or 55 percent) received an adequate work-up based on the intern's diagnostic impression; but only 37 of 98 patients, having received diagnostic X-ray examinations, were informed whether the findings were normal or abnormal; and only 14 of the 38 patients with abnormal X-ray results (or 37 percent) appeared to have received adequate therapy for the conditions indicated. Thus, the study resulted in effective medical care for only 38 patients (or 27 percent). Ineffective care was given to 84 patients (or 60 percent). Neither effective nor ineffective care was given to 19 patients, or the remaining 13 percent.

The study was not conducted in a small rural hospital, nor in the inadequate and shabby facilities often found in major public hospitals. It was conducted in the Baltimore City Hospital emergency room, where it was assumed that the competence and efficiency of the house staff would be optimal.* In terms of staffing ratios, quality of patient care, and evaluation efforts, the assumption was that the Baltimore City Hospital emergency room was the equal of any facility in the city of Baltimore, and perhaps of any in the United States.

At the time of the study, Dr. Brook was a postdoctoral student at Johns Hopkins School of Medicine. Although few doubts were expressed by his superiors about his methodology, the uncritical assumption was that the findings of the study were characteristic of City Hospital, a less prestigious institution than Johns Hopkins. The challenge proved too much for Brook; his next target was the emergency room at Johns Hopkins. Using essentially the same methodology, Brook's work revealed that only 28 percent of 166 patients with gastrointestinal symptoms were given acceptable care, 2 percent less than in the City Hospital (see Brook, 1973). It is a credit to the gentility of Johns Hopkins (or perhaps its relief) that Dr. Brook was graduated shortly thereafter.

In an unpublished study for the National Academy of Sciences, David Kessner, M.D., used "tracer" methods to follow the treatment of one disease condition through the treatment system. His results were not unlike Brook's. He found that treatment was very checkered. And, although he has refrained from generalizing about his results, that is, from drawing inferences about medical

*Ninety to 95 percent of the medical resident staff at that time were affiliated with the highly regarded Johns Hopkins University School of Medicine, and were graduates of American medical schools.

care in general from treatment of the "tracer" condition, generalization seems warranted. John Williamson (1971) employed predictive techniques to assess the physician's skill at relating the processes used to the outcomes of care to the patient. The findings do not foster an image of the physician as seer. Still other significant studies have been undertaken by Mildred Morehead, Barbara Starfield, Laurence Weed, and others (see, for example, Trussel et al., 1972; Starfield and Scheff, 1972). The sobering conclusion is that medicine is not the well-honed instrument it is generally thought to be. Inevitable human error abounds, and this is understandable. Less understandable is medicine's persistent refusal to examine *what* it does for the patient in relation to the result to the patient.

Iatrogenesis: How Patients Get More Than They Bargained For

Every August more tonsils are removed than in any other month of the year. There are a number of reasons why this occurs, but a principal one is that the physicians need to keep busy. Tonsillectomy is the most common surgical procedure performed in Western civilization (National Center for Health Statistics, 1968). The procedure is used for various conditions for which removal of the tonsils appears to be the cure; unfortunately, tonsillectomy often seems to be a ritual. According to Dr. A. Frederick North, Jr., visiting professor of pediatrics at the University of Pittsburgh, "Ninety to ninety-five percent [of the procedures] are unnecessary" (*Christian Science Monitor* 138, p. 98). In a recent study, existing data on the performance of tonsillectomy were scrutinized. No compelling evidence of any long-term benefits was discovered (see Evans, 1968). Under the most favorable conditions, no more than 2 to 3 percent of children require tonsillectomy. Nevertheless, recent data reflect that, in most communities, approximately 20 to 30 percent have their tonsils removed (National Center for Health Statistics, 1968).

A more important issue is what possible risks and dangers are experienced by those who undergo surgery. The mortality rate is low, about 1:1000 patients. Nonetheless, because of the volume of cases, tonsillectomies account for 100 to 300 deaths annually in the United States. Serious complications occur in 15.6:1000 cases per year. Finally, there is some evidence that removal of the tonsils results in the loss to the patient of an invaluable "immunity" mechanism, possibly linked to increased risk of Hodgkin's disease and bulbar poliomyelitis (see Ogra, 1971).

But the most important complications may be emotional. The young tonsillectomy candidate, perhaps five or six years of age, is made captive in a hospital, separated from his or her parents, and surrounded by mysterious figures in white coats. The emotional harm is demonstrable, and the palliative ice cream at the end of surgery hardly compensates. The psychiatric literature contains evidence that childhood tonsillectomy often has profound irreversible and lifelong repercussions (see, for example, Lipton, 1962).

Children's tonsils are not the only targets. Normal ovaries are also often needlessly removed. There is an extensive literature on this subject, most of which has been ignored by practitioners. Two studies are illustrative. The subtitle of the first speaks for itself: "A Study Based on Removal of 704 Normal Ovaries from 546 Patients." (One wonders which of the women lost more than one normal ovary.) In the second study, the investigators established surgical justification based on postoperative or pathological examination in only 54.9 percent of 6,960 cases (Doyle, 1952, 1963).

Still other patients suffer injuries through the administration of drugs or the use of procedures which have unanticipated side effects. Classic examples of calamities in medicine have been the loss or impaired hearing of some patients given chloramphenicol, and the wrenching results of the use of thalidomide.* Moreover, infections contracted in hospitals exceed the rate in the average household, despite elaborate safety and hygiene measures. They include postoperative pulmonary infections, wound infections, burn infections, and tracheotomy infections, to name a few.

Catastrophes occur outside the hospital as well. Some recently concluded research links the deaths of thousands of asthmatics to the inhalation of isoprotermol, a medication for the treatment of asthma, which can be purchased either with a prescription or over the counter. Dr. Paul Stolley of the School of Hygiene and Public Health at Johns Hopkins University, in reviewing research on the question, remarked, "It's the most tragic drug disaster on record. There's nothing else—even thalidomide—that ranks with it" (*Minneapolis Tribune,* October 16, 1972). The physicians who prescribed the drug and the drug company that marketed it undoubtedly expected the drug to relieve a common ailment. But that is not what happened. In England, the deaths of approximately 3,500 asthmatics have been traced to its use.

Adverse results from tonsillectomies and hysterectomies, and infections are the most common iatrogenic phenomena, but there are others. Seymour Handler (1971), in his article, "Bring Back the Mustard Plaster," lists some others. One of the worst dangers for the unsuspecting patient is chemotherapy. Handler includes a table in his article matching modern medicinals with diseases that drugs can introduce:

Drug	Disease
Enteric coated KCI	Small intestine stenotric ulcers
Methysergide	Retroperitoneal fibrosis
Warfarin	Intramural intestinal hemorrhage
Tetracycline	Pediatric tooth discoloration

*In the case of chloramphenicol, routine oral use results in 1:10,000 deaths from anemia. Despite this fact the drug is still prescribed. See California State Department of Public Health, Senate Committee, "Fatal Aplastic Anemia in California, Its Relationship to the Drug Chloramphenicol," November 23, 1962.

Drug	Disease
Nitrofurantoin	Pulmonary infligrates
Long-acting sulfonamides	Stevens-Johnson syndrome
Hydralizine, procainamide	Lopus enythematosus

This list is remindful of Immanuel Kant's observation that "Physicians think they are doing something for you by labeling what you have as a disease." Other iatrogenic procedures and practices listed by Handler include poly-pharmacy, the overprescribing of drugs for some patients. Charlotte Muller (1972), a professor of urban studies at City University of New York, has extensively studied drug prescribing and use patterns. She documents the staggering degree of overmedication, and concludes that it is "one source of reduced human welfare." Handler adds that the diagnosis of "nondisease" or, in other words, the erroneous determination by the physician that a disease is present when it is not, often results in needless restrictions to patients. Damage arising both from faulty diagnostic and therapeutic procedures is another example. Handler also spotlights a new and fascinating problem, psychosemantics, a congeries of anxieties induced in patients by what a physician says or implies (for a comprehensive treatment, see Moser, 1969).

John Pekkanen (1973) examined the links between the pharmaceutical industry and medicine in his book, *The American Connection*. Pekkanen examines drug advertisements addressed to physicians in widely read and respected journals such as the *New England Journal of Medicine* and the *Journal of the American Medical Association*. Amphetamines, tranquilizers like Valium and Librium, are the big sellers. New drugs are introduced to the market with an advertising barrage focused on the physician. Doctors are literally inundated by pharmaceuticals and pharmaceutical ads. Their journals, even the more popular ones like *Medical Economics* and *Medical World News,* are filled with them. Doctors' offices and probably their homes are well stocked with drugs, many proffered free by pharmaceutical companies. And then there are the grinning drug pushers —the detailers of the major pharmaceuticals. Since doctors do not have the time to educate themselves about most drugs, they frequently look to the detailer for their information. Pekkanen (1973, pp. 84-85) puts it this way:

Contrary to their accepted image and contrary to what the public rightly expects, doctors often know very little about the drugs they are prescribing. Too often all they know is precisely what the drug companies want them to know. . . . He relies on the detail men, those ambassadors of good will from the industry. . .

There are unquestionably effective drugs, effectively prescribed. But there are also drugs like isoproternal and thalidomide that kill and maim. There are drugs that dull, like tranquilizers, and others that speed up, like the friendly amphetamine family. Doctors who seek to calm the frenzied patient with tranquilizers and to bolster the will of the overweight patient with amphetamines are not necessarily harming the patients. But physicians who maintain a patient on drugs because they are unwilling to consider alternatives may be.

Iatrogenesis is a larger problem than malpractice. There is ample evidence of malpractice—that is, error due to simple negligence. A study completed in 1973 shows that, conservatively, 7 percent of all patients suffer compensable injuries while hospitalized, but few of these patients do anything about it (U.S. Department of Health, Education, and Welfare, 1973). The word "iatrogenesis" was coined to refer to damage caused by the medical care system itself, often unanticipated, but including more than that arising out of the negligence of practitioners. Infections, overmedication, removal of healthy organs are all included, but a more penetrating example is the diagnosis and treatment of "nondisease."

Among the more common errors made in medicine is diagnostic error. The assumption is that the error arises from a false diagnosis, or from a failure to diagnose. But error also arises when a problem is diagnosed that does not exist. Heart murmurs can be "detected" in up to one-half of a given sample of children. For example, in one investigation, 44.4 percent of 4,039 Nashville schoolchildren had "innocent" murmurs (Quinn and Campbell, 1962). Unfortunately, heart "murmur" is often confused with heart "disease." In a study of 20,800 Seattle schoolchildren, 93 were identified as having heart disease or rheumatic fever. On closer examination, heart disease was discovered in only 18 percent of the 93. Of the remainder—those who did not have any heart abnormality—40 percent or 30 children were "restricted" in their activities. Six of them were severely restricted, ostensibly because they had heart disease. Most of the restrictions were imposed by physicians, but parental zeal was a contributing factor. In this case, therefore, the amount of disability resulting from nondisease *exceeded* the disability due to actual heart disease. Medicine caused more disability than it cured (Bergman and Stamm, 1967).

Damage is done and disease caused by the medical care system for a number of reasons. There is no malice on the part of practitioners or administrators. The medical care system is subject to the same foibles, imperfections, and inefficiencies that plague all large institutions. One of the major differences, however, between the medical care system and many other large institutions lies in its capacity to do harm. An unavoidable conclusion is that the way in which our medical care system has evolved has created conditions that increase the likelihood of damage to patients (for a good treatment of this point, see Andy, 1970).

In *Medical Nemesis,* Ivan Illich (1974) takes the argument to near extremes. He argues that medicine unquestionably injures more than it cures—not just through crude technology, but essentially because it has stripped patients of the tools to take care of themselves. Illich refers to this as "social iatrogenesis."

A medicine trapped in the logic of intervention with elimination of symptoms as its principal objective may act too hastily when the elimination of symptoms appears expedient, may ignore potentially untoward by-products of the means used to treat those symptoms, and, most deplorably, may fail to comprehend the lesson that thousands of deaths represent.

The Placebo: How Patients Get Less Than They Bargained For

The placebo has a long and respected history. The use of chemically inert medications is common practice. In fact, until the last few decades, most medicinals were pharmacologically inert, and, in that sense, the "history of medical treatment until relatively recently is the history of the placebo effect" (see Shapiro, 1959; Evans, 1974). But there is more to the placebo than pills. For example, one use of the placebo is in the treatment of warts. The healer paints the wart with a brightly colored but inert dye and instructs the patient that when the color has worn off, the wart will disappear. It works as often as any other treatment, including surgery.

Shamans and shamanistic ritual can be traced throughout history. Contemporary analysts often discount shamans as healers because of their alleged use of chicanery. For example, a common technique among shamans is the use of blood-stained down, which is expelled from the mouth after "treatment." In many instances, no human tissue was or could have been extracted to "produce" the expectorate. But this is beside the point; since its importance was symbolic, this use of down is no different from the prescription of null medications. Jerome Frank (1961, p. 66), a psychiatrist at Johns Hopkins who has extensively examined the use of placebos, says of it:

The most likely supposition is that it gains its potency through being a tangible symbol of the physician's role as a healer. In our society, the physician validates his power by prescribing medication, just as a shaman in a primitive tribe may validate his by spitting out a bit of bloodstained down at the proper moment.

The placebo may be far more than a symbol. The expectations of some patients about a treatment can alter or even reverse the action of a pharmacological agent. Frank (1961, p. 67) recounts an experiment in which patients subjected to an emetic, an agent designed to cause convulsive stomach contractions and regurgitation, were told that their stomachs would not become upset. The subjects did indeed overcome the drug—they experienced no stomach discomfort.

When disease has a clear emotional base, the effectiveness of the placebo appears to be enhanced. In one study, patients with bleeding peptic ulcers were given a placebo but informed that it was a powerful and effective drug. Other patients were given the same agent but were advised that it was a new and promising experimental drug of undetermined effectiveness. The first group scored 75 percent in their remission rate; the second only 25 percent (Folgyesi, 1954).

The effectiveness of the placebo is not entirely understood, although it appears to be related to the "belief" of the patient in its efficacy. Thoughtful observers, like Frank, think there is more to it. The healer as well as the patient must believe in the efficacy of the treatment, or at least skillfully convey a state of belief to the patient. As Frank (1961, p. 70) puts it:

If the effectiveness of the placebo lies in its ability to mobilize the patient's expectancy of help, then it should work best with those patients who have favorable expectations from medicine and, in general, accept and respond to symbols of healing.

To some patients the healer may be the most effective placebo. The placebo, whether a drug or some other treatment, may serve only as a material symbol of the healer's power.

The placebo effect demonstrates that medicine can cure some patients through its symbolic presence, simply by being there. But at what cost? If cures can be achieved by a fusion of the patient's belief in the treatment and the manifestation of symbols of healing, we must ask if it is possible to use equally effective but less expensive symbols.

Caring: How Patients Get Something But Not Necessarily What They Pay For

It is easy to be too scientific in condemning medicine. For centuries healers have administered to patients, with little impact if measured by the test of effectiveness. Until recently, medicine had few weapons. But medicine worked in the past and still works today, although with mixed results. Medicine has effective technologies—technologies that link what the physician does with what happens to the patient. But healing also occurs without sophisticated technology. A major ingredient has been "caring."

A number of research studies have assessed the Hawthorne effect. Most of the research was designed to ascertain optimal conditions for the production of goods. But the investigators discovered an anomaly—whatever they did, production improved. The conclusion was inescapable. When workers believed that management cared, whether by increasing or decreasing the lighting, for example, they tried harder. (For a comprehensive and critical assessment of the research on the "Hawthorne effect," see Landsberger, 1958.) Of course, there are limits; increasing the temperature in an office to an intolerable level may not be viewed as caring. But the point is well-established—"caring" motivates workers. It motivates patients as well. In fact, it may be a determinative factor in healing. Some patients given placebos respond better to the null "treatment" than those given active drugs. In some studies, groups of patients given placebos had better treatment outcomes than groups treated with active medications.

Again Jerome Frank's analysis is pertinent. The symbols of healing, unadorned with any proven technology, can cure. One of the dangers, then, of too rigorous an examination of medicine—requiring proof beyond a reasonable doubt—is that caring might be lost in the process.

THE IMPACT OF MEDICAL CARE ON HEALTH STATUS

At the turn of the nineteenth century, an observer described medical care in a way that still fits: "There is a great difference between a good physician and a bad one; yet very little between a good one and none at all" (Arthur Young, quoted in Handler, 1971, p. 973). Available evidence and underlying theory both indicate that medical care has considerably less impact on health than is generally assumed. Medical care is effective when applied to certain illnesses. In procedures such as reduction of fractures; treatment of infectious diseases such as diphtheria, tetanus, poliomyelitis, and tuberculosis; and surgery for removal of pathenogenic organs, the physician truly heals. Medical care also heals when it utilizes therapies with which it has been entrusted. Penicillin, sulfa drugs, and antibiotics have expanded the capacity of the medical care system to treat and heal. But there remains much that medicine cannot do. Lewis Thomas (1973), former Dean of the Yale University Medical School and now at the Sloan-Kettering Institute, says:

The genuinely decisive technology of modern medicine is exemplified best by methods for immunization against diphtheria, pertussis, and various virus diseases and the contemporary use of antibiotics and chemotherapy for bacterial infections. The capacity to deal effectively with syphilis and tuberculosis represents a milestone in human endeavor, even though full use of this potential has not yet been made. And there are, of course, other examples: the treatment of endocrinologic disorders with appropriate hormones, the prevention of hemolytic disease of the newborn, the treatment and prevention of various nutritional disorders, and perhaps just around the corner, the management of Parkinsonism and sickle-cell anemia. There are other examples, and everyone will have his favorite candidate for the list, *but the truth is that there are not nearly as many as the public has been led to believe. . . .*

It is commonly understood that medical care cannot cure cardiovascular disease, most cancers, arthritis, multiple sclerosis, stroke, advanced cirrhosis, and the common cold, to name a few. Of course, there are some exceptions. The Papanicolaou test for cervical cancer has proven utility (but see Cochrane, 1972), and the means have been found to treat some forms of skin cancer. But cancers and heart disease cannot presently be cured.

Paradoxically, some diseases that are both preventable and treatable continue to strike large numbers of people. Allen Chase (1972) in *The Biological Imperatives* lists a number of preventable diseases which either kill or debilitate large numbers of people simply because resources have not been allocated to their control. Included are hookworm disease, which afflicts approximately 600 million people; ascariasis, another worm infestation; schistosomiasis; trachoma, which causes irreversible blindness; and endemic goiter. The fact that most of these diseases are rampant in underdeveloped areas does not make them irrelevant.

Even in the United States there are diseases that could be more effectively treated, or possibly even prevented. An example is illness affecting the digestive system. According to Dr. J. Edward Berk, Chairman of the Department of Medicine at the University of California at Irvine, more than half of the population of the United States registers frequent complaints about digestion. Roughly 15 to 20 percent of all illnesses reported afflict the digestive tract—the stomach, intestines, biliary passages, liver, and pancreas (*Los Angeles Times,* November 6, 1972). The data are probably understated. Because of nonspecific symptoms, many cases of peptic ulcer and gallstones, for example, remain undetected. Nevertheless, digestive disease ranks second only to circulatory disorders as a cause of workdays lost per year. It ranks first as a cause of hospitalization (unpublished data, National Center for Health Statistics). Although digestive disease causes this much sickness, the number of gastroenterologists is inadequate, according to Dr. Berk. And research funds are disproportionately spent in other areas, particularly those that have strong lobbies, such as cystic fibrosis and muscular dystrophy.

Despite its limitations and despite its questionable priorities, the medical care system continues to grow and consume more and more resources. This is partly because we do not yet know enough about medicine's effectiveness. But we know some things—we are just beginning to ask the right questions. Some of the most trenchant thinking about the effectiveness of medical care has been done by A. L. Cochrane (1972) in his assessment of the British National Health Service. In *Effectiveness and Efficiency,* Cochrane concludes that the National Health Service has had little to do with improving mortality and morbidity rates. He acknowledges the effectiveness of some medications for some conditions; strikes a loud note for preventive measures such as immunization and curtailment of population growth and cigarette smoking; expresses doubt about some tried and true measures, including the pap smear and the coronary care unit; and, almost hesitatingly, argues that further development of medical therapies should be deferred until definitive proof of their effectiveness is available. To read Cochrane is to conclude with him that little of medical care is effective and that health will never be the exclusive product of medical care—there are too many other factors.

When somebody gets the flu, the advice given by both the professional practitioner and the amateur diagnostician is the same—wait it out. A great deal of disease is self-limiting.* The human body, for reasons that are not completely understood, strives for equilibrium. This is the result of selective evolutionary pressures, which cut both ways. First, man can develop resistance to many diseases.† Tuberculosis is an example. But, mysteriously, some diseases never strike

---

*One major study, for example, followed 176 cases of confirmed cancer that regressed without treatment. See Eversa and Cole (1966).

†See, for example, McKeown (1971), who traces the rise and fall of disease conditions as they are influenced by social and environmental factors.

some cultures at all. Several researchers have established the rarity of cancers, vascular disorders, and other degenerative diseases among primitive populations. Disease patterns vary greatly around the world. Unique geographical and cultural factors affect both the incidence and control of certain diseases.

In recent history, human beings adapted to new environmental conditions. In the nineteenth century, at the height of the Industrial Revolution, thousands of migrants were compressed into urban industrial sinks. Sickness and death resulted. But despite the human loss, enormous in some cases, people in most affluent countries have adapted to urban conditions (and, of course, the conditions have been improved as well). To use a concrete example, the devastating disease known as "consumption" in the nineteenth century is now understood to have been pulmonary tuberculosis. Although the virulence of the bacilli is as great now as it was then, our adaptive response has come to blunt its severity. In short, both the types of disease and the patterns of disease reflect prevalent conditions in a given culture. To quote René Dubos (1968, p. 78):

Without question, nutritional and infectious diseases account for the largest percentage of morbidity and mortality in most underprivileged countries, especially in those just becoming industrialized. Undernutrition, protein deficiency, malaria, tuberculosis, infestation with worms, and a host of ill-defined gastrointestinal disorders are today the greatest killers in these countries, just as they used to be in the Western world one century ago. In contrast, the toll taken by malnutrition and infection decreases rapidly wherever and whenever the living standards improve, but other diseases then become more prevalent. In prosperous countries at the present time, heart diseases constitute the leading cause of death, with cancers in the second place, vascular lesions affecting the central nervous system in the third, and accidents in the fourth. Increasingly also, persons who are well fed and well sheltered suffer from a variety of chronic disorders, such as arthritis and allergies, that do not destroy life but often ruin it.

The insignificance of medical care in improving health status cannot be overemphasized. Increased longevity, reductions in maternal and infant mortality, and other related improvements are not owed to medicine. Diseases associated with industrialization—largely infectious disorders—were tamed in developed cultures. The result was a steady improvement in health. But no new gains have been reported. If anything, due to our incapacity to adjust to the stresses of postindustrial society, health status is tapering. John Powles (1973), in a paper on the ebbs and flows in health and disease patterns, summarizes the point:

Industrial populations owe their current health standards to a pattern of ecological relationships which serves to reduce their vulnerability to death from infection and to a lesser extent to the capabilities of clinical medicine. Unfortunately, this new way of life, because it is so far removed from that to which man is adapted by evolution, has produced its own disease burden. These diseases of maladaption are, in many cases, increasing.

Social factors are even more underrated than the environment. John Cassel (1972), a noted epidemiologist at the University of North Carolina, has argued for more research focused on the relationship between disease rates and social phenomena such as industrialization, stress, and congestion. He points to the major shifts in disease patterns which have been portrayed and concludes: "Despite intensive research, the explanation for the genesis of these changes in disease patterns have proved so far to be relatively unsatisfactory."

The Comparative Impact of Other Factors on Health Status

It is a sad commentary on biomedical research that more attention has not been given to the *relative* impact on health of many variables, including medical care. It is generally agreed that contaminated food, degraded air and water, garbage and filth, and drafty, cold housing can cause illness. But the assumption has not been pinned down by research. Consequently, a reallocation of resources has not been undertaken. But there has been some work.

Economists have contributed more than their share. A 1969 study focused on the "production function" in health—its effectiveness in terms of what it is supposed to do. The study revealed that factors associated with income and education have a significant impact on health status (Auster, Leveson, and Sarachek, 1969; see also Fuchs, 1966). The wealthier and more educated a person is, the healthier he is likely to be. Table 12.1 illustrates the relationship between family income and health status. The effect of education on health was illustrated by a National Bureau of Economic Research study that examined interstate differen-

TABLE 12.1

HEALTH STATUS BY FAMILY INCOME—PERSONS AGED 45-64

Family income	Restricted activity days per person per year	Bed disability days per person per year	Work loss days among currently employed persons per person per year	Percentage of persons with one or more chronic conditions	
				Limitation in amount or kind of major activity	Unable to carry on major activity
Under $3000	38.6	12.9	9.9	22.7	7.4
$3000-$3999	24.5	7.5	7.7	14.9	3.7
$4000-$6999	20.0	6.2	7.7	10.4	2.1
$7000-$9999	17.4	5.5	5.8	7.7	1.1
$10,000 and over	15.4	5.2	5.4	5.9	0.8

Source: U.S. Department of Health, Education, and Welfare, Public Health Service, *Age Patterns in Medical Care, Illness, and Disability, United States—July, 1963-June, 1965.* Series 10, no. 32, National Center for Health Statistics (Washington, D.C.: HEW, 1966).

tial and age-adjusted death rates. One finding was that as large a reduction in mortality is associated with the expenditure of one more dollar for education as an additional dollar spent on medical care (Fuchs, 1968). These findings have been dramatically corroborated by the Institute of Medicine of the National Academy of Sciences in a study that used anemia as a "tracer" condition (a disease "followed" through the medical care system to examine its detection and treatment in order to generalize about the detection and treatment of other conditions). The study demonstrated that the education level of the patients was more highly correlated with health than with the source of medical care (*Drug Research Reports,* 1972). The study has to be read carefully—all it demonstrated is that education is a proxy for health; it correlates with health, but does not necessarily cause it.

Another economist, Charles T. Stewart, Jr., has examined the relative importance of different allocations of resources to health. In comparing treatment, prevention, information, and research, he found that both literacy (as a proxy for information) and potable water (as a proxy for prevention) had high impacts on life expectancy in all nations in the Western hemisphere. Neither research nor treatment were significantly correlated. The data showed virtually the same results for the United States alone (Stewart, 1971).

Finally, the economist Eli Ginzberg (1969), in *Men, Money, and Medicine,* discussed the impact of nutrition on both physical and mental health. Ginzberg approvingly quotes an earlier report stressing the importance of nutrition for physical development:

a diversified enriched diet will probably contribute to the health of the population . . . more than any other specific addition to medical resources, such as an increase in the number of doctors or the number of hospital beds. (*Journal of the Mount Sinai Hospital of New York,* 1953)

But Ginzberg points out, paradoxically, that "for the first time in our history more people die prematurely because they eat too much than too little" (1969, p. 23). This irony is reflected in other research as well. Victor Fuchs (1973), in an unpublished paper, points out that affluence frequently leads to excessive consumption, even engorgement of some goods, such as rich foods, that adversely affect health. Morbidity data reflect this well; the least healthy members of our population are white males over 55, the population cohort most likely to overconsume, overwork, and underrest.

A link between nutrition and health has also been established by studies contrasting the impact on health of nutrition and medical care. The sites were poor villages in the underdeveloped world. In one village, only improved medical care was introduced; in another, only nutrition was enriched; in a third, both medical care and diet were enhanced. The results show that nutrition was far more significant in improving health than the provision of medical care (Taylor and Scrimshaw, 1968).

Little cost-benefit or cost-effective research has been focused on the medical care system. (What little work there is was reviewed by Grosse, 1972.) A few studies have assessed the relative benefits of selective disease control programs and maternal and child health care programs. In both cases the results, while tentative and crude, tend to prove the worth of certain disease detection programs. In general, programs that provide increased services for mothers and children in areas that have traditionally had few medical services have the greatest payoff. But, despite this, few low-cost, high-benefit programs have been established. Fluoridation programs, which are relatively inexpensive, produce benefits (in terms of reduced numbers of cavities) in more than 300,000 children for an expenditure of $10 million. Treatment-oriented programs for the same amount of money potentially benefit only 18,000 to 44,000 children (Grosse, 1972, p. 98).

Little evidence of impact of mental health services exists. No cure is known for schizophrenia, the most prevalent psychosis, although proponents of megavitamin treatment profess to have had some success. The use of tranquilizers and shock therapy has also had some impact on reducing hospitalization rates. But rehospitalization rates are no better than with other therapies (see, for example, Tuma and Tuma, 1965). There are also claims for the effective treatment of depression. The overall record is mixed at best.

There is, however, some evidence that social and environmental factors may play a role. In *Mental Health,* a series of epidemiologic studies are reviewed (U.S. Department of Health, Education, and Welfare, 1969, pp. 193-97). The factors purportedly related to mental health included poor housing, congestion, poverty, and nutritional deficiencies. Although not all the studies confirm the hypothesis of the authors, the conclusion is reached that two of the studies "suggest strongly that improvement in social environment probably does have a favorable effect on mental health" (p. 195).

There is a hard issue here. The fact that treatment is emphasized over prevention is not entirely the fault of medicine. In the case of maternal and child health, flouridation programs, and other similar programs, the choice of whether to fund or not to fund is a political decision. In this sense the choice of treatment over prevention can be said to be a choice made by the public. But, given the power and mystique of medicine, it is also true that the public's choices about health matters are strongly influenced by physicians and, to a lesser extent, other health professionals. Medicine has chosen treatment over prevention, and it continues to defend its choice. Prevention programs are starved at least in part because medicine wants too much of the loaf. But the problem cannot be camouflaged by making medicine the only villain. Prevention programs are also starved because medical care is often a "life and death" matter. No arguments and no logic will convince terrified parents that the resources needed to treat their child would be more rationally allocated to prevention. This is a major reason why prevention programs are crippled. Medicine could do far more to inform public opinion, but the problem would remain. This is why I argue that our basic conceptions about health must change if medicine is to change. The public's value preferences are real; only when those value preferences change will medicine change.

In combination, then, the empirical evidence and the theory seem convincing; medical care has a limited impact on health and is most effective when applied to certain identifiable conditions where there is evidence about its effectiveness. But when contrasted with all the other factors that demonstrably affect health, medicine plays a minor role, despite being cast for lead.

REFERENCES

Audy, J. R. "Man-Made Maladies and Medicine." *California Medicine* (November 1970): 48.

Auster, R.; Leveson, I.; and Sarachek, D. "The Production of Health; An Exploratory Study." *Journal of Human Resources* 4 (Fall 1969).

Bergman, A. B., and Stamm, S. J. "The Morbidity of Cardiac Non-Disease in Schoolchildren." *New England Journal of Medicine* 276 (May 4, 1967): 1008.

Brook, R. H., et al. "Effectiveness of Non-Emergency Care via an Emergency Room." *Annals of Internal Medicine* 78 (1973).

Bunker, J. P. "Surgical Manpower." *New England Journal of Medicine* 282 (January 15, 1970).

Cassel, J. C. "Health Consequences of Population and Crowding." Paper presented at the AMA Congress of Environmental Health, Los Angeles, 1972.

Chase, A. *The Biological Imperative.* New York: Holt, Rinehart & Winston, 1972.

Cochrane, A. L. *Effectiveness and Efficiency.* London: Nuffield Provincial Hospitals Trust, 1972.

Codman, E. A. "The Product of the Hospital." *Surgery, Gynecology and Obstetrics* 18 (1914): 491-96.

Doyle, J. C. "Unnecessary Ovariectomies." *Journal of the American Medical Association* 148 (1952).

Doyle, J. C. "Unnecessary Hysterectomies: Study of 6,248 Operations in 35 Hospitals in 1948." *Journal of the American Medical Association* 151 (1963): 360-65.

Drug Research Reports 15 (November 22, 1972): 6.

Dubos, R. *Man, Medicine and Environment.* New York: Praeger, 1968.

Evans, F. "The Power of a Sugar Pill." *Psychology Today* (April 1974).

Evans, H. E. "Tonsillectomy and Adenoidectomy: Review of Published Evidence for and against T. & A." *Clinical Pediatrics* 7 (February 1968): 71-75.

Eversa, T. D., and Cole, W. H. *Spontaneous Regression of Cancer.* Philadelphia: W. B. Saunders, 1966.

Folgyesi, F. A. "School for Patients." *British Journal of Medical Hypnotism* 5 (1954): 5.

Frank, J. *Persuasion and Healing.* New York: Schocken Books, 1961.

Fuchs, V. "The Contribution of Health Services to the American Economy." *Milbank Memorial Fund Quarterly* 44 (October 1966).

Fuchs, V. *The Service Economy.* New York: National Bureau of Economic Research, 1968.

Fuchs, V. "Some Economic Aspects of Mortality in Developed Countries." Paper presented to the International Economic Association Conference on Economics of Health and Medical Care, Tokyo, 1973.

Ginzberg, E. *Men, Money, and Medicine.* New York: Columbia University Press, 1969.

Grosse, R. N. "Cost-Benefit Analysis of Health Services." *Annals of the American Academy of Political and Social Science* 399 (January 1972): 89.

Handler, S. "Bring Back the Mustard Plaster." *Minnesota Medicine* 54 (December 1971): 973-79.

Illich, I. *Medical Nemesis.* London: Calder & Boyars, 1974.

Journal of the Mount Sinai Hospital of New York 19 (March/April 1953); 734.

Landsberger, H. A. *Hawthorne Revisited.* Ithaca, N.Y.: Cornell University Press, 1958.

Lewis, C. E. "Variations in Incidence of Surgery." *New England Journal of Medicine* 281 (October 16, 1969): 880-84.

Lipton, S. D. "On Psychology of Childhood Tonsillectomy." *Psychoanalytic Study of the Child* 17 (1962): 363-417.

McCleery, R. S., et al. *One Life–One Physician.* New York: Public Interest Press, 1971.

McKeown, T. *Time Trend Studies.* London: Oxford University Press and Nuffield Press, 1971.

Moser, R. H. *Diseases of Medical Progress: A Study of Iatrogenic Disease* (3rd ed.). Springfield, Ill.: Charles C Thomas, 1969.

Moses, L., and Mosteller, F. "Institutional Differences in Post-Operative Death Rates." *Journal of the American Medical Association* 162 (October 13, 1956).

Muller, C. "The Over-Medicated Society: Forces in the Marketplace for Medical Care." *Science* 176 (May 5, 1972): 488.

National Center for Health Statistics. *Statistics of the Bureau of Health and Vital Statistics* 7 (February 1968).

Ogra, P. L. "Effect of Tonsillectomy and Adenoidectomy on Nasopharyngeal Antibody Response to Poliovirus." *New England Journal of Medicine* 284 (January 14, 1971): 59-64.

Pekkanen, J. *The American Connection.* Chicago: Follett, 1973.

Powles, J. "On the Limitations of Modern Medicine." *Science, Medicine and Man* 1 (1973): 1-30.

Quinn, R. W., and Campbell, E. S. "Heart Disease in Children: Survey of School Children in Nashville, Tennessee." *Yale Journal of Biology and Medicine* 34 (1962): 370-85.

Shapiro, A. K. "The Placebo Effect in the History of Medical Treatment: Implications for Psychiatry." *American Journal of Psychiatry* 116 (1959): 293.

Starfield, B., and Scheff, D. "Effectiveness of Pediatric Care: The Relationship Between Process and Outcome." *Pediatrics* 49 (April 1972).

Stewart, C. T., Jr. "Allocation of Resources to Health." *Journal of Human Resources* 6 (1971): 105.

Taylor, C. E., and Scrimshaw, N. *Interactions of Nutrition and Infection.* Geneva: World Health Organization, 1968.

Thomas, L. "Guessing and Knowing." *Saturday Review* 55 (January 1973).

Trussel, R. E., et al. "A Study of the Quality of Hospital Care Secured by a Sample of Teamster Family Members in the New York Area." New York: School of Public Health and Administration Medicine, Columbia University, 1972.

Tuma, M., and Tuma, N. "Schizophrenia–An Experimental Study of Five Treatment Methods." *British Journal of Psychiatry* 111 (June 1965): 505-10.

U.S. Department of Health, Education, and Welfare. Public Health Service. *Mental Health.* Washington, D.C.: HEW, 1969.

U.S. Department of Health, Education, and Welfare. *Report of the Secretary's Commission on Medical Malpractice.* Washington, D.C.: HEW, 1973.

Williamson, J. "Evaluating Quality of Patient Care." *Journal of the American Medical Association* 218 (October 25, 1971).

Selection by Lewis Thomas

The common theme running through almost all the criticisms leveled at the American health care system these days is the charge of inadequacy or insufficiency. There are not enough doctors and nurses, and those around lack sufficient interest and compassion; there are not enough clinics, and those around lack sufficient time to see everyone; there are too few medical schools, medical centers, and specialized hospitals, with inequities in their distribution around the country; most of all, there is not enough money, not enough commitment.

And yet, the system has been expanding with explosive force in the last quarter century. It has been nothing short of a boom. In 1950, the total national expenditure in health care was estimated at $10 billion. By 1972, it had risen to over $70 billion. In 1974, it was $110 billion. This year it will at least exceed $130 billion, and it will be still larger if a national health insurance program emerges. According to some more or less official estimates it could exceed $250 billion by the 1980s.

Whatever the defects, it cannot be claimed that the nation has been failing to react. Any enterprise that amplifies itself over a twenty-five-year period in this exuberant fashion is surely making a try. It is, whatever else, a massive effort to improve.

The question is: What are we improving? What, in fact, have we been trying to accomplish with these vast sums?

An alien historian would think, from a look just at the dollar figures for

Reprinted by permission from "On the Science and Technology of Medicine," *Daedalus* (Winter 1977), pp. 35-46.

each of those years, that some sort of tremendous event must have been occurring since 1950. Either (1) the health of the nation had suddenly disintegrated, requiring the laying on of new resources to meet the crisis, or (2) the technology for handling health problems had undergone a major transformation, necessitating the installation of new effective resources to do things that could not be done before, or (3), another possibility, perhaps we had somehow been caught up in the momentum of a huge, collective, ponderous set of errors. If any of these explanations is the right one, we ought at least to become aware of it, since whatever we are improving will involve, in the near future, an even more immense new bureaucracy, an even larger commitment of public funds, regulations that will intervene in every aspect of the citizen's life, and, inevitably, still more expansion. This paper will deal with the arguments around each of these three possible explanations.

THE HEALTH OF THE NATION, 1950-1975

There is, to begin with, no real evidence that health has deteriorated in this country, certainly not to the extent indicated by the new dollars spent each year for health care. On the contrary, we seem to have gotten along reasonably well.

There is perhaps more heart disease, but this is to be expected in a generally older population living beyond the life expectancy of fifty years ago. Heart disease is, after all, one of the ways of dying, and death certificates do not usually distinguish between heart failure as the result of time having run out and other forms of heart disease, except by noting age. The total numbers have increased somewhat, and perhaps there are also somewhat more cases of coronary occlusion in middle-aged men, but we have not suddenly been plagued, just since 1950, by new heart disease in anything like frightening numbers.

Cancer, stroke, kidney disease, arthritis, schizophrenia, cirrhosis, multiple sclerosis, senility, asthma, pulmonary fibrosis, and a few other major diseases are still with us, but the change in incidence per capita is not sufficient to account for the move from a $10 billion enterprise to a $130 billion one.

Aging is not in itself a health problem, although a larger number of surviving old people obviously means proportionately more people with the disabling illnesses characteristic of the aged. However, the increased number of such patients since 1950 is not great enough to account for much of the increased investment.

Meanwhile, there has been a general improvement in the public health with respect to certain infectious diseases which were major problems in the twenty-five-year period prior to 1950. Lobar pneumonia, scarlet fever, erysipelas, rheumatic fever, subacute bacterial endocarditis, typhoid fever, poliomyelitis, diphtheria, pertussis, meningococcal meningitis, staphylococcal septicemia, all of which filled the wards of municipal and county hospitals in the earlier period, have become rarities. To be sure, new sorts of bacterial infection have appeared in hospital communities, as complications of other therapy in most instances, but the total number of these is a small figure alongside the infectious diseases of the pre-antibiotic, pre-immunization period.

On balance, then, no case can be made for a wave of new illnesses afflicting our population in the years since 1950. If anything, we are probably a somewhat healthier people because of the sharp decrease in severe infectious disease.

But this is not the general view of things: the public perception of the public health, in 1975, appears to be quite different. There is now a much more acute awareness of the risk of disease than in earlier periods, associated with a greater apprehension that a minor illness may turn suddenly into a killing disease. There is certainly a higher expectation that all kinds of disease can be treated effectively. Finally, personal maladjustments of all varieties—unhappiness, discontent, fear, anxiety, despair, marital discord, even educational problems—have come to be regarded as medical problems, requiring medical attention, imposing new, heavy demands for care. In addition, there are probably many more people in this country requiring specialized rehabilitation services for disabilities resulting from physical trauma (Korea and Vietnam veterans, automobile- and industrial-accident victims, etc.).

HEALTH CARE TECHNOLOGY, 1950-1975

Has the effective technology for medical care changed in the past twenty-five years to a degree sufficient to explain the increased cost? Is there in fact a new high technology of medicine?

Despite the widespread public impression that this is the case, there is little evidence for it. The most spectacular technological change has occurred in the management of infectious disease, but its essential features had been solidly established and put to use well before 1950. The sulfonamides came to medicine in the late 1930s, penicillin and streptomycin a few years later, and the major advances in the control and cure of infectious disease occurred during the 1940s. There has been no quantum leap in anti-infectious technology since 1950. Several new virus vaccines have been developed. The antibiotics have come into more widespread use (probably with considerable overuse and waste); a multiplicity of new variants of antibiotics and chemotherapeutic agents has appeared on the market, but one would not expect that the rational use of this technology, even allowing for the high cost of development and marketing, would have proven to be anything like the previous cost of hospital care in the absence of such a technology. A typical case of lobar pneumonia, pre-antibiotic, involved three or four weeks of hospitalization; typhoid was a twelve-to-sixteen-week illness; meningitis often required several months of care through convalescence; these and other common infectious diseases can now be aborted promptly, within just a few days. The net result of the anti-infection technology ought to have been a very large decrease in the cost of care.

There have been a few other examples of technology improvement, comparable in decisive effectiveness, since 1950, but the best of these have been for relatively uncommon illnesses. Childhood leukemia and certain solid tumors in children, for example, can now be cured by chemotherapy in a substantial proportion of cases, but there are only a few thousand of these per year in the country. Endocrine-replacement therapy has become highly effective and relatively inexpensive ("relative" considering the cost of caring for untreated endocrine abnormalities) for a variety of disorders involving the adrenals, pituitary, parathyroid, ovary, and thyroid; in particular, the biochemical treatment of thyroid dysfunction has improved markedly. Hematology has offered new and effective replacement treatment for certain anemias. Immunologic prophylaxis now prevents most cases of hemolytic disease of the newborn. Progress in anesthesia, electrolyte physiology, and cardiopulmonary physiology has greatly advanced the field of surgery, so that reparative and other procedures can now be done which formerly were technically impossible.

But the list of decisive new accomplishments is not much longer than the contents of the above paragraph.

We are left with approximately the same roster of common major diseases which confronted the country in 1950, and, although we have accumulated a formidable body of information about some of them in the intervening time, the accumulation is not yet sufficient to permit either the prevention or the outright cure of any of them. This is not to suggest that progress has not been made, or has been made more slowly than should reasonably have been expected. On the contrary, the research activity since 1950 has provided the beginnings of insight into the underlying processes in several of our most important diseases, and there is every reason for optimism regarding the future. But it is the present that is the problem. We are, in a sense, partway along, maybe halfway along. At the same time, medicine is expected to do something for each of these illnesses, to do whatever can be done in the light of today's knowledge. Because of this obligation, we have evolved "halfway" technologies, representing the best available treatment, and the development and proliferation of these are partly responsible for the escalating costs of health care in recent years. Associated with this expansion, the diagnostic laboratories have become much more elaborate and complex in their technologies; there is no question that clinical diagnosis has become much more powerful and precise, but at a very high cost and with considerable waste resulting from overuse.

This way of looking at contemporary medicine runs against the currently general public view that the discipline has by this time come almost its full distance, that we have had a long succession of "breakthroughs" and "major advances," and that now we should go beyond our persistent concern with research on what is called "curative" medicine and give more attention to the social aspects of illness and to preventive medicine.

It does not, in fact, look much like the record of a completed job, or even of a job more than half begun, when you run through the list, one by one, of the diseases in this country which everyone will agree are the most important ones. A handy index for this sort of exercise is the annual *United States Vital Statistics Report,* in which are tabulated the ten causes of death, as well as the commonest nonfatal illnesses requiring attention from the health care system.

The questions to be asked are the following: For how many of these illnesses do we now possess a decisively effective technology for cure or prevention, directed at a central disease agent or mechanism, comparable to the treatment, say, of pneumococcal lobar pneumonia with penicillin? Are we failing to employ effective measures because of deficiencies in the health care system? To what extent do present mortality and morbidity rates simply reflect the absence of any known technology that works?

In the following section, these questions are explored. It should be emphasized here that we will not be discussing the availability of medical treatment in general. Obviously, there is a great deal that can be done for patients with the diseases considered below in the way of supportive care, the amelioration of symptoms, and sometimes the extension of life. In some conditions, this amounts to what might be called partial control of the disease, but this is not the question at hand. What we are examining here is the capacity of medicine to cure outright or to prevent completely—in situations analogous to lobar pneumonia or poliomyelitis.

Listed below are the ten leading causes of death from disease in the United States in 1974:

Cardiovascular disease (39 percent of total deaths in 1974): In general, cardiovascular disease lacks any decisive, conclusive technology with the power to turn off, reverse, or prevent disease. There are two possible exceptions: rheumatic heart disease is known to be preventable when the antecedent streptococcal infection can be quickly terminated by early antibiotic treatment or prevented by prophylaxis; some forms of congenital heart disease can be completely corrected by surgery. Except for these, the other therapies now available are directed at secondary results of already established disease: coronary care units and specialized ambulances, designed primarily for coping with cardiac standstill and arrythmias, anticoagulant treatment to prevent extension and recurrence (largely given up in recent years), digitalis and diuretics for myocardial failure, drug therapy to inhibit arrythmias, and surgical replacement of already damaged coronary arteries or valves.

As to coronary disease, it is believed in some quarters that dietary lipids are an etiologic factor. It is also proposed that lack of exercise, excessive emotional stress, and various usually unstipulated environmental influences are somehow implicated in pathogenesis. The evidence for these beliefs is still inconclusive. In any event, intervention to correct them would involve grand-scale, societal reforms of living habits. Meanwhile, the actual pathologic events which cause the coronary lesions remain unknown. Until these are elucidated in some detail, a direct approach to coronary disease must await the future.

Hypertension is a separate disease state, frequently associated with cardiac disease. This will be considered below.

Cancer (19 percent of total deaths in 1974): Up to now, the technologies available for the treatment of cancer are all in the "halfway" category, in the sense that they deal with the already established disease and represent efforts to destroy, by one means or another (surgery, radiation, chemotherapy, immunotherapy), existing cancer cells. There are no methods for reversing the neoplastic process in cells or for preventing their emergence from normal cells. Prevention would be possible for a few types, if exposure to the known environmental carcinogens, e.g., cigarettes, asbestos, and certain industrial chemicals, could be eliminated. But prevention in the sense of eliminating the biological steps involved in the transformation of cells is not yet feasible.

Cerebrovascular diseases (11 percent of total deaths in 1974): Stroke results from disease of the arteries of the brain, usually associated with atherosclerosis or hypertension. Since no therapy exists for preventing or reversing atherosclerosis, this class of strokes is neither preventable nor reversible. Hypertension is considered below.

Once stroke occurs, therapy is limited to efforts at minimizing the extent of disability, largely a matter of retraining, rehabilitation, and speech therapy. No treatment exists for preventing the recurrence of stroke. Anticoagulant therapy, once attempted on a large scale, is no longer in general use.

Kidney disease (10.4 percent of total deaths in 1974): The major forms of kidney disease responsible for most cases of renal failure and death are chronic glomerulonephritis and pyclonephritis.

At the present time, no effective treatment exists for chronic glomerulonephritis, beyond measures aimed at compensating for the loss of renal function, e.g., electrolyte adjustment, chronic dialysis and, in a relatively few cases, kidney transplantation. Some cases are perhaps prevented by early treatment of antecedent streptococcal infection, but the initial cause in most instances is unknown. The essential lesion is a deposit of an antigen-antibody complex within the walls of glomerular capillaries, followed by injury to the vessels probably mediated by leucocytic lysosomes and complement. A direct therapeutic approach to these events cannot be conceived until more detailed scientific information becomes available.

Chronic pyelonephritis can probably be prevented in some instances by early treatment of the acute infection, but in most cases the kidney lesions develop gradually and unobtrusively, and once established they are not reversible. It is believed by some that bacterial protoplasts are involved in etiology, perhaps also with an associated immunologic injury to the tissues; even if this is so, currently available antimicrobial therapy is not effective.

Pulmonary disease (approximately 4.5 percent of total deaths in 1974):

Included under this heading, in the *Vital Statistics Report,* are influenza and pneumonia, bronchitis, emphysema, and chronic obstructive lung disease.

Almost all cases of primary bacterial and mycoplasmal pneumonia are treatable and curable by use of the appropriate antibiotic.

Influenza can be prevented in some cases by immunization, provided the antigenic strain is recognized early enough in an outbreak to prepare vaccine. Once it has occurred, there is no therapy for the influenza viral infection itself. Bacterial superinfections, when they occur, are reversible except in the occasional cases of sudden, overwhelming infection to which pregnant women and debilitated elderly people are most prone. Antibiotic treatment of uncomplicated influenza is ineffective and probably hazardous.

Bronchitis, emphysema, and chronic pulmonary obstructive disease are still unsolved etiologic problems. Cigarette smoking and air pollution are suspected as causes, but the actual mechanisms underlying the injury to lung tissue remain unknown. Although technologies exist for the improvement of aeration by the damaged lungs, and thus for some prolongation of life, there are no measures available for stopping or reversing the progress of disease.

Diabetes mellitus (1.9 percent of total deaths in 1974): Although the discovery of insulin fifty years ago made possible the survival of most diabetics who would otherwise have died in diabetic coma, the blood-vessel disorder which is a major aspect of the disease is unaffected by insulin and remains a mystery. Hence, the disabilities and deaths of diabetics, mostly in middle-age and later, are now due to chronic kidney disease and the occlusion of arteries in one or another part of the body. Virtually nothing is known about the cause of vascular lesions, and there is no therapy to stop or reverse the process.

Cirrhosis of the liver (1.8 percent of total deaths in 1974): The chief cause of cirrhosis is unquestionably alcohol taken in excess and over a long period of time. If alcoholism could be prevented, cirrhosis would become a relatively rare affliction. The hepatic lesions are to some extent reversible, and the disease can sometimes be stopped and even reversed in its early stages by simple abstention.

This, however, represents about the total of today's effective therapy. The mechanism of hepatic cell injury by alcohol is not understood, nor is the process by which the liver becomes progressively atrophic and fibrosed. Nutritional deprivation, believed a few years back to play a central role, is no longer thought to be centrally involved. Once the disease is firmly established, there is no known method for turning it around. Surgical measures have been developed for reducing ascites (that is, fluid accumulation in the abdomen) and the back pressure of portal blood, with some ameliorative effort on the symptoms of cirrhosis, but the injury to the liver itself is unalterable.

Perinatal disease (1.5 percent of total deaths in 1974): Much of the infant mortality in the earliest days of life is associated with prematurity, and obstructive disease of the lungs accounts for much of this. At the present time, there is no effective therapy for this pulmonary disease, caused by hyaline, membranous deposits which occlude the alveolar walls. The mechanisms leading to these deposits are unknown.

Bacterial and viral infections account for a majority of other neonatal deaths. The bacterial infections are treatable with antibiotics, but often occur abruptly in overwhelming form. The viral infections are untreatable.

Hemolytic disease of the newborn, formerly a common cause of death, is now preventable by immunologic treatment during pregnancy; some cases can be cured by total blood replacement and transfusions.

Congenital malformations and deficiencies (0.7 percent of total deaths in 1974): Although surgical measures are available for the correction of some types of congenital malformation, such as cardiac and intestinal anomalies, most of them are untreatable. A few of the highly disabling and fatal enzyme deficiencies can be recognized during early pregnancy and thus prevented by abortion. The biochemical and genetic nature of these rare disorders is currently under investigation in many laboratories, and there is some optimism that methods for reversing the defects will eventually be found.

Peptic ulcer: Few human ailments have been subjected to as great a variety of medical and surgical treatments over the years as peptic ulcer, often with enthusiastic predictions of success, but always replaced by new and different therapies. The main problem hampering decisive progress is that the mechanism that produces peptic ulcers is not understood, and therefore there is no basis for devising a genuinely rational method of treatment or prevention. This is not to say that it is not a treatable condition, of course. There are many ways in which the symptoms and the progress of the disease can be alleviated. Nevertheless, it must be ranked as an essentially unexplained disorder.

The foregoing list accounts for approximately 80 percent of all deaths in this country. It does not, of course, account for the major part of the work of physicians, nor the greatest element of cost for the health care system. We are afflicted, obviously, by a great (but it must be said, finite) array of nonfatal illnesses varying in severity and duration, and it is here that the greatest demands for technology are made. For the purposes of this paper, some of the commonest of these self-limited or nonfatal diseases are listed below:

Acute respiratory infections: These and the acute gastroenteric infections and intoxications (see below) make up the great majority of transiently disabling illnesses with which people are afflicted in a year's turning.

The common cold and the array of other respiratory viral infections including influenza (sometimes called "grippe") are essentially untreatable. The measures employed for alleviating discomfort—bed rest, aspirin, a good book— are no different today from what one's grandmother would have prescribed. There is, in short, no medical technology for such illnesses. The administration of antibiotics, antihistamines, vitamin C, and various other "cold remedies" probably have no effect other than reassurance. There is a general apprehension that such illnesses may lead to other, more severe, respiratory infections, such as pneumonia, if not monitored by a physician, but there is in fact no evidence for this. By and large, people with these illnesses get better by themselves, usually within a day or two. The most frequent complications are the result of untoward reactions to unnecessary therapy, most often the antibiotics used in the hope of preventing complications.

Gastrointestinal infections: The general run of acute gastrointestinal ill-nesses, usually caused by a virus or salmonella infection or by staphylococcal toxin, are common, self-limited, and entirely without hazard. Intervention by medicine would be desirable, since these are unpleasant experiences for the af-flicted, and there are in fact several symptomatic measures for partial relief, but the illnesses are usually so short in duration that no therapy is necessary. As in the case of acute respiratory infections, grandmother's advice is as good as any, maybe better.

Arthritis: Both rheumatoid arthritis and osteoarthritis, which account for more than five million illnesses each year, are unexplained, mystifying diseases for which no therapy beyond analgesic drugs is available. Rheumatoid arthritis is currently believed by a consensus of clinical investigators to be caused by an unknown infectious agent, probably with a still unidentified immunopathologic component. The partial relief provided by salicylates and related drugs, and by gold salts, are still unexplainable. In approximately 35 percent of all cases the disease subsides spontaneously and vanishes. Prolonged, chronically disabling forms of arthritis can be partially benefited by surgical removal of inflamed synovial (joint) tissues. Prolonged hospitalization and various forms of rehabilita-tive care are required in some cases. In the absence of information concerning etiology, it is probable that treatment will remain at a symptomatic, empirical level not very different from the measures of fifty years ago.

Osteoarthritis remains totally unexplained. Surgical treatment is useful in some (notably hip) cases; otherwise therapy is limited to analgesic drugs.

The neuroses: It is frequently said that at least 75 percent of the patients seeking help in doctors' offices or clinics have complaints for which there is no "organic" explanation. Some of these patients are not really ill, but simply in need of reassurance that they do not have one or another disease which they are worried about. Others are beset by family, economic, or various other social problems which seem temporarily insoluble, and for which they seek advice. Still others, an unknown number, are disabled by classical psychoneuroses.

The possible therapeutic approaches to such problems have not changed significantly in the past quarter century. Counseling, comforting, and what is called psychotherapy are essentially the same procedures as in earlier times, without any real elements of technology, nor is there any statistical evidence for their effectiveness. An immense store of so-called "tranquilizer" drugs has been provided by pharmaceutical research in recent years, but there is little informa-tion as to the efficacy of its contents. They may provide transient symptomatic relief, but it is unlikely that they alter the underlying processes of these illnesses.

In short, there is no real technology available for the treatment of "functional" illness, psychoneurosis, or the various forms of social maladaptation. It seems safe to say that nothing much has happened since 1950 to alter the situation one way or the other.

The psychoses: Schizophrenia and the manic-depressive psychoses account for the greatest part of mental illness requiring hospitalization and prolonged ambulatory care. Drug therapy evolved since 1950 has greatly improved the "manageability" of schizophrenia, but it has not much changed the disease itself. The manic-depressive psychoses are improved in some instances by pharmacologic treatment, including lithium, and also in some by electric shock. All forms of psychosis remain unexplained, however, in terms of identifiable mechanisms attributable to dysfunction in the central nervous system, and therapy directed at underlying processes has not advanced beyond what was available before 1950.

Parkinsonism: The introduction of L-Dopa as therapy for Parkinsonism in the mid-1960s by Cotzias and his associates represents a milestone in neurological medicine. Although not all patients are uniformly benefited, and some become refractory or display untoward reactions to the drug, many do well and have their lives transformed.

Essential hypertension: In some respects, hypertension is a paradigm illustrating a central dilemma in today's health care system. Drugs are now available with the capacity to reduce blood-pressure levels to normal. At the same time, however, the actual mechanisms of the disease remain without explanation, and it is not yet known whether the reduction of blood pressure has any effect on the underlying vascular disturbance. There is now some evidence, still incomplete, that prolonged treatment with antihypertensive drug decreases the incidence of stroke as a complication of hypertension. There may also be an effect on the incidence of coronary occlusion, although the evidence for this is less conclusive. There appears to be no doubt that drug treatment can prolong survival in patients with malignant hypertension.

On the basis of these observations, it has been proposed that large-scale screening programs be set up, so that all of the 10 million or more young, potentially vulnerable people with hypertension in this country can be identified and treated. This means that great numbers of patients with essential hypertension will be placed on lifelong treatment with complex pharmacologic agents, necessarily persuaded to stay under treatment because of the threat of a fatal outcome. At the same time it is a certainty that many patients with essential hypertension, if not treated, would nevertheless be able to look forward to the statistical probability of a normal life span. Indeed, there are reasons to believe that essential hypertension is a normal state of affairs for some people. The difficulty is that there is no way to predict which patients will eventually have cardiac, cerebral, or renal complications associated with hypertension; in the absence of such knowledge, all hypertensives must be treated. Meanwhile, the disease itself remains an enigma. If a mass screening and therapy program is launched it will be done in the hope that treating a symptom of disease will have long-range beneficial effects. Moreover, it will involve drug therapy, with certain predictable side effects, and perhaps still others unpredicted thus far, aimed at the protection of a minority of the patients to be treated.

THE COST OF WORRY IN THE HEALTH CARE SYSTEM

Nothing has changed so much in the health care system over the past twenty-five years as the public's perception of its own health. The change amounts to a loss of confidence in the human form. The general belief these days seems to be that the body is fundamentally flawed, subject to disintegration at any moment, always on the verge of mortal disease, always in need of continual monitoring and support by health care professionals. This is a new phenomenon in our society.

It can be seen most clearly in the content of television programs and, especially, television commercials, where the preponderance of material deals with the need for shoring up one's personal health. The same drift is evident in the contents of the most popular magazines and in the health columns of daily newspapers. There is a public preoccupation with disease that is assuming the dimension of a national obsession.

To some extent, the propaganda which feeds the obsession is a result of the well intentioned efforts by particular disease agencies to obtain public money for the support of research and care in their special fields. Every mail brings word of the imminent perils posed by multiple sclerosis, kidney disease, cancer, heart disease, cystic fibrosis, asthma, muscular dystrophy, and the rest.

There is, regrettably, no discernible counterpropaganda. No agencies exist for the celebration of the plain fact that most people are, in real life, abundantly healthy. No one takes public note of the truth of the matter, which is that most people in this country have a clear, unimpeded run at a longer lifetime than could have been foreseen by any earlier generation. Even the proponents of good hygiene, who argue publicly in favor of regular exercise, thinness, and abstinence from cigarettes and alcohol, base their arguments on the presumed intrinsic fallibility of human health. Left alone, unadvised by professionals, the tendency of the human body is perceived as prone to steady failure.

Underlying this pessimistic view of health is a profound dissatisfaction with the fact of death. Dying is regarded as the ultimate failure, something that could always be avoided or averted if only the health care system functioned more efficiently. Death has been made to seem unnatural, an outrage; when people die—at whatever age—we speak of them as having been "struck down," "felled." It is as though in a better world we would all go on forever.

It is not surprising that all this propaganda has imposed heavy, unsupportable demands on the health care system. If people are educated to believe that they may at any moment be afflicted with one or another mortal disease and that this fate can be forestalled by access to medicine, especially "preventive" medicine, it is no wonder that clinics and doctors' offices are filled with waiting clients.

In the year 1974, 1,933,000 people died in the United States, a death rate of 9.1 per 1,000, or just under 1 percent of the whole population, substantially lower than the birth rate for the same year. The life expectation for the whole population rose to 72 years, the highest expectancy ever attained in this country. With figures like these, it is hard to see health as a crisis, or the health care system, apart from its huge size and high cost, as a matter needing emergency action. We really are a quite healthy society, and we should be spending more time and energy in acknowledging this, and perhaps trying to understand more clearly why it is so. We are in some danger of becoming a nation of healthy hypochondriacs.

For all its obvious defects and shortcomings, the actual technology of health care is not likely to be changed drastically in the direction of saving money—not in the short haul. Nor is it likely that changes for the better, in the sense of greater effectiveness and efficiency, can be brought about by any means other than more scientific research. The latter course, although sure, is undeniably slow and unpredictable. While it is a certainty, in my view, that rheumatoid arthritis, atherosclerosis, cancer, and senile dementia will eventually be demystified and can then become preventable disorders, there is no way of forecasting when this will happen; it could be a few years away for one or the other, or decades.

Meanwhile, we will be compelled to live with the system as we have it, changing only the parts that are in fact changeable. It is not likely that money problems can induce anyone—the professionals or the public at large, or even the third-party payers—to give up the halfway technologies that work only partially when this would mean leaving no therapeutic effort at all in place. For as long as there is a prospect of saving the lives of 50 percent, or even only 33 percent, of patients with cancer by today's methods for destroying cancer cells, these methods must obviously be held onto and made available to as many patients as possible. If coronary bypass surgery remains the only technical measure for relieving untractable angina in a relatively small proportion of cases, it will be continued, and very likely extended to larger numbers of cases, until something better turns up. People with incapacitating mental illness cannot simply be left to wander the streets, and we will continue to need expanding clinics and specialized hospital facilities, even though caring for the mentally ill does not mean anything like curing them. We are, in a sense, stuck with today's technology, and we will stay stuck until we have more scientific knowledge to work with.

But what we might do, if we could muster the energy and judgment for it, is to identify the areas of health care in which the spending of money represents outright waste, and then eliminate these. There are discrete examples all over the place, but what they are depends on who is responsible for citing them, and there will be bitter arguments over each one before they can be edited out of the system, one by one.

The biggest source of waste results from the general public conviction that contemporary medicine is able to accomplish a great deal more than is in fact possible. This attitude is in part the outcome of overstated claims on the part of medicine itself in recent decades, plus medicine's passive acquiescence while even more exaggerated claims were made by the media. The notion of preventive medicine as a whole new discipline in medical care is an example of this. There is an arguably solid base for the prevention of certain diseases, but it has not changed all that much since the 1950s. A few valuable measures have been added, most notably the avoidance of cigarette smoking for the prevention of lung cancer; if we had figured out a way of acting on this single bit of information, we might have achieved a spectacular triumph in the prevention of deaths from cancer, but regrettably we didn't. The same despairing thing can be said for the preventability of death from alcohol.

But there is not much more than this in the field of preventive medicine. The truth is that medicine has not become very skilled at disease prevention— not, as is sometimes claimed, because it doesn't want to or isn't interested, but because the needed information is still lacking.

Most conspicuous and costly of all are the benefits presumed to derive from "seeing the doctor." The regular complete checkup, once a year or more often, has become a cultural habit, and it is only recently that some investigators have suggested, cautiously, that it probably doesn't do much good. There are very few diseases in which early detection can lead to a significant alteration of the outcome: glaucoma, cervical cancer, and possibly breast cancer are the usually cited examples, but in any event these do not require the full, expensive array of the complete periodic checkup, EKG and all. Nevertheless, the habit has become fixed in our society, and it is a significant item in the total bill for health care.

"Seeing the doctor" also includes an overwhelming demand for reassurance. Transient upper-respiratory infections and episodes of gastroenteritis account for most of the calls on a doctor because of illness, and an even greater number of calls are made by people who have nothing at all the matter with them. It is often claimed that these are mostly unhappy individuals, suffering from psychoneuroses, in need of compassionate listening on the part of the physician, but a large number of patients who find themselves in doctors' offices or hospital clinics will acknowledge themselves to be in entirely good health; they are there because of a previous appointment in connection with an earlier illness, for a "checkup," or for a laboratory test, or simply for reassurance that they are not coming down with something serious—cancer, or heart disease, or whatever. Or they may have come to the doctor for advice about living: what should their diet be?, should they take a vacation?, what about a tranquilizer for everyone's inevitable moments of agitation and despair? I know a professor of pediatrics who has received visits from intelligent, well-educated parents who only want to know if their child should start Sunday school.

The system is being overused, swamped by expectant overdemands for services that are frequently trivial or unproductive. The public is not sufficiently informed of the facts about things that medicine can and cannot accomplish. Medicine is surely not in possession of special wisdom about how to live a life.

It needs to be said more often that human beings are fundamentally tough, resilient animals, marvelously made, most of the time capable of getting along quite well on their own. The health care system should be designed for use when it is really needed and when it has something of genuine value to offer. If designed, or redesigned, in this way, the system would function far more effectively, and would probably cost very much less.

CONCLUSION

If our society wishes to be rid of the diseases, fatal and nonfatal, that plague us the most, there is really little prospect of doing so by mounting a still larger health care system at still greater cost for delivering essentially today's kind of technology on a larger scale. We will not do so by carrying out broader programs of surveillance and screening. The truth is that we do not yet know enough. But there is also another truth of great importance: we are learning fast. The harvest of new information from the biological revolution of the past quarter century is just now coming in, and we can probably begin now to figure out the mechanisms of major diseases which were blank mysteries a few years back as accurately and profitably as was done for the infectious diseases earlier in this century. This can be said with considerable confidence, and without risk of over-promising or raising false hopes, provided we do not set time schedules or offer dates of delivery. Sooner or later it will go this way, since clearly it can go this way. It is simply a question at this stage of events of how much we wish to invest, for the health care system of the future, in science.

13

National Health Insurance

Selection by Karen Davis

Evaluating the possible alternative approaches to national health insurance requires decisions about a multitude of issues. A plan must be designed so that it not only meets today's needs but also is flexible enough to adjust to the demands of changing medical technology. Deciding which of the many possible features of a national health insurance plan should be included is not always a clear-cut choice. In most cases, some tradeoff must be made between one set of advantages and another. An attempt is made in this chapter to clarify the tradeoffs involved in most of the major features of national health insurance plans.

WHO SHOULD BE COVERED?

The first choice to be made in designing a national health insurance plan is the extent of population coverage. National health insurance aims primarily at assisting people with low incomes or high medical bills; yet a national health insurance plan that attempts to meet only their needs may fail to do so. Demands on the medical care system by higher-income people who are excluded from the plan but covered under private insurance may divert resources away from the poor. Physicians may find treatment of higher-income patients financially more attractive than serving the poor, and subject to fewer constraints on

Reprinted by permission from "Basic Issues in National Health Insurance," *National Health Insurance: Benefits, Costs and Consequences* (Washington, D.C.: Brookings Institution, 1975), pp. 56-79.

their methods of practice. The supply of resources available to low-income persons is thus inevitably interlocked with patterns of medical care for others.

One approach to national health insurance would limit population coverage to those who have made contributions to the social security system, on the assumption that people feel better if they believe, whether correctly or incorrectly, that they have "paid" for their benefits through systematic contributions. Thus, they are collectively more willing to submit to higher tax rates than they would be if the link between costs and benefits were not so direct. But excluding those outside the social security system would frequently exclude those who are most in need of assistance, thus undermining one of the basic goals of the plan.

One group that would be excluded if coverage were linked to the social security system consists of young adults who are no longer in school but have not yet found jobs. They would not be eligible for insurance under their parents' coverage, nor could they have their own policies. While this group is generally healthy, an accident or serious illness could result in burdensome medical bills that would inflict serious hardships on them or their parents.

Another approach to national health insurance would provide coverage under employer group plans, with separate plans for the poor, the aged, and those not eligible for coverage under an employer group plan. However, if few subsidies are provided for the latter group, the cost of coverage to them can be quite high. Under one such plan, a part-time worker earning $7,500 a year would have to pay an annual premium of $600. Self-employed workers, families with a disabled head, unemployed workers, or workers employed on a temporary or part-time basis would frequently be excluded from coverage because of the high cost of obtaining insurance without employer or government contributions. This would particularly affect families with incomes between about $5,000 and $10,000—those who are neither poor enough to qualify for governmental assistance nor sufficiently well to do to afford the full cost of the insurance.

An approach that provides coverage through employer groups can either require employers and employees to accept the plan or introduce some element of voluntarism. If employees may decline the plan, employers may exert some pressure on them to do so to minimize the cost to the employer. Compulsory coverage with substantial employer contributions, however, may place serious financial strains on employers who do not currently have good health insurance plans for workers.

Thus, while universal coverage does have disadvantages, the major goals of national health insurance cannot be achieved so long as there are segments of the population that do not have adequate protection against the high cost of medical care. Universal coverage without regard to family composition, employability, or social security contribution history seems to provide the most equitable solution.

WHAT SHOULD BE COVERED?

Several considerations affect the choice of the range of medical services that should be covered under national health insurance. High priorities include: (1) medical services that reduce mortality or increase productivity, hence benefiting society as a whole; (2) medical services that can add substantially to the financial burden of medical care for an individual; (3) medical services that are so essential they will be sought regardless of the cost; (4) medical services that constitute acceptable lower-cost substitutes for covered services. The decision to include any given type of medical service in the benefit package, however, is separate from the decision to make the service available to all or a portion of covered persons free of any direct charge. Considerations bearing on that issue will be considered in the next section.

A number of medical services have been identified as having high social benefits because they reduce mortality or increase worker productivity. Prenatal care for women and immunizations and other basic care for babies are frequently cited. Mental health care, while its efficacy is somewhat more controversial, can have substantial benefits not only for those receiving care but for society as a whole through improved worker productivity, reduction in crime or antisocial behavior, and reduced dependence of the patient or family on public resources.

Items that can be quite costly include not only hospitalization and specialist physicians' fees but also lower-cost services that are required in great volume, such as weekly allergy shots, drugs for the proper management of chronic illness, and the periodic surveillance by a physician of conditions such as diabetes and hypertension. Some dental services and cosmetic surgery, despite their high cost, are typically excluded from coverage on the grounds that they are amenities that add to the enjoyment of life but are not essential to good health; as such they should be available only to those willing to pay for them, just as are sailboats, color television sets, and vacations abroad.

Since there is rarely only one possible treatment method for any given medical problem it is important that choices be made among alternatives on the basis of the expected benefits in relation to cost. Covering only a limited range of services alters this calculation by reducing the net cost of some services to the patient but not others. For example, procedures may be carried out in a hospital that could be done in a hospital outpatient department or physician's office with recuperation at home. Nursing home care for the elderly may come to be preferred over services rendered in the home by family or home health nurses. If prescription drugs are covered but not nonprescription drugs, more costly drugs may be used where others are equally efficacious. If insurance coverage is restricted to physician services, patients may not use less trained personnel for some services that can be adequately performed by them. Obviously, there must be a cut-off point for coverage, but it should be established on the basis of the degree of substitutability likely to occur, the cost savings of substitution, and the efficacy or quality of substitute forms of care.

There are some services that may be required for some groups of the population but not others. For example, residents of sparsely populated areas may need transportation assistance in order to receive needed medical services. Groups with lower levels of education may require "outreach" services to inform them of available care and of the importance of early medical intervention. These services might be more appropriately rendered by being offered to special groups through supplementary health programs.

SHOULD PATIENTS SHARE IN COSTS?

One of the more controversial issues in national health insurance is what role there should be for direct payments by patients. Plans commonly specify deductible amounts requiring the patient to pay all of the cost up to some figure and have coinsurance provisions requiring the patient to pay a fraction of all expenses above the deductible—the total called cost-sharing amounts. For example, a policy may require a family to pay (within the calendar year) all of the first $150 of medical expenses for each of three family members and then pay twenty-five cents of every additional dollar of medical expenses beyond that.

Cost-sharing provisions raise several important questions. Should all patients share in the cost of all services, or should some patients or services be exempt from cost sharing? If patient charges are included in a plan, how high should they be? Should they be the same for all patients regardless of income or financial resources? If the plan does not cover all expenses, should patients be permitted, or even encouraged, to purchase supplementary private insurance to cover the remainder?

Although lack of any cost sharing is increasingly recognized as inflationary and conducive to inefficient and wasteful use of resources, uniform cost-sharing provisions fall heavily upon the poor and substantial, unlimited cost sharing can cause heavy financial burdens for even the nonpoor (Davis, 1974, pp. 206-15). One option would be to relate the amount of payments required of patients to their incomes and to set ceilings on how much any family would have to pay. While such a solution has obvious merit, it adds to the administrative complexity of the plan and requires the accumulation of sensitive data banks on income as well as health problems. Furthermore, little empirical evidence is available for judging the consequences of any given schedule of income-related cost-sharing requirements. This makes it important to preserve flexibility so that changes can be made in the plan over time as experience is gained.

Perhaps the best way to develop criteria to weigh the cost-sharing options is to review the basic goals of national health insurance. Clearly, substantial cost sharing by lower-income patients will deter them from seeking needed medical care and thus undermine the first major goal of national health insurance. An elderly couple struggling to make ends meet on social security payments of $3,000 a year cannot reasonably be expected to pay $150 for each deductible, 25 percent of the cost of additional hospital and medical bills, and all of the cost of excluded services such as eyeglasses, hearing aids, dentures, and prescription drugs. But an elderly couple with an income of $15,000 from a good retirement plan may be able to meet the cost-sharing amounts without undue burden. Thus, reducing or eliminating cost-sharing requirements for the lowest-income families is important in achieving the goals of national health insurance but is not necessary for all families.

It should be recognized that not all costs of medical care are direct ones. Use of medical services normally entails some time and transportation costs as well. These costs alone may be sufficient to curb any abuses of excessive care. Adding to these costs with even nominal cost-sharing amounts may deter use of needed medical services, particularly by the poor. Since the poor tend to live in areas with few medical resources, the time and travel costs required of them may be substantial. Furthermore, the preference of many physicians for treating higher-income patients undoubtedly acts as a restraint on excessive use of services by the poor even without any direct monetary costs. It has sometimes been argued that making medical care free for everyone would give the poor an advantage since those who are willing to wait would eventually obtain the needed care and the cost of time to the poor is cheap. However, many working poor are unlikely to have generous sick leave provisions and so may lose income while obtaining medical care. Lower-income families are less likely to have an adult at home with time to seek out medical care for children. These indirect costs of medical care are sufficiently important for most poor people that adding direct monetary costs to their burden seems unjustified.

The second goal of national health insurance—preventing financial hardship for all families—clearly requires that a ceiling be placed on patient contributions, so that a family's payments will never exceed a fixed sum, such as $1,000, or a fixed percentage of income, such as 10 percent. If low-income families are not required to contribute toward their medical care, some mechanism for increasing the ceiling gradually as income rises must be devised. For example, families with incomes below $5,000 might not be required to pay any of their medical bills, families with incomes between $5,000 and $10,000 required to contribute up to 20 percent of their income in excess of $5,000, and families with incomes above $10,000 required to pay a maximum of $1,000. Thus, a family with a $5,000 income would pay nothing; a family with a $7,500 income would pay a maximum of $500; and a family with a $10,000 income or above would pay a maximum of $1,000.

Justification for Substantial Direct Patient Payments

While such sums may still seem sizable, there are strong justifications for retaining substantial direct payments by patients in a national health insurance plan. First, cost sharing reduces the cost of the plan, which must be financed through taxes or other sources. Plans that contain no deductible and coinsurance provisions would thus require massive increases in payroll and income taxes to finance expenditures that are currently made in the private sector. This would move into the federal budget private outlays for normal medical expenses that are now being made by middle- and upper-income groups with little financial strain. Furthermore, the large tax increases necessary to finance such a program might force the nation to give up other high-priority objectives. Experience with Medicare also suggests that even with adequate financing of medical care services budgetary funds would still be required for special programs to ensure access to medical care for minority groups and rural residents. Attempting to finance the entire cost of medical care through the federal budget, therefore, may impede other social programs as well as restrict budgetary outlays for medical care.

Second, cost sharing reduces (but does not eliminate) the need for administrative control over the use of medical services. Deductible and coinsurance amounts give patients and physicians an incentive to choose alternative forms of care: care on a less costly outpatient basis versus inpatient hospital care, care from family physicians rather than specialists, greater use of physician extenders and nurse practitioners for services not requiring a physician. In addition, it is important that the advantages of making additional units of medical care services available be weighed against the resources that must be devoted to providing them. While an extra day of hospital care, a follow-up visit to the physician, or an extra battery of laboratory tests may contribute to improved health, the resources required to provide these incremental services may have greater social value if diverted to other uses. Considerable evidence has accumulated that the presence or absence of cost-sharing provisions in insurance plans can have a substantial effect on the amount and mix of medical services. For evidence, see Scitovsky and Snyder (1972), Peel and Scharff (1973), Newhouse and Phelps (1974), Feldstein (1973), Ginsburg and Manheim (1973), and Kaplan and Lave (1971). For studies indicating that patient payments have adverse effects on utilization of services by the poor, see Hall et al. (1973), Beck (1974), and Greenlick et al. (1972). For dissenting points of view on the effect of patient payments, see Hardwick, Shuman, and Barnoon (1972).

In the absence of such financial incentives to weigh the cost of medical services to society, regulatory bodies must be established to review the necessity of hospitalization, the appropriateness of the length of hospital stay, and the efficacy of laboratory tests and ancillary services. Controls on the numbers of specialists, family physicians, other health personnel, and health facilities must be created and enforced. Unfortunately, the administrative expertise and accumulated knowledge required for such an undertaking is not yet available, nor is the question resolved of who should serve on such regulatory bodies.

In addition to providing important automatic incentives for the appropriate utilization of medical services, cost sharing can help reduce the charges that physicians and hospitals set for their services. This is especially important if the national health insurance plan contains no effective mechanism for placing a lid on reimbursement levels. For example, a physician who charges $5 to a patient without insurance may charge $20 when the patient pays only 25 percent of the bill, and substantially more when the patient pays none of the bill. Similarly, hospitals have increased charges as insurance coverage has grown, and hospital administrators have had no difficulty in finding ways to spend the increased revenues. Competition among health care providers, which admittedly works far from perfectly even in the absence of insurance, will not work at all without some direct patient payments, since patients have no reason to select a physician charging lower fees even if he or she provides exactly the same care with regard to convenience, quality, sensitivity, and all the other dimensions of this very personal service. Nor will either patient or physician have any incentive to select a lower-cost hospital, all other considerations being equal. In short, direct controls on costs are very difficult to enforce without providing some incentives for those who actually make the decisions.

These pressures for additional services and demands for higher reimbursement by providers could greatly increase the cost of medical services. A recent study by Newhouse, Phelps, and Schwartz (1974) estimates that absence of any cost sharing would increase the demand for hospital inpatient services by approximately 5 to 15 percent (the low estimate reflects the already extensive third-party payment for hospital costs). Increased demand for ambulatory services would be much more dramatic—approximately 75 percent—since present coverage of such services is limited.

Some increase in demand for services, particularly by lower-income people, is desirable; in fact, national health insurance would be a failure if it left existing patterns of medical care utilization unchanged. Increases in demand of this magnitude, however, may cause strains on the medical system. Newhouse notes that most of the increased demand for ambulatory services could not be fulfilled because of the limited supply of physicians and other providers. Inflationary pressures would build up, patients would experience longer delays in receiving appointments, and physicians might change the character of services provided (such as reducing time spent with each patient) and be more selective about the types of patients served. Physicians might even decide to work fewer hours, since with rising fees they would be able to earn higher incomes from seeing fewer patients.

Feldstein and Friedman (1975) have attempted to estimate the increase in prices that would be induced by greater insurance coverage. They consider replacing current coverage with a plan that contains a deductible of $50 each for hospital care and medical services, a coinsurance rate of 20 percent, and a maximum ceiling on patient contributions of 10 percent of family income. Based upon studies of the way hospitals and physicians respond to insurance coverage, they estimate that this type of coverage would increase prices by 40 percent. The inflationary impact of complete removal of patient payments would be even greater.

One way to resolve the dilemma of encouraging greater utilization of medical services by the poor without greatly increasing inflationary pressures would be to relate any cost-sharing provisions to income. Lower-income persons would have minimal or no direct costs, while others would be required to participate more fully in the cost of care. The following is illustrative of an income-related cost-sharing schedule. A family of four with an income below $5,000 would be excused from any direct payments. Families with incomes between $5,000 and $7,500 would be required to pay the first $50 of medical expenses for each of three family members and 20 percent of all expenses above that, with a ceiling on family payments set at 20 percent of income in excess of $5,000. Families with incomes between $7,500 and $10,000 would be required to pay the first $100 of medical expenses above that, also with a ceiling of 20 percent of income in excess of $5,000. Finally, families with incomes above $10,000 would be required to pay the first $150 of medical expenses for each of three family members and 25 percent of all medical expenses above that, with a total ceiling of $1,000 on family contributions. Figure 13.1 illustrates the maximum family payments that would be required and average expenditures families at various income levels would make if they incurred total medical expenditures of $1,000.

Cost-sharing provisions that are related to income have other desirable consequences. Experience with Medicare and Medicaid has illustrated that when lower-income people are not required to pay deductible and coinsurance amounts and higher-income people are, a more uniform utilization of medical care services among income classes results (Davis and Reynolds, 1975). Relating cost sharing to income in a systematic way should thus help eliminate major disparities among income classes in the use of services for people with comparable health problems. Income-related cost-sharing provisions are also a mechanism for reducing the adverse work incentives that might be created by an abrupt termination of benefits as income rises. That is, termination of benefits at, say, a family income of $5,000, may discourage a second family member from seeking a job or even discourage the primary earner from moonlighting or undertaking overtime work.

Limitations of Cost-Sharing Provisions

While the arguments for substantial cost sharing are many, there would inevitably be some ill effects. A complex schedule of payments is frequently difficult to understand, with the result that many people may not take advantage of the benefits available. This danger is minimized if the plan assumes responsibility for paying providers and billing patients for their share.

If cost sharing is related to income, some administrative mechanism must be devised for obtaining income information in a way that protects the individual from as much infringement of privacy as possible. One alternative would be

FIGURE 13.1
FAMILY COST SHARING IN NATIONAL HEALTH INSURANCE
UNDER AN ILLUSTRATIVE INCOME-RELATED PLAN

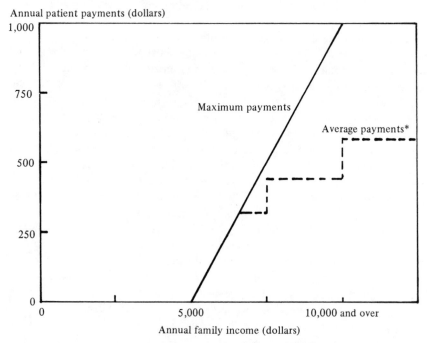

Annual patient payments (dollars)

Annual family income (dollars)

*Based on a family of four with family member medical expenses of $550, $250, $150, and $50.

for the Internal Revenue Service to issue a health "credit card" coded with the appropriate income information. Patients would charge services to the card and the administering agency would then pay the medical care provider and bill the patient for his or her share of the bill.

Imposition of cost-sharing amounts may also discourage some needed medical care, deter patients from seeking early treatment for a serious symptom, or cause patients to forgo beneficial preventive care. Preventive services of proven efficacy, however, can be exempted from deductible amounts if payment for such services can be shown to deter even high-income people from seeking this form of care.

The merits of cost-sharing provisions may be eroded in two ways: first, many people may purchase supplementary private insurance to pick up the deductible and coinsurance amounts; second, the importance of fixed cost-sharing amounts may be reduced over time by inflation in medical care costs. Under national health insurance there is no rationale for subsidizing the purchase of supplementary insurance. Any contributions by an employer to supplementary insurance should be counted as taxable income to the employee and not as a legitimate business expense of the firm. Deductions for health insurance and medical expenses under the personal income tax should also be eliminated. The real value of cost-sharing amounts can be retained by escalator clauses that automatically adjust deductible and maximum liability amounts to changes over time in average health expenditures per capita.

Unfortunately, the complete ramifications of cost sharing are not well known. Very little is known about how the use of supplementary private insurance would vary with different income-related cost-sharing schedules; even less is known about how such schedules would affect the mix of essential and marginal care. A national health insurance experiment was recently initiated by the U.S. Department of Health, Education, and Welfare to find answers to some of these questions, but even preliminary results will not be available for a couple of years. For a description of the experiment, see Newhouse (1974). In the meantime, experience with Medicare emphatically suggests that uniform cost-sharing provisions will lead to wide disparities in utilization among income classes but that reduced cost sharing for lower-income people can allow them to adopt patterns of medical care utilization similar to those of middle- and upper-income persons with similar health problems (see Davis and Reynolds, 1975; Peel and Scharff, 1973). Given the unknown consequences of either including or omitting cost sharing, retention of cost sharing, with the flexibility to alter schedules over time as experience is gained, seems to be the best approach.

HOW SHOULD THE PLAN BE FINANCED?

A decision about the appropriate method or methods of financing health insurance must weigh a number of objectives: (1) avoiding a regressive tax structure; (2) preventing adverse effects on employment; and (3) minimizing any windfall gains to those currently financing medical care. These objectives, however, are not absolute and may be altered by the mix of financing for other public goods and services.

Equity in Financing

A method of financing is considered to be regressive if its cost represents a higher fraction of income for lower-income than for higher-income families. In the case of national health insurance, the cost is the sum of premiums and taxes (whether payroll or other federal and state taxes) paid by the family, either directly or indirectly.

The distribution of insurance benefits by income classes under the plan may influence the degree of progressivity or regressivity deemed appropriate. (This point has been made by Feldstein, Friedman, and Luft, 1972. Many of the concepts discussed in this section are explored in greater detail there.) Differences in benefits among income classes may arise either because family composition varies by income class (for example, many low-income families are one- or two-person elderly families) or because the benefits of the plan vary directly with income. The plan may require lower cost sharing by lower-income families, thus diverting a larger than proportionate share of benefits to the poor. The poor may also receive more benefits because of their greater incidence of medical problems. The actual distribution of benefits, however, will also depend on variations in total medical expenditures by income class. That is, cost-sharing provisions are less of a deterrent to the use of medical services by higher-income families, and medical resources are more readily available to them. Therefore, higher-income families may have greater total medical expenditures, which offsets somewhat the lower proportion of the total bill paid by the insurance plan. In comparing the progressivity or regressivity of two plans that differ in their distribution of benefits as well as costs, it is useful to examine the distribution of *net benefits*—that is, insurance benefits less premiums or taxes paid into the plan—among income classes.

Another measure of the distributional effects of a national health insurance plan would have to include medical expenditures not covered by the plan. If lower-income families are not required to make any direct payments while higher-income families must pay most of their medical expenses directly, the cost of medical care will fall more heavily on higher-income families. The average total payment, including direct patient payments as well as premiums and taxes paid, indicates the complete cost of medical care to the family. If the total level of medical care varies by income, this measure of cost does not apply to a constant amount of medical care. Thus, some families with a higher average total payment may obtain more medical care for their contribution than a family with lower average total payment.

Financing for most national health insurance plans is based upon premiums, payroll tax revenues, and federal and state general revenues. Financing by premiums paid directly by employers or private individuals to private insurance companies has the effect of limiting the federal budgetary cost of the plan. If the premium is mandatory, however, this lower budgetary cost is largely illusory because the compulsory premium contribution is actually no different from a tax assessed on the employer for purposes of providing the benefits. In fact, if a firm responds to this premium by lowering cash wages or raising them less than it would otherwise, the premium is borne by the employee. In this case, it becomes a regressive tax, representing a much higher share of income for low-income groups. For example, if the total premium cost were $600, workers with incomes of $15,000 would pay 4 percent of their incomes for the premium while workers with incomes of $6,000 would pay 10 percent of their incomes.

The payroll tax, while not a progressive source of financing like the income tax, is markedly less regressive than a fixed premium per family. For example, if the insurance plan were financed by a 4 percent tax on the first $20,000 of family earnings, all families earning below $20,000 would pay a constant 4 percent rather than the higher percentage that low-income workers would pay with a fixed premium. Reform of the payroll tax could further mitigate its regressive nature. One step in this direction would be to make the tax applicable to all earnings. Its burden on two-worker and low-income families could be further lightened by providing rebates or subsidies to low-income workers. If the payroll tax were combined with a tax on unearned income (dividends, interest, rent, capital gains, transfer payments, and so forth), the overall tax burden could be made more proportional to total income. Heavy reliance on the progressive personal income tax as a method of financing would make such reform less urgent.

The cost of health insurance should not only be fairly borne by families of varying incomes, but families with the same income should be treated equally. Making all sources of income subject to taxes is one means of achieving this end. Special difficulties arise, however, in plans that rely on premiums as a method of financing. Policies sold by private health insurance companies typically have higher premiums for small groups, the self-employed, and groups that include some poor health risks. Thus, a family may find that its cost is higher because of the type of employment or nature of the group to which it belongs even though it receives the same benefits as another family with the same income. Even when payroll or general taxes are used, a family living in an area with limited medical resources and low medical prices may receive lower payments from the plan than a family with the same income and premiums that lives in an area with ample medical resources of high quality and specialization.

Employment Effects

The way in which national health insurance is financed can also have important effects on the demand and supply of labor. An employer may be unable to shift the cost of a premium to workers if wages are already at the minimum wage level. For these low-wage employers, the premium is much the same as an increase in the minimum wage, thus raising the cost of workers to the firm. If the increase in cost is substantial, some low-wage employers may either go out of business or substantially reduce their labor force.* Employers would also have a

---

*An excellent discussion of the adverse economic effects of premiums is contained in a criticism by the Department of Health, Education, and Welfare of the administration's original national health insurance proposal:

Employer mandated health insurance coverage would have the following economic effects:

1. The income distribution consequences would be regressive with regard to both the financing and to a lesser extent, the benefit structure. NHISA [the former administration plan] would be financed by a fixed tax per employee that is unrelated to earnings. Thus, the proportion of earnings that would be devoted to NHISA premiums would be greatest among low income workers. . . .

2. The economic effect on the labor market of mandated coverage is identical

strong incentive to hire part-time workers, secondary family earners, or those who decline the insurance.

In addition to influencing employer preferences among employees or the employment opportunities offered to different types of workers, a health insurance plan may affect people's willingness to work by imposing high marginal tax rates on additional earnings. Marginal tax rates on income net of medical expenses are affected by a reduction in benefits and an increase in costs as income rises.* In some plans, reduction in benefits and increases in costs may more than offset additional earnings, so that the marginal tax rate exceeds 100 percent. A working family that finds itself with less money to spend on nonmedical expenses after a pay raise, after working overtime, or after a second earner enters the labor force may feel resentful and reluctant to work as hard.

Windfall Gains

Finally, the choice of methods of financing should depend to some extent on current sources of payment. In 1975, it is estimated that employers will contribute $20 billion to employee health insurance plans, and state and local governments will contribute $6.3 billion to public health insurance plans (U.S. Department of Health, Education, and Welfare, 1974, p. 3). If no consideration were given to these payments, employers and state governments would gain from the plan. If the balance between federal and state government expenditures is desirable, a continuing contribution from the states may be in order. While reductions in contributions by employers to health insurance plans might eventually result in higher wages, some windfall gains to employers may occur if they are relieved of responsibility for currently scheduled payments. To avoid such gains, employers could be required to contribute to premiums or payroll taxes at least the amount they currently pay under private health insurance plans. Gradual reductions could be implemented over time if continuing employer contributions were not required.

---

to that of an increase in the minimum wage of an amount equivalent to the employer's share of premiums. . . . The dislocation occurs for those marginal workers who are at the minimum wage. A strong equity argument can be made that, if the Federal government wishes to mandate coverage, it ought to help pay for it.
3. Since small employers as a group offer their employees less generous health insurance benefits than large employers, they would be most affected by the requirement to offer a minimum benefit package. (Hearings before the Senate Committee on Labor and Public Welfare, 93rd Congress, 1st session, 1973)
   *If the family is more concerned with premiums and taxes and not as aware of reductions in medical benefits as income rises, the marginal gross tax rate—defined as the increase in costs as income rises—may be a more appropriate measure of work disincentive.

WHAT ROLE SHOULD PRIVATE INSURANCE COMPANIES
AND STATE GOVERNMENTS HAVE?

A wide range of administrative arrangements in a national health insurance plan is possible. Private health insurance companies could be charged with selling plans, underwriting coverage, and making profits. Alternatively, their role could be limited to that of administrative agents of a public plan, simply processing claims and making payments but not setting premiums and underwriting coverage. Or they could be totally replaced by a publicly administered plan. Similarly, state governments could be charged with regulating health insurance companies, establishing methods of paying medical care providers, and guaranteeing quality standards, either with or without general federal guidelines, or the federal government could assume all of these roles. States could participate in the subsidy of medical care for low-income persons, or all costs could be assumed federally.

Private Health Insurance Industry

The private health insurance industry has grown from an infant industry in 1940 to one with an estimated sales volume of $32.5 billion in 1975 (U.S. Department of Health, Education, and Welfare, 1974, p. 3). Insurance companies, acting as administrative agents for the Medicare program, will also cover another $13 billion of medical care expenditures in 1975. In addition, several states contract with private insurance companies for the administration of Medicaid claims. Any national health insurance plan that does not have a role for private companies could result in substantial displacement effects.

Administrative expenses under the Medicare and Medicaid programs have been considerably lower than for private health insurance plans, averaging 5 percent of benefit expenses in recent years. A valid comparison with private plans is difficult, however, because of the population covered. For one thing, the elderly tend to have larger average claims, so the administrative cost per dollar of benefits is low. Medicaid covers a population with greater than average health problems, so the average claim size may be greater there as well. Government plans may not capture all types of costs included in private plans, particularly capital costs, but they also provide additional services to the community such as ensuring quality and safety standards and enforcing discrimination provisions. The health insurance industry points to the experience of several large groups—such as the privately run federal employees indemnity benefit plan, where operating expenses are 3 percent of benefits, and other large groups that cover 50,000 or more employees, where expenses average 2.9 percent of benefits—to suggest that private plans could have much lower administrative costs if the size of their groups were comparable to those of the Medicare and Medicaid programs (*National Health Insurance,* vol. 4, 1974, p. 1528). A recent unpublished study by the Department of Health, Education, and Welfare, however, shows that administrative expenses of the Medicaid program have been 30 percent higher in states that contract with private insurance companies for administration rather than administering the program directly.

The performance of private health insurance companies has been varied and difficult to assess. For the most part, the industry has had great difficulty in staying ahead of rapidly rising medical prices, so that profits do not appear to be high. During the period of price controls beginning in late 1971, private health insurance companies appear to have experienced more rapid increases in premium income than in claims expenses (Mueller, 1974). However, since private insurance companies are not required to report income from investment of reserves, no measure of overall profitability of the industry is available. As shown in table 13.1, Blue Cross-Blue Shield plans averaged a net income of 4.0 percent

TABLE 13.1

FINANCIAL EXPERIENCE OF PRIVATE HEALTH INSURANCE
ORGANIZATIONS, 1972

(millions of dollars)

						Net income	
Type of plan	Total income	Subscrip- tion or premium income	Claims expense	Operat- ing expense	Net under- writing gain	Amount	As per- cent of premium income
Blue Cross-Blue Shield	10,079	9,923	8,991	689	243	399	4.0
Blue Cross	7,175	7,067	6,501	365	201	309	4.4
Blue Shield	2,904	2,856	2,490	324	43	90	3.2
Insurance com- panies	n.a.†	10,905	9,120	2,334	−548	n.a.	n.a.
Group poli- cies	n.a.	8,309	7,754	1,113	−558	n.a.	n.a.
Individual policies	n.a.	2,596	1,366	1,220	10	n.a.	n.a.
Independents*	1,517	1,499	1,381	112	5	24	1.6
All plans	n.a.	22,327	19,492	3,135	−300	n.a.	n.a.

*These include community, employer-employee-union, private group clinic, and dental service corporation plans.

†Not available.

Source: Mueller (1974, p. 32). Figures are rounded.

of premium income in 1972. Claims and operating expenses of other insurance companies exceeded premium income in 1972, but these losses may have been made up by income on investments.

The cost of insurance, measured as the difference between premium payments and benefit expenditures, has varied from plan to plan. Table 13.2 shows

TABLE 13.2
OPERATING EXPENSES AND RETENTIONS OF
PRIVATE HEALTH INSURANCE ORGANIZATIONS, 1972

	Operating expense as percent of premium income	Operating expenses per enrollee (dollars)	Retentions as percent of premium income
Insurance companies			
Blue Cross	5.2	5.05	8.0
Blue Shield	11.3	5.07	12.8
Type of plan			
Group policies	13.4	13.05	6.7
Individual policies	47.0	24.45	47.4
Independent	7.5	9.77	7.8
All plans	14.0	..	12.7

Source: Mueller (1974, pp. 32, 37, 38).

that in 1972 operating expenses as a percent of premium income averaged 5.2 percent in Blue Cross plans, 11.3 percent in Blue Shield plans, 13.4 percent in other group plans, and 47.0 percent in other individual insurance plans. This measure of cost, however, is sensitive to the size and frequency of claims and the mix of services insured. Differences in operating expenses per enrollee are not so marked, averaging $5 per enrollee in both Blue Cross and Blue Shield plans, $13 in other group plans, and $24 in other individual plans. Low operating expenses, however, may result in excessive benefit expenses if claims are not carefully reviewed. Thus low operating expenses do not necessarily imply efficient operation.

In spite of the conflicting evidence about the relative efficiency of public and private insurance administration, it is clear that over a billion dollars of marketing costs could be saved by federal administration of a national health insurance plan. Complete elimination of the industry, however, would cause substantial dislocation, and an intermediate role as administrative agent seems justified. Competitive bidding for this role should help to weed out the most inefficient carriers. Reform of the industry to make it more responsive to consumers and less responsive to the wishes of medical care providers should also help to curb some of the abuses that have occurred in the Blue Cross-Blue Shield plans (Law, 1974).

State Governments

The major roles that have been proposed for state governments in national health insurance are to regulate the private insurance industry, establish standards for participation and payment methods and levels for medical care providers, and administer and subsidize coverage for low-income families.

Combining some of these roles can create dilemmas for state governments. For example, if a state is charged with establishing fee levels for physicians, it must trade off pressures to set higher fees that would attract physicians to the state against the lower fees that would minimize the cost of the low-income plan. If experience with Medicaid is any guide, those states with the most limited medical resources would also have the least attractive physician reimbursement levels, while the states that could afford to heavily subsidize care for the poor are likely to have the most generous reimbursement levels, even though they are also likely to have the least need for additional health manpower.

Since newly trained medical manpower is largely mobile from state to state, a federal reimbursement policy would seem to be indicated. Experimentation with other roles for state governments, with appropriate federal guidelines, might also be a worthwhile undertaking.

WHAT ROLE SHOULD CONSUMERS HAVE?

An often forgotten component of a national health insurance plan is a clearly defined role for consumers. Although consumers have frequently had little say in the formulation and operation of a plan, their participation on a number of levels should help to ensure that the system is flexible and responsive to the needs of those it is designed to serve. (For a discussion of the emerging role of consumers in health care organizations, see Sheps, 1972.)

First, it is important that grievance processes be established so that consumers may channel complaints quickly and efficiently and without substantial legal expenses. Periodic hearings should also be held to uncover deficiencies in the coverage or operation of the plan. Second, consumers should be guaranteed representation on all important policy-setting or advisory boards. Preferably, these positions would be elected ones, thus minimizing the danger that the so-called public members are really appointed by those with vested interests in the plan. Finally, safeguards for patient privacy are essential in any plan collecting massive amounts of sensitive medical information. Patients should have a right to examine their own records, and patient approval of the release of any medical information should be required. If the plan requires income information, this should be obtained in a manner that does not reveal personal income to medical care providers, other patients, or private companies.

HOW SHOULD HOSPITALS, PHYSICIANS, AND OTHER PROVIDERS BE PAID?

One of the most difficult issues to resolve in a national health insurance plan is how to pay providers of services. Since cooperation of hospitals, physicians, and other providers is essential to the success of the plan, any substantial reduction in their relative incomes or change in their modes of practice may thwart the objectives of the plan. Yet one important objective of national health insurance is to limit rises in medical costs and encourage more efficient use of resources. Solutions to this dilemma are not easily found.

The first issue is whether reimbursement or payment by the insurance plan should constitute total payment for services, or whether physicians, hospitals, and others should be permitted to charge some patients, or all patients, more than the plan allows.

The Medicare program has permitted physicians to determine on each claim whether or not to accept assignment—that is, to accept the allowed charge as payment in full. On approximately 57 percent of the claims, physicians do accept assignment, but this fraction has been declining in recent years as Medicare has sought to tighten the level of reimbursement. In fiscal 1973, the difference between billed and allowed charges on unassigned claims under Medicare amounted to $214.3 million. This amount represents one-eighth of aggregate private expenditures by the aged for physicians' services (*National Health Insurance*, Vol. 2, 1974, pp. 601-02). Thus, experience with Medicare suggests that if given an option many physicians may choose to charge more than the allowed reimbursement, thus undermining the objectives of the plan, which are to ensure that medical care is not unduly expensive for those with limited means, to eliminate the financial burden of medical care for all, and to restrain cost increases.

More physicians may choose to accept assignment if they must select one fee basis for all patients, if they are relieved of bad debts and billing costs, and if they are offered other inducements such as free malpractice insurance.* However, under any plan that greatly increases inflationary pressures—and one study has estimated that demand for ambulatory services would increase by 75 percent under a full-coverage plan (Newhouse, Phelps, and Schwartz, 1974)—many physicians would be tempted to set fees at more than the allowed charge. Requiring physicians to accept assignment for certain classes of patients, such as the poor and elderly, so as to protect those who cannot pay from the financial consequences of nonassignment, may well simply reduce the supply of physician services available to them. Physicians, finding that they can earn higher incomes from other patients, may refuse to take patients for whom assignment is required or may give them lower-quality care. Such practices could reinforce the tradition of two-class medicine that national health insurance should help to eliminate.

Even if the physician is required to accept the reimbursement level established by the plan as allowable, several choices among reimbursement methods may be made. Physicians could be reimbursed on the basis of customary or usual fees according to a preestablished fee schedule, on a salary basis, or on a capita-

*Free malpractice insurance was proposed by Wilbur J. Cohen in testimony before the House Committee on Ways and Means. See *National Health Insurance*, vol. 7 (1974, p. 2762).

tion basis. Each method of reimbursement has its own set of incentives, and abuses can occur under any method. Physicians paid on a fee basis may increase the number of services provided, such as by repeat office visits or additional tests and procedures, in order to increase their incomes. Physicians paid on a salary or capitation basis may try to restrict the number of services provided and the time spent with each patient in order to increase leisure time. Usual and customary fee reimbursement probably has the greatest inflationary potential, and it preserves the incentives now operative for the distribution of medical personnel. A uniform national payment plan, on the other hand, would provide positive incentives for physicians to locate in lower-cost areas, which are frequently areas with a shortage of medical services, rather than in areas with a surplus of services where demand from high-income patients has led to high monetary rewards for physicians. Fee schedules, if developed by the medical profession, may reward those with the greatest power in the profession, such as specialists and physicians affiliated with medical schools and penalize physicians engaging in primary care or family practice.

There are also a number of methods possible for reimbursement of institutional providers. Reimbursement methods that would determine payment in advance of the provision of services, and independently of cost experiences, have been suggested. However, experience with such methods in Canada has shown them to be largely ineffective in containing costs (Evans, 1975). Other proposals would gear reimbursement to the level of all hospitals of a given type in a given geographical area, rather than to the actual cost experience of the individual hospital. Still others would devise formulas taking into account the diagnostic mix of patients served, the level of services provided, and adjustment for quality differences (Lave, Lave, and Silverman, 1973). Unfortunately, only limited experience has been obtained under any of these methods, and little is known about the efficacy of any one procedure. Experiments currently being conducted by the Social Security Administration and others should make possible more informed judgments about appropriate institutional reimbursement methods.

HOW SHOULD THE PLAN CHANGE OVER TIME?

Since answers to all the basic questions about the most appropriate form of national health insurance cannot be formulated before enactment of a plan, it is important that any plan adopted be flexible enough that it can be altered as experience is gained. Mechanisms for collecting appropriate data on performance and for feeding this information back into improved design are important features to be included in any plan.

It can be anticipated, however, that several features of the plan will require automatic adjustment over time—namely, those that are sensitive to overall changes in prices and incomes in the economy. Deductible amounts, for example, should be adjusted upward over time at the same rate as the average level of expenditures on medical services in order to preserve the original cost-sharing relationships. Income classes should also be adjusted upward as money incomes rise over time. Reimbursement of providers should likewise be tied to experience. Rather than tying physician *fees* to an appropriate economic index, tying *average physician expenditures* under the plan to an index would prevent physicians from increasing incomes by proliferating services.

REFERENCES

Beck, R. G. "The Effects of Co-payment on the Poor." *Journal of Human Resources* 9 (Winter 1974): 129-42.

Davis, K. "Lessons of Medicare and Medicaid for National Health Insurance." *National Health Insurance—Implications* (Hearings before the Subcommittee on Public Health and Environment of the House Committee on Interstate and Foreign Commerce, 93rd Congress, 1st and 2nd sessions, 1974). Brookings Institution Reprint 295.

Davis, K., and Reynolds, R. "The Impact of Medicare and Medicaid on Access to Medical Care." *The Role of Health Insurance in the Health Services Sector,* edited by R. N. Rosett. New York: National Bureau of Economic Research, 1975.

Evans, R. G. "Beyond the Medical Marketplace: Expenditure, Utilization and Pricing of Insured Health Care in Canada." *The Role of Health Insurance in the Health Services Sector,* edited by R. N. Rosett. New York: National Bureau of Economic Research, 1975.

Feldstein, M. S. "Econometric Studies of Health Economics" (Discussion Paper 291). Cambridge, Mass.: Harvard Institute of Economic Research, 1973.

Feldstein, M. S., and Friedman, B. "The Effect of National Health Insurance on the Price and Quantity of Medical Care." *The Role of Health Insurance in the Health Services Sector,* edited by R. N. Rosett. New York: National Bureau of Economic Research, 1975.

Feldstein, M. S.; Friedman, B.; and Luft, H. "Distributional Aspects of National Health Insurance Benefits and Finance." *National Tax Journal* 25 (December 1972): 497-510.

Ginsburg, P. B., and Manheim, L. M. "Insurance, Copayment, and Health Services Utilization: A Critical Review." *Journal of Economics and Business* 25 (Winter 1973): 142-53.

Greenlick, M. R., et al. "Comparing Medical Care Services by a Medically Indigent and a General Membership Population in a Comprehensive Prepaid Group Practice Program." *Medical Care* 10 (May/June 1972): 187-200.

Hall, C. P., Jr., et al. "The Effects of Cost-Sharing in the Medicaid Program: Final Report." Philadelphia: Temple University, 1973.

Hardwick, C. P.; Shuman, L.; and Barnoon, S. "Effect of Participatory Insurance on Hospital Utilization." *Health Services Research* 7 (Spring 1972): 43-57.

Kaplan, R. S., and Lave, L. B. "Patient Incentives and Hospital Insurance." *Health Services Research* 6 (Winter 1971): 288-300.

Lave, J. R.; Lave, L. B.; and Silverman, L. P. "A Proposal for Incentive Reimbursement for Hospitals." *Medical Care* 11 (March/April 1973): 79-90.

Law, S. A. *Blue Cross—What Went Wrong?* New Haven: Yale University Press, 1974.

Mueller, M. S. "Private Health Insurance in 1972: Health Care Services, Enrollment, and Finances." *Social Security Bulletin* 37 (February 1974): 32.

National Health Insurance, vols. 2, 4, 7 (Hearings before the House Committee on Ways and Means, 93rd Congress, 2nd session, 1974).

Newhouse, J. P. "A Design for a Health Insurance Experiment." *Inquiry* 11 (March 1974): 5-27.

Newhouse, J. P., and Phelps, C. E. *On Having Your Cake and Eating It Too: Econometric Problems in Estimating the Demand for Health Services.* Santa Monica, Calif.: Rand, 1974.

Newhouse, J. P.; Phelps, C. E.; and Schwartz, W. B. "Policy Options and the Impact of National Health Insurance." *New England Journal of Medicine* 290 (June 13, 1974): 1345-59.

Peel, E., and Scharff, J. "Impact of Cost-Sharing on Use of Ambulatory Services Under Medicare, 1969." *Social Security Bulletin* 36 (October 1973): 3-24.

Scitovsky, A. A., and Snyder, N. M. "Effect of Coinsurance on Use of Physician Services." *Social Security Bulletin* 35 (June 1972): 3-19.

Sheps, C. G. "The Influence of Consumer Sponsorship on Medical Services." *Milbank Memorial Fund Quarterly* 50, no. 4 (October 1972): 41-69.

U.S. Department of Health, Education, and Welfare. *Estimated Health Expenditures Under Selected National Health Insurance Bills* (A Report to the Congress). Washington, D.C.: HEW, 1974.

Selection by Roger M. Battistella and John R. C. Wheeler

INTRODUCTION

In comparison with other countries, the United States, a country generally respected for its political and technological innovations and for its unexcelled standard of living, has been very slow to enact a social program for safeguarding families against the threat of economic insecurity arising from the costs of illness and health care. Some insight into why a national health insurance program has been so slow to develop may be found in the historical influence which ideology has had in shaping U.S. social policy. In addition to describing the evolution of national health policy legislation, this paper seeks to assess the prospects for the future in terms of what seems feasible, given the interplay of social, political, and economic forces conditioning government action.

NATIONAL HEALTH INSURANCE: EVOLUTION OF AN IDEA

If, in the course of economic history, the practice of unfettered free enterprise was a short-lived aberration, nowhere did the idea take root more firmly than in the United States. In the company of collateral doctrines disseminated from England (laissez-faire, social Darwinism, and the Protestant ethic), free enterprise, reinforced by the challenge of a vast, unsettled western frontier, provided the ideological glue for the structuring of economic and social relationships constituting the core of American culture. This historical background supports our current popular belief that the free market should solve the economic problems of allocation, production, and distribution, and that governmental

This selection, "Ideology, Economics, and the Future of National Health Insurance," was revised especially for this volume.

373

intervention can be justified only in the event of some malfunctioning of the market system. The key concepts in our modern ideology are that government action is *intervention* into the operation of our preferred mechanism for solving the problems of society and that such action must hence be *justified* in terms of a breakdown in the preferred mechanism. Our reliance on the market has been and continues to be so fundamental that the development of social programs external to the market has been slow indeed. As a general rule, the United States has consistently been among the last countries in the industrialized world to implement programs in such areas as unemployment insurance, old age pensions, disability insurance, income supports, public housing, etc. (For a scholarly review of the origins and significance of free enterprise values in shaping U.S. social policy, see Mencher, 1967.) The feature which differentiates national health insurance from other social programs is that the implementation lag has been far longer. (A comparative chronology of social service programs may be found in U.S. Social Security Administration, 1974.)

That private financing of the costs of health care has survived for so long is due to a combination of factors. First of all, so long as medicine remained technologically simple and inexpensive, the gainfully employed and the middle class were able to keep pace with health care costs through advances in income and the expansion of private health insurance. Second, the especially close identification which medicine has had with free enterprise, and the effective manner in which the American Medical Association has appealed over the years to the xenophobic suspicions of public opinion toward foreign-inspired ideas and competing ideologies, have impeded governmental intervention in the financing and delivery of health care. These factors, in combination with the patchwork strategy of meeting the most pressing social needs, have made possible the persistence of the private sector as the chief element in the financing of the cost of health care.

HISTORICAL HIGHLIGHTS

The grip of free enterprise ideology in shaping health policy is manifested in the protracted struggle for national health insurance which extends as far back as 1912, when it was an important issue in the presidential campaign of Theodore Roosevelt. (On the history of U.S. health policy and the struggle for national health insurance, see, for example, Davis, 1955; Anderson, 1968; Falk, 1973.) During this lengthy period there were bursts of activity in the following years: (1) from 1915 to 1920, when a model bill drafted by the American Association for Labor Legislation was introduced into many state legislatures; (2) from 1927 to 1933, when the Committee on the Cost of Medical Care, in its desire to find an American solution to the problem of health care financing, rejected as politically untenable the principle of compulsory public insurance prevalent in Europe at the time in favor of a private-voluntary approach; (3)

from 1934 to 1935, when, in the midst of a serious economic depression and in the face of bitter controversy over socialized medicine, the President's Committee on Economic Security tabled for further study the question of national health insurance in advancing its recommendations for enactment of the Social Security Act; (4) from 1938 to 1939, when a national health conference convened by President Franklin Roosevelt to study the question of health financing recommended approval of a national program, prompting Senator Robert F. Wagner of New York to introduce in the Congress the first of a series of bills implementing one or more parts of the conference's recommended program; (5) in 1943, when President Roosevelt, in a message to the American people, called for a program of adequate medical care and protection from the problem of economic insecurity; and (6) from 1946 to 1952, when President Truman pushed repeatedly for adoption of a nationwide program of compulsory social insurance. In seeking to attain his objective, President Truman convened a second national health conference in 1948 and in 1951 set up a Presidential commission to further study and make recommendations on the health needs of the nation. The conflict and controversy accompanying these moves was intense and highly acrimonious.

The American Medical Association, which had from 1924 pursued a strategy of minimizing the publication of dissenting opinions and of attacking individual dissenters as socialists and communists, launched a massive nationwide campaign which had as its objective stopping the agitation for compulsory health insurance by enrolling the people in sound voluntary health systems. Toward this end, a campaign fund of $2,250,000 was amassed by a special assessment of $25 upon every member, and the services of a prominent public relations firm, which had earlier worked for the California Medical Association to defeat Governor Earl Warren's proposal for a state compulsory health insurance law, were obtained. With the defeat of several prominent Congressmen who had supported national health insurance and the Republican landslide in the presidential election of 1952, the issue of universal compulsory health insurance receded. In the place of division and conflict there arose a consensus which favored making voluntary health insurance the nation's major line of defense in the struggle against economic insecurity due to the unpredictability of illness and the cost of health care. This consensus was born of practicality and the conclusion that government-sponsored health insurance did not have the voter appeal usually attributed to it.

The consensus proved highly favorable to the growth of voluntary health insurance, which had its beginnings as an important social force in the depression of the 1930s, when hospitals were threatened with fiscal insolvency. An additional stimulus occurred in World War II, when the freezing of wages established fringe benefits like health insurance as a significant element of collective bargaining. The tendency in the postwar years has been for employers to pay for larger shares of premiums as a condition of employment for workers. (Employers paid two-thirds of the cost of premiums for their workers in 1975 and roughly two-fifths of employers now contribute all of the cost of premiums. See U.S. Public Health Service, 1976, p. 31.) The proportion of the civilian resident population possessing some form of voluntary hospital insurance increased from less than 10 percent in 1940 to 87 percent in 1973. Over the same period coverage for surgical expenses increased from 4 percent to 81 percent (U.S. Department of Health, Education, and Welfare, 1976, p. 185). This impressive growth in voluntary health insurance notwithstanding, it became apparent with experience and study that certain population groups, such as the poor and the aged, because of the combination of inability to pay premiums, high rates of illness, and escalating medical costs, required special assistance. In the face of such need among population groups outside the reach of private insurance, the federal government initiated a number of responses culminating in the Medicare and Medicaid programs. (On the political and legislative history of Medicare and Medicaid, see, for example, Harris, 1966; Feingold, 1966.)

Medicaid is a component of the federal-state public assistance program which, following its inception as part of the Social Security Act of 1935, has evolved to become the backstop of economic security for the poor. First, federal aid was granted to the states in 1950 permitting direct payment to medical vendors (doctors, hospitals, and others) providing health care to recipients. As in other parts of the public assistance program, the states were given the option to participate selectively and to set separate standards for each of the four eligible groups (the aged, the blind, the permanently and totally disabled, and families with dependent children). Second, federal aid in the vendor payments program was expanded in 1960 to permit special grants to the states for medical assistance for the aged. Popularly named after its Congressional sponsors, Senator Robert Kerr and Congressman Wilbur Mills, the Kerr-Mills program broke new ground in introducing a specific federal-state program for health and expanding the concept of indigency to encompass persons who were self-sustaining except when it came to meeting the cost of health care—the medically indigent. Finally, the Social Security Act Amendments of 1965 provided for the gradual replacement of the separate vendor payment program by a single uniform statewide medical care program (Medicaid) on behalf of all persons eligible for public assistance, and widened the concept of medical indigency further to include the nonaged. Through a series of incremental improvements the program was designed to eventually provide low-income persons with comprehensive benefits and to eliminate class distinctions among hospital and physicians' services by enabling the poor to receive their care from the same sources as the middle class. Unexpectedly high expenditures, however, have led both state and federal governments, which share fiscal responsibilities, to back away from the initial Medicaid benefits and eligibility standards, with the result that there has been a shift back toward the pre-1965 welfare situation. The unpopularity of Medicaid, stemming from the lumping together of the "deserving" and "nondeserving" poor (notably unmarried black women and out-of-wedlock children), and from the inefficient administration and cheating intrinsic to a highly decentralized, loosely controlled, and complex system of services, has provided a convenient justification to cut back. Ironically, the widespread requirement for local government to participate with the state government in financing the nonfederal share of the cost of services has resulted often in some of the most severe complaints against Medicaid among people in low-income areas who are most in need of services. (See, for example, U.S. Department of Health, Education, and Welfare, 1976, pp. 127-30.)

In the case of the aged not on welfare rolls, a succession of studies in the 1950s and early 1960s painted a startling picture of quiet suffering. As revealed in the Beveridge Report in England over a decade previously, a remarkably large number of the elderly appeared to prefer destitution and silent poverty rather than submit to the indignity of applying for welfare and public assistance. To a generation steeped in the values of hard work, thrift, self-sufficiency, and the perception of poverty as a sign of moral failure, the means test was a dreadful form of humiliation. In addition to the problem of insufficient retirement income, the evidence pointed to the cost of health care as a principal threat to the peace of mind and economic security of the elderly. These shocking disclosures produced an outpouring of public sympathy which, following almost ten years' effort, resulted in 1965 in the passage of the Medicare Act, which had as its most important feature a program of compulsory social insurance for hospital care for the aged and the establishment for the first time, albeit on a limited basis, of the principle that health care is a right. Together with compulsory hospital insurance, Medicare made available to aged persons government-subsidized voluntary physicians and surgeons insurance. (However, due to increases in coinsurance and deductible payments and the failure of benefits to keep pace with inflation, the reduction in the level of protection provided by Medicare parallels the erosion of Medicaid—declining from roughly 40 percent of the health costs of the elderly in 1969 to only 35 percent in 1974. See U.S. Department of Health, Education, and Welfare, 1976, p. 120.)

THE CURRENT SCENE

The result of this lengthy historical contest between forces for social reform and those in support of the status quo is that the United States now has four separate schemes for financing the cost of health care: (1) nonprofit and commercial health insurance for the gainfully employed and their dependents, financed individually and/or by employer contributions; (2) public assistance payments from federal and state revenues for the indigent and medically indigent in Medicaid; (3) government-subsidized voluntary physicians and surgeons insurance for the aged in Part B of Medicare; and (4) compulsory social insurance for hospital care for the aged in Part A of Medicare. Despite the imaginative compromises represented by this pluralistic approach, experience has shown that conditions are far from satisfactory. The signs point increasingly to the need for more fundamental changes.

Governmental health policy in the 1970s appears to revolve around two highly interrelated issues: (1) the supposed imminence of some form of national health insurance; and (2) the need to counteract pressures toward rising health expenditures. The experience with Medicare and Medicaid has inspired the feeling that something must be done about the latter issue before we deal with the former issue. (See, for example, Klarman, 1977; U.S. Public Health Service, 1976, pp. 29-37.) However, the interrelatedness of the two is such that the existence of rapidly rising costs is precisely what generates demands for national health insurance. (Following the implementation of Medicare and Medicaid, federal health outlays have more than doubled, and they now comprise roughly 12 percent of the government's budget—subordinate in magnitude only to defense, national debt interest payments, and income security programs. See Council on Wage and Price Stability, 1976a, p. 29.) There has been a persistent secular trend of higher costs and expenditures, because of (1) the rise in consumer demands for more and better services; (2) the growth in high-risk groups at both ends of the population pyramid (i.e., the young and the aged); (3) the shift in disease patterns toward more complex and intractable forms of chronic illness; (4) the explosion of sophisticated but highly expensive biomedical technology; and (5) the rapid inflation in medical care prices. (See, for example, National Leadership Conference, 1977.)

Inflation has made the job of providing adequate coverage more difficult. It calls for a lot of running just to stay even, let alone move ahead. Consider the following: since the introduction of Medicare and Medicaid programs in 1965, physicians' fees have been increasing on the average at a rate of about 6 percent and hospital charges at a rate of 12 percent—in both cases approximately doubling the rates prevailing in the five-year period prior to 1965. Because it is by far the largest and most expensive health care item, the increase in the cost of hospital care represents a special cause for concern. The cost per day of care in a community hospital rose from roughly $16 in 1950 to $175 in 1976—a fivefold jump even after adjustments for general price inflation are made. (A convenient collection of data on health care costs and finances may be found in Gibson and Mueller, 1977.) Much of the increase is thought due to the proliferation of sophisticated but costly new services (e.g., cardiac care units, kidney dialysis, cobalt therapy). Because of the improved ability of hospitals to purchase new equipment following advances in voluntary health insurance and the provision of public financing to low-income populations (i.e., Medicare and Medicaid), new services have been introduced without careful analysis of their relative benefits and costs. Many represent overlap and duplication; even when utilized fully, some services are put to uses which are medically questionable or unnecessary. (For analyses of hospital costs, see Feldstein and Taylor, 1977; Baron, 1974; Elnicki, 1974; Jeffers and Siebert, 1974; Waldman, 1972.)

Although almost all Americans now have some form of private or public coverage against the cost of health care, the depth of coverage is far from complete. Currently all forms of third-party payment (i.e., private insurance and public payments) cover only about two-thirds of total health expenditures; the remaining one-third comes out of consumers' pockets. Notwithstanding increases in the share of total health expenditures paid for by government and private health insurance, the average direct payment by families was three times as great in 1974 as in 1950, due to rising prices and greater consumption of health care services (U.S. Public Health Service, 1975, p. 58). Under a strictly private health insurance system, comprehensive coverage (no coinsurance or deductibles) would cost $2,000 or more for a typical family of four in 1978.* Such an amount clearly is beyond the reach of many families, indicating that private health insurance can probably not be expected to meet the need for adequate protection against the cost of health care. It seems unlikely that premiums of that magnitude can be financed out of payroll deductions, especially in a period when the take-home pay of employees is being eroded by general inflation and employers are beginning to worry that the growth in fringe benefits is imposing a heavy burden on the cost of doing business. (See Council on Wage and Price Stability, 1976b, pp. 1-3.) Hence, the future of private health insurance as the principal mechanism for financing the cost of health care is in doubt; some form of governmental subsidization or at least mandating of private health insurance is required.

A measure of the degree to which the inevitability of some form of national health insurance has come to be accepted is the fact that the coalition of support for the idea, once razor thin, now encompasses virtually every important interest group in the nation. The coalition ranges the political spectrum from Liberals and Democrats to Republicans and Conservatives. Support for national health insurance comes from such groups as major purchasers of health care, providers of health services, and consumers. (See, for example, Margolis, 1977.) Though all favor national health insurance, each group does so for its own reasons, colored by ideology, self-interest, and varying concepts of the public interest.

Major purchasers under collective bargaining are concerned principally with the cost of doing business, of which health insurance premiums are a large and growing part—estimated to average nearly 4 percent of payroll in 1975, excluding Medicare contributions (*Health Security News*, 1977). Organized labor, under pressure from its members to increase take-home pay, is worried about the

*Estimates originally prepared in the late 1960s indicating a range from $800 to $1,000 were adjusted conservatively over a ten-year period to reflect a 10 percent annual rate of increase in medical care expenditures. See Reed and Carr (1968); U.S. Senate Committee on Finance (1970, p. 135). Another way of arriving at the $2,000 estimate is to note that per capita health care expenditures are currently substantially above $500 per year. Hence, comprehensive health insurance coverage for four people must surely exceed $2,000 in premiums.

effect of rising health insurance premiums on management's ability and willingness to provide pay and nonhealth fringe benefit increases. Both management and labor would no doubt welcome any opportunity to transfer part of the cost of financing health care from payroll to general revenues and appear to be eager supporters of any proposal designed to rationalize health care organization and slow down present rates of cost increases. Providers of care, such as hospitals, see national health insurance as a means for assuring income needed to meet escalating operating costs. Physicians look to it as a device for assuring adequate compensation for their services and for preserving fee-for-service principles in a time of increasing consumer and purchaser criticism of rising physicians' fees. Suppliers of health services, such as pharmaceutical manufacturers, hospital supply firms, and equipment manufacturers, are interested in opportunities to make money in a market with profits already totaling billions of dollars. Insurance companies, both nonprofit and commercial, see national health insurance as an instrument for assuring their relative position in the health market. Faced with intensive competition by commercial plans underwriting on an experience basis, Blue Cross and Blue Shield are increasingly looking to government to stabilize and improve their position in the health field. Commercial insurance companies also look to government as a vehicle for expediting more general market ambitions and for increasing profits by subsidizing the salaries of staff engaged in the marketing more profitable lines of insurance while at the same time fulfilling responsibilities in a program of national health insurance. Middle-class consumers are worried about the shrinking protection provided by health insurance and increased payroll deductions necessary just to hold the line on benefits, let alone expand them. The rising cost of care is a special problem for low-income families and the poor who possess little or no insurance protection. Consumers in general are becoming worried about problems of access and quality resulting from personal shortages, inadequate regulation, and absence of planning controls. They are also critical of the lack of responsiveness on the part of health professionals and health care organizations to personal and community needs. In this regard, the poor have been especially vocal in requesting a larger voice in program decisions affecting them.

Many of the above groups have developed their own proposals for national health insurance. Despite differences in concerns and motives which can be expected to have a powerful effect on the type and degree of change, the strength of the coalition suggests that some change is forthcoming (Davis, 1975, pp. 80-128).

Although in the later 1970s we have come to the point where some sort of national health insurance program appears inevitable, we have simultaneously arrived at the understanding that resources, including those devoted to the provisions of medical care, are truly scarce. The fact that we are spending over 8.5 percent of our Gross National Product on health care has begun to shift health policy in the direction of attempts to control health care expenditures. Especially as a result of our experiences with Medicare and Medicaid, the fear is that without some governmental control over the allocation of resources to and within the health care sector, expenditures for health care might rise to unbearable levels. Hence, we have seen in recent years a body of health care legislation which implicitly rejects the market solution to resource allocation which prevailed until a few years ago. This legislation, while continuing the move away from market decision making, nonetheless contains vestiges of the antigovernment bias characteristic of our social history. In light of our earlier discussion about the influence of ideology on health policy, these actions should be appraised as much in terms of what they do not do as in terms of what they do.

As part of PL 92-603, the Social Security Amendments of 1972, the Professional Standards Review Organization program was established. It has as its explicit objective the evaluation of services provided to beneficiaries of federal health care programs in terms of the necessity for care received, the appropriateness of the level of care, and the adequacy and quality of service provided. The implied objectives are to contain utilization, and thereby cost of health services, and to assure that the services purchased are medically necessary and appropriate. (See, for example, Little, 1973, pp. 2-26.) Hence, the PSRO program is essentially a cost and quality control measure. As such, it appears to be an intrusion by the government into the medical care market, contrary to the historical development of health policy. However, a closer look at the PSRO system reveals it to be a device designed to keep the government out as much as possible. The original idea for the program came from the American Medical Association. Furthermore, the administration of the program is solely in the hands of physicians. Finally, the philosophical foundation for the programs, according to Senator Bennett, its sponsor, is that the profession of medicine can police itself better than can government. However, even allowing for its ideological and organizational character, the PSRO program does constitute a significant erosion of the freedom of the individual physician. Furthermore, it signifies an implicit rejection of the market as the mechanism for allocating health care resources.

The second major piece of recent health policy legislation, the Health Maintenance Organization Act, PL 93-22, assisted in the establishment and expansion of a particular type of health care financing and delivery institution. "The HMO has a limited membership who pay predetermined sums of money to a specific provider group which is obligated to deliver a specific set of comprehensive health services" (Roy, 1972, p. 13). Hence, the HMO Act is an attempt to join the delivery with the financing of services in order to improve the availability of care and provide incentives for the control of costs. It does so by controlling the access of both consumers and providers to high-technology, high-cost care. The economic incentives favor ambulatory care over hospital care and encourage doctors in their decision making to weigh whether the expected benefits are sufficient to justify the costs. A second objective is to make federal expenditures more predictable for fiscal planning purposes by substituting prospective payment for retrospective payment. Again, in this Act there are elements of anti-government bias as well as further evidence of a rejection of the free market solution. The former is manifested in the fact that, while government is providing financial and statutory nurturing, the HMOs themselves are nonetheless private organizations, competing with conventional health insurance companies for business. Therefore, the HMO Act is an attempt to encourage the use of private resources in a different kind of health delivery setting. Although it cloaks unconventional organizations in a conventional value system, it must also be recognized as an additional intrusion by government into the actual organization of health care delivery, and hence another example of lack of satisfaction with the medical care market. The transformation of medical practice from solo fee-for-service to prepaid group practice inevitably moves in the direction of greater management control and planning at the expense of the autonomy of entrepreneurially oriented individual practitioners.

As a final piece of recent health policy legislation which demonstrates the current ambivalence regarding governmental involvement in health care, we turn to the National Health Planning and Resources Development Act, PL 93-641, which called for major reorganization of the federal health planning programs by setting up local Health Services Areas with Health Systems Agencies empowered to advise state authorities concerning the addition or elimination of facilities. (For a review of the legislative background and provisions, see U.S. Department of Health, Education, and Welfare, 1977, pp. 1-28.) Again, the Health Systems Agencies are private, nonprofit entities, reflecting our national aversion to governmental intervention. By their very nature, however, planning agencies represent a rejection of market decision making; that is, a planning system is the antithesis of a market system. In order to determine how far down the road we have moved from the free market to the planned system in health care, however, we shall have to wait to see how much power the planning agencies and their associated governmental authorities are able to exercise.

The evidence seems clear that, while the ideology of competition and the free market continues to exercise considerable influence over the formulation of national health policy, its grip is becoming weaker. Dissatisfaction with the private financing and organization of the health care system, as manifested in national health care legislation, particularly since the mid-1960s, seems to be signalling a move toward more government involvement. In the next few years, the relative strengths of the market ideology, and of the dissatisfaction with the results of a system based on that ideology, will determine what kind of national health insurance we will have.

MAJOR PROPOSALS FOR NATIONAL HEALTH INSURANCE

There are presently several national health insurance bills before the 95th Congress, many of which have been under consideration for several years. Five of these bills have sufficient political sponsorship that some of their features may be incorporated into the program that wins approval. These are: (1) The Health Security Bill introduced by Senator Kennedy and supported by organized labor and the Committee for National Health Insurance; (2) the Comprehensive Health Insurance Bill, which was sponsored by the Nixon Administrations; (3) The National Health Care Bill supported by the Health Insurance Association of America; (4) The Health Care Insurance Bill (Medicredit) supported by the American Medical Association; and (5) the Catastrophic Health Insurance and Medical Assistance Reform Bill sponsored by Senators Long and Ribicoff and others (Margolis, 1977, p. 33; Davis, 1975, pp. 80-128).

When assessed in relation to the magnitude of consumer economic security needs and the disorganization in the structure and delivery of health care, all of the proposals appear surprisingly modest and conventional. With the exception of the Kennedy plan, which goes much further than the others, no appreciably new departures in financing are contemplated. If anything, the primary objectives seem to be aimed at (1) resuscitating and building on the present pluralistic foundation and (2) the preservation of the bias toward private insurance.

The attachment to familiar values of pluralism and private financing is seen most clearly in the Nixon proposal, which in effect is three separate programs. First, at the core of this plan is the *requirement* that all employers purchase private health insurance or membership in an HMO for their employees and their dependents, with employers eventually paying 75 percent of the premium. To assure a uniform floor of protection, it calls for nationwide minimum benefit standards and close federal regulation of the private health insurance industry. The second component of the Nixon plan is an assisted health insurance plan for low-income persons and others not eligible for either the employer-financed plan or Medicare. It would be paid for through income-related premiums from enrollees and federal and state contributions. The third component is an expanded Medicare program with additional benefits and very little change in financing structure.

The commercial health insurance industry's proposal would keep both Medicare and Medicaid and introduce tax incentives for employers and individuals to purchase standard private insurance protection. Like the Nixon plan, it would use federal subsidies for the purchase of private insurance for the poor and near-poor. The major difference between the two schemes is that the Nixon plan would use the power of the federal government to set uniform nationwide standards, whereas the private insurance companies prefer to work through the separate administrative machinery of the fifty state governments.

The American Medical Association plan favors a voluntary health insurance approach in which the federal government would pay for the purchase of health insurance for the poor. All others would be given income tax credits towards the purchase of private health insurance.

The catastrophic program advanced by Senators Long and Ribicoff would simply add a fifth layer to the four layers of financing currently operating in the United States. Its chief target is the relief of the middle class through catastrophic insurance financed out of social security taxes. Benefits would begin following the expiration of conventional voluntary health insurance benefits. Hospital benefits would start following sixty days of hospitalization with a $15-a-day coinsurance. Medical coverage would commence after families had spent $2,000 during the year and there would be a coinsurance of 20 percent. The principal shortcoming of catastrophic insurance is that, in the absence of effective planning controls over the supply and distribution of new services, it might have the effect of financing continuing overlap and duplication of sophisticated and expensive technologies.

The Health Security plan is the only one which would do much to rationalize and streamline the present complex pattern of financing in the United States. It would replace voluntary health insurance and the Medicare program with a single universal program of social insurance funded jointly on a fifty-fifty basis from employer-employee payroll taxes and general revenues, with 36 percent of the total coming from employers. Because of the exclusion of such benefits as dentistry for adults and custodial psychiatric and nursing home services, together with some drugs, it would pay on the average about 70 percent of personal health care expenditures. Persons not able to pay for the remaining 30 percent out of their own pockets would continue to fall back on the Medicaid welfare system. In contrast, all of the other plans reviewed here can be expected to provide protection in the range of 30 to 50 percent, judging from a rough extrapolation of the experience of the voluntary insurance and Medicare models on which they are based. For most Americans the changes are that the cost of health care will continue to be a major source of worry and threat to economic security.

In matters of organization and delivery the most notable of the proposed changes involves a gradual movement, through use of various fiscal incentives and removal of legal obstacles, toward (1) the consolidation of health services, and (2) forward payment of providers on a per capita arrangement in place of prevailing retrospective payment of fees and charges. The collective purpose of these changes is to promote more stable budgetary planning at the national level, while simultaneously encouraging stronger management and greater efficiency at the level of day-to-day operations. The proposals of former President Nixon, Senator Kennedy and, to a limited extent, the private health insurance industry, are geared to moving physicians out of the predominant solo fee-for-service form of practice into groups called health maintenance organizations. Each group would be expected to provide a comprehensive range of services to persons opting for the group in place of competing solo physicians and other groups. The strategy is to create a climate of competition, while tilting the balance in favor of group practice through generous construction and equipment grants along with attractive incomes for physicians. The hope is that by encouraging prevention and early detection of disease and the use of more careful cost-effectiveness weighing of alternative modes of treatment, costs can be lowered by capturing illness in its early stages and by discouraging unnecessary hospitalization. The inducement to physicians to cooperate is provided by the substitution of per capita payment for fees and by the opportunity to share in any end-of-year surplus in the group's budget. A frequently mentioned but unpublished objective is to cut hospital admissions by anywhere from one-fourth to one-third. In the light of the experience of a number of prepaid group practice plans which have been in existence for over thirty years such a target seems feasible (see Council on Wage and Price Stability, 1976b, p. 8; Donabedian, 1969).

Recently, the Carter Administration has received and is reportedly viewing somewhat favorably a national health insurance proposal written by Professor Alain Enthoven of Stanford University under a commission from HEW. The Enthoven proposal represents a departure from the proposals discussed above in that it relies heavily upon consumer choice as a mechanism for promoting competition and keeping costs down. The consumer would be given tax credits or vouchers for health insurance premiums paid and would be allowed to choose between traditional insurance and HMOs. Also, consumers would be able to choose not to participate. The proposal envisages differential subsidies based upon ability to pay. In addition to the consumer choice element, the proposal contains other provisions designed to control costs. Enthoven estimates that the plan, as written, would cost the government about $23 billion. Interestingly, this proposal can be viewed as still another attempt by government to use the leverage of its purchasing power to control cost and to influence the market sector to serve social objectives.

FUTURE PROSPECTS

Mindful of the trillion dollar economy which makes it among the richest countries in the world, foreign observers are understandably bewildered when they hear that the United States government takes the position that it cannot afford to pay for improvements in those social services which, like health, are so important for making life tolerable, if not pleasant. This curious contention is the result of the combination of an inequitable and obsolete tax system and a still powerful popular prejudice against public spending.

At every level, government in the United States is confronted with a paradox: people are demanding more and better public services while simultaneously demanding tax relief and more private consumption. The bias against public spending has been instrumental in the decision of the federal government to distribute the gains of economic growth in the form of tax cuts rather than improved social services. Since 1961, federal income taxes have been cut five times, resulting in a loss of receipts totalling at least $70 billion annually (Leckachman, 1977, p. 90). This amount, although short by nearly 25 percent of the amount of public financing required by the most comprehensive health insurance scheme before the Congress currently, is sufficient to provide Americans with substantially increased protection against the cost of health care. Another manifestation of the bias against public spending is that Americans feel their taxes are oppressive when, in fact, they are among the most lightly taxed industrial nation in the world. In 1970, the total U.S. tax collections equalled only 31 percent of national income, compared to 36 percent for Canada, 38 percent for West Germany, 41 percent for Britain, and 46 percent for Sweden (Statistical Office of the European Communities, 1972, p. 33).

It is no wonder that economic planners and Congressmen expert in fiscal affairs are carefully scrutinizing the estimates of what the leading national health insurance proposals will wind up costing the economy, and especially the government. The results of a recent study, commissioned by the Department of Health, Education, and Welfare and conducted by Gordon R. Trapnell Consulting Actuaries, are presented in table 13.3. They indicate that by 1980 the Health Security proposal would cost the federal government an additional $103 billion, while the proposal sponsored by the commercial health insurers would cost the federal government only about $8 billion more. Interestingly, the difference in total private and public expenditures between the two programs is not that pronounced —approximately $14 billion. While it is true that it is always the taxpayer who pays in the end, the central issue is from which pocket. Until taxpayers come to appreciate the importance of maintaining a harmonious and balanced relationship between private consumption and public spending, it is doubtful whether any truly comprehensive scheme of national health insurance providing close to 100 percent protection can be enacted. In the prevailing climate, even Senator Kennedy's proposal for 70 percent coverage and fifty-fifty financing from general revenues and social insurance taxes may seem overly ambitious and radical.

The reliance on economic growth to reconcile consumer desires for more and better social services with the desire of taxpayers to pay less may also hinder the chances of enacting a nationwide uniform system of comprehensive health insurance on a par with, or more progressive than, the Kennedy plan. Policy makers are openly worried by the long-term trend of health expenditures rising in relation to gross national product—a trend that will put health consumption at as much as 12 percent of the gross national product in 1990, if unchecked (Council on Wage and Price Stability, 1976a, p. 9). The fear is not only that health care may swamp the rest of the economy, but that it, together with other services such as education (which have attained the status of major industries both in terms of total outlays and numbers of persons employed), may act as a brake on the high productivity gains in the industrial and agricultural sectors where employment is declining. (For additional insights into the concerns of policy makers at the federal level, see, for example, Schultze, 1976, pp. 323-70.)

Because of the conquest of many of the acute-communicable diseases of young people, the aging of the population, and the growing dominance of

TABLE 13.3
COST IMPLICATIONS IN 1980 OF ALTERNATIVE NATIONAL HEALTH INSURANCE PROPOSALS

Personal health care expenditures	No NHI program	Alternative national health insurance proposals				
		Long and Ribicoff	Nixon Administration	Health Insurance Assoc.	American Medical Assoc.	Health Security
Total U.S. health expenditures	$223.5	$233.5	$234.8	$243.5	$243.8	$248.3
Additional expenditures resulting from adoption of proposal*		+9.8	+11.3	+11.0	+20.3	+24.8
Federal government health expenditures†	59.3	74.9	68.7	67.0	82.0	189.4
Additional expenditures resulting from adoption of proposal		+15.6	+9.4	+7.7	+22.7	+103.1
Health expenditures covered by all insurance (private and public)‡	127.5	145.2	152.3	153.6	161.2	191.4
Covered by the national health insurance program‡		80.4	121.5	125.9	140.0	181.7
Additional insurance resulting from adoption of proposal		+17.7	+24.8	+26.1	+33.7	+63.9

*Represents the additional costs that would result from the national health insurance programs, for example, from increased use of health services.

†Represents total federal expenditures for personal health care including health insurance programs and military, VA and PHS facilities.

‡The national health insurance program is defined to include the plans established under the proposal, and the Medicare and residual Medicaid programs if they are retained under the proposal. The total for health insurance includes the NHI program and other coverage not required under some programs, for example, health coverage for federal employees and additional insurance benefits, beyond those provided by law, purchased by employers and individuals.

Note: All expense data in the body of the report are in constant 1976 dollars. The data in this table have been adjusted to 1980 price levels using the official inflation estimates of the Council of Economic Advisors.

Source: U.S. Department of Health, Education, and Welfare, "A Comparison of the Cost of Major National Health Insurance Proposals." Washington, D.C.: HEW, 1976.

chronic degenerative disease patterns, health expenditures have come to decline in significance as a form of investment. More and more, they represent a costly form of consumption. Although innovation in biomedical technology has been impressive, costs are shooting upwards, while the marginal economic benefits to society may be declining. The practical pressures for flexibility in the management of the national economy may indicate a preference for some national health insurance measure which would improve the existing situation while bringing costs under better control. Too high a proportion of the gross national product going to consumption of health services may interfere with economic measures aimed at raising the standard of living while avoiding the social and political conflicts which arise when claims for resources are met by open and direct redistribution among competing interests. In the name of economy and efficiency, policy makers may opt for a pluralistic-selective scheme like that advocated by former President Nixon, rather than a single uniform plan based on egalitarian principles.

In sizing up the future prospects, it is also necessary to consider the feelings of providers and other groups with a stake in a constantly expanding and growing health sector. Among persons mindful of the fact that Britain is the only advanced industrialized country in the Western world in which the proportion of gross national product going to health has not grown appreciably over the past twenty years, there is apprehension about the potentially adverse effects of over-relying on a single instrument of raising money and becoming too dependent on centralized governmental authority. In addition to having the lowest growth rate in expenditure, Britain also spends less of its gross national product for health than does any other highly developed country, contrary to the popular image of profligacy associated with the "welfare state." At a time when government is taking a closer look at what it is getting in return for the larger amounts of money it is spending on health, and when the general economy is exhibiting signs of instability, the best way of assuring an expanding influx of money into the health field may center on a strategy of diversification as a hedge against economic decline and stagnation. (For a comparison of health spending between the U.S. and Britain, together with the practical arguments for pluralistic financing, see McNerney, 1971, pp. 137-74.)

CONCLUSIONS

In summing up the implications of the interplay of political and economic factors, it does not appear that any major breakthrough in health care financing can be expected in the short run. In particular, the chances for national health insurance structured along the lines of a single nationwide system seem very remote. While many of the ideological barriers to governmental involvement in the medical care market have been overcome because of extreme dissatisfaction with the functioning of the system, more practical constraints remain in the shape of public resistance to higher taxes and competing priorities in the federal budget. The predisposition in government to keep spending in line with budgetary constraints points to a phasing-in approach to national health insurance and a less than total federal role in the financing of health services. The combination of resource scarcity and strong national bias against the public sector suggests, moreover, a substantial role for the private sector in the delivery of health services. In addition, the stake which providers have in avoiding dependence on a single source of funds and in maintaining a constantly expanding health economy indicates a reinforcement of the present quadripartite system and a continuation, through greater governmental subsidy, of the historic bias for private financing and private administration of the delivery of services.

Nationalization is both ideological anathema and impractical. The situation overall favors a substantial but limited increase in federal financing and the use of governmental purchasing power to guide decentralized and predominantly private sector machinery to assure that social goals are better met through planning, monitoring, and evaluation. While there will be an expansion of services in accord with the principle that access to them is a right, the economic and political realities point to incremental progress based on principles of pluralism and selectivity rather than principles of universalism and egalitarianism.

REFERENCES

Anderson, O. W. *The Uneasy Equilibrium*. New Haven: College and University Press, 1968.

Baron, D. P. "A Study of Hospital Cost Inflation." *Journal of Human Resources* 9 (Winter 1974): 33-49.

Council on Wage and Price Stability. *The Problem of Rising Health Care Costs*. Washington, D.C.: Executive Office of the President, 1976a.

Council on Wage and Price Stability. *The Complex Puzzle of Rising Health Care Costs: Can the Private Sector Fit It Together?* Washington, D.C.: Executive Office of the President, 1976b.

Davis, K. *National Health Insurance: Benefits, Costs and Consequences*. Washington, D.C.: Brookings Institution, 1975.

Davis, M. M. *Medical Care for Tomorrow*. New York: Harper & Brothers, 1955.

Donabedian, A. "An Evaluation of Prepaid Group Practice." *Inquiry* 6 (March 1969): 3-27.

Elnicki, R. A. "Hospital Productivity, Service Intensity, and Costs." *Health Service Research* 9 (Winter 1974): 270-92.

Falk, I. S. "Problems, Proposals and Programs from the Committee on the Cost of Medical Care to the Committee for National Health Insurance." *Milbank Memorial Fund Quarterly, Health and Society* 51 (Winter 1973): 1-32.

Feingold, E. (ed.). *Medicare: Policy and Politics*. San Francisco: Chandler, 1966.

Feldstein, M., and Taylor, A. *The Rapid Rise of Hospital Costs* (A Staff Report of the Council on Wage and Price Stability). Washington, D.C.: Executive Office of the President, 1977.

Gibson, R. H., and Mueller, M. S. "National Health Expenditures, Fiscal Year 1976." *Social Security Bulletin* 40 (April 1977): 3-27.

Harris, R. *A Sacred Trust*. New York: American Library, 1966.

Health Security News. "Health Benefits Costly to Business." *News* 6 (May 9, 1977): 2.

Jeffers, J. R., and Siebert, C. D. "Measurement of Hospital Cost Variation: Case Mix, Service Intensity, and Input Productivity Factors." *Health Services Research* 9 (Winter 1974): 293-307.

Klarman, H. E. "The Financing of Health Care." *Daedalus* 106 (Winter 1977): 215-34.

Leckachman, R. *Economists at Bay*. New York: McGraw-Hill, 1977.

Little, A. D., Inc. *PSRO: Organization for Regional Peer Review*. Cambridge, Mass.: Ballinger, 1973.

Margolis, R. J. "National Health Insurance—The Dream Whose Time Has Come." *New York Times Sunday Magazine* (January 9, 1977): 12.

McNerney, W. J. "Financing and Delivery of Health Services in Britain—Impressions and Questions." *Programs and Progress in Medical Care*, edited by G. McLachlan. London: Nuffield Provincial Hospital Trust, 1971.

Mencher, S. *Poor Law to Poverty Program*. Pittsburgh: University of Pittsburgh Press, 1967.

National Leadership Conference. *Controlling Health Care Costs*. Washington, D.C.: National Journal, 1977.

Reed, L. S., and Carr, W. "The Benefit Structure of Private Health Insurance Organizations, 1968" (Research and Statistics Report no. 31). Washington, D.C.: Social Security Administration, 1969.

Roy, W. R. *The Proposed Health Maintenance Organization Act of 1972*. Washington, D.C.: Science and Health Communications Group, 1972.

Schultze, C. L. "Federal Spending: Past, Present and Future." *Setting National Priorities: The Next Ten Years*, edited by H. Owen and C. L. Schultze. Washington, D.C.: Brookings Institution, 1976.

Statistical Office of the European Communities. *Basic Statistics of the Community*. Luxembourg: European Economic Community, 1972.

U.S. Department of Health, Education, and Welfare. Bureau of Health Planning and Resources Development. *Trends Affecting U.S. Health Care Systems* (Publication no. HRA 76-14503). Washington, D.C.: HEW, 1976.

U.S. Department of Health, Education, and Welfare. *Papers on the National Health Guidelines: Baselines for Setting Health Care Goals and Standards* (Publication no. HRA 77-640). Washington, D.C.: HEW, 1977.

U.S. Public Health Service. *Forward Plan for Health, FY 1977-81* (Publication no. OS 76-50024). Washington, D.C.: HEW, 1975.

U.S. Public Health Service. *Forward Plan for Health, FY 1978-82* (Publication no. OS 76-50046). Washington, D.C.: HEW, 1976.

U.S. Senate Committee on Finance (HR 16311). *Administration Revision of the Family Assistance Act of 1970* (91st Congress, 2nd session, 1970).

U.S. Social Security Administration. *Social Security Programs Throughout the World, 1973* (Publication no. SSA 74-11801). Washington, D.C.: Government Printing Office, 1974.

Waldman, S. *The Effect of Changing Technology on Hospital Costs* (Research and Statistics Note no. 4-1972). Washington, D.C.: HEW, 1972.